A Holistic Conceptualization of Stress and Disease

Stress in Modern Society: No. 7

Other titles in This Series:

STRESS IN MODERN SOCIETY
Number 7

A Holistic Conceptualization of Stress and Disease

Benjamin H. Newberry, Ph.D.
Department of Psychology,
Kent State University

Janet E. Jaikins-Madden, Ph.D.
Department of Psychology,
Kent State University

Thomas J. Gerstenberger, Ph.D.
Department of Psychology,
State University of New York at Potsdam

AMS PRESS
New York

Library of Congress Cataloging-in-Publication Data

Newberry, Benjamin H.
    A holistic conceptualization of stress and disease / Benjamin H.
Newberry, Janet E. Jaikins–Madden, Thomas J. Gerstenberger.
       (Stress in modern society : no. 7)
    Includes bibliographical references and indexes.
    ISBN 0-404-63258-0
      1. Medicine, Psychosomatic. 2. Holistic medicine. 3. Stress
(Psychology) I. Jaikins–Madden, Janet E. II. Gerstenberger.
Thomas J. III. Title. IV. Series.
      [DNLM: 1. Disease—etiology. 2. Holistic Health. 3. Stress.
Psychological—complications. WM 172 N534h]
RC49.N493 1991
616.08—dc20
DNLM/DLC
for Library of Congress   86-82021
                                           CIP

AMS Press, Inc.
56 East 13th Street
New York, N.Y. 10003

MANUFACTURED IN THE UNITED STATES OF AMERICA

To
Deborah
Margaret
and Andrea

Contents

Preface

This monograph developed from long conversations among the three of us about the psychobiology of disease and particularly about the literature on stress and cancer. It has been apparent for many years that such psychologically relevant factors as stress can influence pathologic processes, but the explosion of knowledge in biology and the increasing sophistication of the behavioral sciences are providing new lenses through which researchers can regard these phenomena. We are able, if not forced, to glimpse some of the intricacy in the connections between body and mind.

One thing our growing acuity allows us to sense is the sheer number of connections—connections among events at the biologic level, among events at the psychologic level, and across whatever boundary one might like to assume exists between the biologic and psychologic domains. Although it may not be literally accurate, the idea that everything affects everything else seems a reasonable approximation to the truth. Moreover, the same kinds of interconnectedness are seen at various levels of analysis from the cellular to the social, something reminiscent of the self-similarity which is found in the world of fractal geometry.

From interconnectedness as premise there follows the need for a holistic approach to stress and disease. Holism can hardly be an immediate agenda, however. That would, if taken seriously, bar us from concluding anything about anything until we knew everything about everything. Indeed, in retrospect the authors have come to question the term "conceptualization" in the title of this monograph. To us, that term connotes more rigor and completeness than we can claim. In fact, a rigorously holistic conceptualization of anything involving living organisms can probably be managed only when the number of variables is quite small.

If we cannot realistically take holism as a prescriptive framework for the study of stress and disease, we can at least take it as an attitude. A holistic attitude merely requires that we acknowledge the tentativeness of our conclusions and keep one eye on the range of phenomena known to be plausible. The reader will quickly come to see that the question of plausibility is an important one for this monograph. The number of relevant variables is huge, and many of them are difficult to investigate. Thus it is very helpful to focus on reasonable extrapolation from what is known and the possibilities suggested by that sort of extrapolation. Naturally, speculation about what is plausible is no substitute for hard data, but a holistic viewpoint keeps reminding us that no limited set of data can substitute for a sense of what might be over the research horizon.

A large number of people have contributed to the present authors' sense of what is plausible. Too many have provided us with "Aha!" experiences for us to list them here, though their names appear in the references. (One advantage of not naming them is that they cannot be held responsible for any odd uses we may have made of their ideas and findings.) We apologize to the many authors whose work we lacked the space to cite, and also to those whose work has been more crucial to the field than our few citations of them would suggest.

We wish to thank Bernard H. Fox, Donna H. Laribee, Oneida H. Levine, Deborah L. Newberry, and Beth G. Wildman, who read parts or all of the manuscript. They made helpful suggestions and provided some comforting comments as well. Without them, the book's accuracy would have been less and its Tedium Quotient would have been higher. (Naturally, we must accept the blame for the remaining inaccuracies and tedium.) Many thanks are due the American Studies Center and the Faculty of Psychology of the University of Warsaw, who provided one of us (B.H.N.) with space, time, and inspiration during part of the writing. Finally, we want to acknowledge the immense assistance provided to us by Diane Poston and Patricia John. It is difficult to decide whether their skill or their patience was the more important factor in getting the manuscript produced.

1:

Introduction

Will a high-pressure life shatter your health or hasten your demise? If so, how? If not, why not? The notion that "stress" affects disease is quite popular. (In some ways it might be too popular.) Scores of books and hundreds of scientific articles present the stress-disease theme. The idea or something similar to it has been around for a long time, but it has gained force from the accumulation of a great deal of reputable supporting evidence.

Current preoccupations with taking positive steps to maintain health may be playing a role in the popularity of the stress-disease connection. It is not rare to find the topic mentioned in the popular media and in professional continuing education. In a recent journal we came across an advertisement for a videotape on stress management techniques (price over $450.00), and at the top of the ad in large print was a newspaper quotation to the effect that stress plays a role in a wide variety of illnesses. Readers will doubtless have seen blandishments of this sort. We are all exorted to "manage" our stress, and one benefit is said to be a reduced risk of illness.

As it is usually presented, the basic stress-disease proposition is thus rather simple: stress is said to potentiate the development of disease in general—to initiate pathology, speed the course of established disorders, and probably hasten the deaths of many. This principle is often taken as established beyond doubt, particularly in popular and semi-scientific accounts. Even technical discussions often make the general stress-exacerbates-disease assumption without qualification.

1

Assertions that stress has no effect on some physical disorder are uncommon. That stress could exert a protective effect sometimes seems to be literally unthinkable. The task for researchers is usually seen as one of filling in the details of exactly how stress promotes various disorders. The details are customarily presumed to be intricate, but their study is not expected to challenge the general principle.

However, contrary to the impression often given, the available data on stress and disease are quite complex and often at least superficially contradictory. If one looks at the topic without the popular preconceptions, the complexity and contradictions turn out not to be very surprising. Living organisms are enormously complicated. They exist in enormously complicated environments and interact with those environments in enormously complicated ways.

There is, therefore, little a priori reason for thinking that stress-disease relationships should be simple. Why should incipient breast cancer respond to the loss of a loved one in the same way that incipient arthritis might respond to the stress of medical school exams? They might respond similarly, but it would hardly be surprising if they did not. (It would not be surprising if stress actually slowed the development of these disorders.) As we shall see, it is beyond doubt that stress *can* promote disease, but when this will occur is still very much in question. We hope to present an overview of stress and disease that considers a variety of possibilities, not merely the most popular one.

PURPOSE AND SCOPE OF THIS BOOK

Our goal is to provide a balanced and broad presentation of the stress-disease field. By balanced, we mean a presentation that relies more on the empirical findings than upon poorly substantiated preconceptions as to what is important. By "broad," we mean a presentation which recognizes that the stress-disease question involves phenomena at numerous levels of analysis, from the biochemical to the cultural. Our chief guiding assumption is that the links between stress and disease are complex—or at least that they have not yet been shown to be simple and must at present be assumed to be complex. The degree of complexity seems so great as to warrant the term "holistic".

We would like this volume to be read by individuals with many demands on their time. Unfortunately, the large quantity of relevant information and the interdisciplinary nature of the area make extreme brevity difficult to achieve.

A staggering number of topics is germane to the stress-disease question. Everything from adenylate cyclase to Zen deserves discussion (though, alas, we shall not get to Zen). For stress to affect disease, the person's situation must directly or indirectly alter cellular and chemical processes that contribute to pathology. The physical environment, the forces shaping the psychosocial environment, the processes by which persons interpret their circumstances, the biological systems that link the brain to pathophysiology, the pathophysiology itself, and the logic of inquiry into complex phenomena all must ultimately be considered. No one person could master all of this information, but the greater the gaps in one's knowledge the more likely one is to miss important connections or accept unwarranted conclusions. It is not difficult to find cases in which stress-disease data have been misinterpreted and the misinterpretations have had more influence than the data themselves. We hope not to add to this problem.

It is clear that the stress-disease question crosses the traditional boundaries among the psychosocial and biomedical sciences. It is part of the field of behavioral medicine, a field that is by definition interdisciplinary (e.g., Miller, 1981). There is therefore a question of shared background. If social and biomedical scientists are to cooperate in understanding behavioral aspects of health and illness, they must be able to talk to each other with some comprehension.

They need to develop some familiarity with each others' jargon and concepts. (The general public could use more sophistication, too.) These needs pose problems in writing general discussions of the field. It is unsafe to assume very much prior knowledge on the part of readers. To write for psychosocial scientists as though they had all of the necessary biomedical background would risk befuddling or misleading some, and the same would hold true for assuming that biomedical readers had the requisite behavioral science background. On the other hand, to explain everything fully would take an encyclopedia, not a monograph.

To the extent that we can do so without being offensively oversimple, we shall try to write about biomedical topics as though for behavioral scientists and to write about psychosocial topics as though for biomedical scientists. We have in mind readers who have some training in either a biomedical or a behavioral area but who are just beginning to venture into the psychobiology of disease. Several devices are used to make topics accessible to such readers. Among them are brief introductory paragraphs, brief interpolated definitions, and the repetition of abbreviations, as well as occasional sections which are frankly introductory. We hope by such means to assist readers who are unfamiliar with any particular topic without irritating too much those with more knowledge about it. One consequence of attempting to accomodate disparate specialists may be to make the volume useful to people who are in neither the biomedical nor the behavioral sciences. We would be pleased if this were the case.

We must emphasize that this monograph is not a review of the stress-disease field in the traditional sense. The amount of pertinent information is so great that we could not hope to locate, let alone read, assimilate, or discuss all of it. We shall concentrate on the critical *ideas* (hence "conceptualization" in the title) and critiques of those ideas, along with enough detail about mediating processes and recent stress-disease findings to give readers a serviceable sense of the field's status and direction. In many places we draw upon reviews and discussions of particular topics rather than citing the primary literature. Were we to do otherwise, the reference list would be prohibitively long.

There are numerous relevant topics which we mention only in passing or do not discuss at all. These neglected topics include the early history of the stress-disease question; brain function; numerous peripheral biologic systems important to stress or disease; development and aging; mental disorders; the statistics of complex correlational research; properties of psychometric instruments used in stress-disease research; and stress management. It is not that these things are unimportant, only that we would be even more uncomfortable leaving out other topics. We would like to offer a theoretical integration of the stress-disease area, but the available information does not permit it. We shall mention theoretical generalizations from time to time, but we shall often have to criticize them.

OVERVIEW

In this section we outline the order in which we take up the several aspects of the stress-disease field and preview the relevance of each topic. To a great extent the order in which we consider topics is arbitrary. Everything is the context for everything else, and to understand how anything fits in, one needs a grasp of the rest.

The book can be regarded as having two parts. The first attempts to set out the context in which stress effects need to be viewed, to provide background for readers unfamiliar with the range of biologic and psychologic factors involved, and in the process to establish that stress effects upon disease are plausible. The second part, consisting of a long final chapter, examines some of the recent research dealing specifically with associations between stress and disease.

Some readers might question the amount of space we devote to background and context. We can only reply that we think it necessary given the nature of the topic and the way in which it is often discussed. The amount that is still unknown about stress and disease is so great that context is at least as important as the specific research findings in many cases. The stress-disease data are made more convincing by a knowledge of why stress effects are plausible, and yet at the same time the background information produces some valuable skepticism about overgeneralizations and premature conclusions.

Complexity in any set of phenomena makes those phenomena difficult to study scientifically. How does one tease out cause and effect when hundreds of subtle factors may need to be considered simultaneously and when nearly all of the elements involved enter into reciprocal relationships in which one element influences itself through its effects on other elements? The scientific approach seems best suited to phenomena that are simple even if they are subtle. Science strives, and rightly so, for generalizations which apply broadly. Its best methods are analytic; they study one or a few factors at a time and those in isolation.

Science becomes more clumsy as it is asked to deal with greater numbers of details simultaneously and to do so in situations which do not permit strict controls. Imagine asking a physicist to predict exactly where a particular snowflake would fall in a blizzard (Miller, 1959). The physicist could not do it, though the principles operating are well understood and reasonably simple. It is sobering to realize how much trouble the physical sciences have in predicting even mildly complex events. It is even more sobering to recognize that very simple, determinate systems can generate apparent randomness ("chaos") (Gleick, 1987; R. Jensen, 1987). Noting its limits is not a criticism of the scientific approach, for no other approach has shown itself able to do as well. But it does mean that there are real methodologic difficulties in coming to firm conclusions about something like stress effects on health. Later in this chapter, we consider some of those problems.

In addition to rather practical methodologic issues, there are conceptual questions which both reflect the complexity of the stress-disease question and contribute to it. One of these deals with the term "holism" and its usefulness. If one ignores the anti-analytic quality that sometimes seems to characterize holistic pronouncements, the term captures rather well the nature of the causal networks that relate stress and disease.

A more serious conceptual problem is the meaning of stress. Stress includes such a variety of poorly related, quantitative phenomena that no scientifically precise definition can be given unless that definition is too restrictive and arbitrary to capture what stress researchers actually study. The concept of disease is also tricky, though not as tricky as stress.

Notice that, to the extent that we do not know what stress and disease are, it is difficult to discover whether one influences the other, if not meaningless to ask. Fortunately, the extent of confusion is not quite paralyzing, and it is possible to make reasonable inquiries into stress effects on illness.

After dealing as best we can with the conceptual puzzles of stress and disease, we turn to more concrete illustrations of what holism implies for stress-disease relations. In Chapters 2 and 3, we deal with some of the biologic and psychologic changes which occur when organisms are confronted with stressful situations. These changes carry stressors' impacts to the sites at which pathology develops, and discussing them is therefore essential to any treatment of the stress-disease question. As the number of relevant variables and the intricacy of their interrelationships become apparent in this discussion, so, we believe, will the appropriateness of the term holism.

We hope that these chapters will give the non-biologically oriented reader a sense of the variety of physiologic factors which need to be considered in tracing the paths from stress to disease. In a parallel way, we want the non-behaviorally oriented reader to see that numerous psychoneural factors influence biologic processes and that an appreciation of individuals' psychologic situations is necessary to a full understanding of their diseases.

Chapter 4, entitled, "A General Schematic for Stress-Disease Relationships," builds upon what is covered under stress responses and attempts to provide a broad perspective on the types of links that can occur between stress and illness. The pertinent variables are put into seven general classes (physical environment, social environment, genome, phenotypic organism, pathologic processes, overt behavior, and disease outcome) and the causal connections among those classes of factors are explored. Each of the seven variable classes (and many of the hundreds of specific variables in each class) is seen to serve as both cause and effect. Therefore, at this very molar level just as at the micro-level of internal processes, it is apparent that a network of interactive, reciprocal influences is operating. Stressors' effects upon disease can involve direct alterations in the biologic microenvironments of pathologic processes, changes in the individual's exposure to exogenous agents, others' responses to the individual, and the individual's own responses to illness. It becomes clear that stress should be capable of producing nearly any type of effect on disease.

Finally, having provided some context and background, we will address the stress-disease findings themselves. Even considering just relatively recent research, there are more studies than we can discuss. There are significant amounts of information and speculation on a variety of specific disorders, as well as a large number of studies reporting illnesses or symptoms in the aggregate. For each specific disease that we take up, we shall discuss first the pathologic processes and then the information on the relevance of stress.

Overall, the data clearly indicate that stress and related factors can affect disease, but they also indicate that much remains unknown. Even in the study of the Type A personality and ischemic heart disease, an area held up as the prime example of how important it is to include stress-relevant factors in accounting for disease, there are contradictory findings. It appears to be at least a bit premature to prescribe stress reduction to the public with assurances that a general improvement in physical health will result. Of course, we do not need improvments in physical health to justify reducing human distress and misery.

CONCEPTUAL QUESTIONS

This section treats several subjects which need to be considered before more substantive topics are taken up. Three conceptual issues—the meanings of holism, stress, and disease—affect how one approaches the whole stress-pathology question. The final section of the chapter deals with methodologic issues, albeit in a very rudimentary manner. A clear perception of why it is difficult to come to firm conclusions about stress and disease can be extremely helpful in resisting the temptation to accept oversimple generalizations.

Holism

The idea of holism appears frequently in comparisons of personality theories. It is at least implicit in many discussions of psychosocial factors and health and is, of course, central to the field of holistic medicine. Smuts (1926/1961) has taken credit for the term.

For him, holism had a literally cosmic philosophic significance as a creative tendency or force. As our title implies, we find the notion of holism useful in thinking about stress and disease, although we use the word with some reservations and without Smuts' awesome attributions. Few extensive, precise discussions of holism seem to have appeared recently in behavioral or biomedical sources. Nevertheless, the basics of the term's use are clear enough for our purposes. Two chief features can be found in descriptions of what holism means. One is an insistence that complex wholes such as living entities function by the dynamic actions of their constituent parts and also have transcendent attributes. The second feature is the notion that analytic approaches are inapplicable to the study of such wholes.

MULTIFACTORIAL, INTERACTIVE, RECIPROCAL RELATIONSHIPS

A set of entities (of "parts") can have properties which are difficult to predict from knowledge of the parts. The parts can influence each other or "cooperate" in bringing about the functioning of the whole (e.g., Smuts, 1926/1961, p. 107). Given that organisms are wholes in this sense, holism implies that studying one or a few of their sub-functions is not likely to explain anything completely.

In psychology, Hall and Lindzey (1978, pp. 23-24) have put this by saying that a holistic position encompasses both an "organismic" perspective and a "field" perspective. That is, to be understood any act must be viewed in the context of every other aspect of the organism (its other behaviors and its internal processes) and in the context of all elements of the organism's environmental field.

Our thesis is that biologic phenomena, including disease, need to be looked at in this same way. This emphasis on a multiplicity of possible influences on disease is hardly unique to us. The adjective *biopsychosocial* has been employed (e.g., Schneiderman & Tapp, 1985; Schwartz, 1982) to indicate that factors from many levels of analysis are needed to explain health and disease. Psychosomatic medicine (e.g., Lipowski et al., 1977) is based on a similar idea.

Systems theory has provided a good expression of holism as applied to disease (e.g., Schwartz, 1982; Tapp & Warner, 1985). General systems theory is a metatheory; it claims to consist of principles that apply to widely divergent phenomena. Tapp and Warner (1985) list the basic properties of systems in this technical sense. Several of these properties are of immediate concern to us.

Systems have boundaries such that the whole which makes up any system can be identified. They are organized hierarchically, any system consisting of lower level systems and also being a part of a higher level system. Any element of a system is capable of affecting all other elements directly or indirectly. Systems maintain their characteristics over time despite potentially disruptive external influences. (That is, they incorporate negative feedback mechanisms which maintain near-steady states by sensing and compensating for deviations from preset values of particular variables—everyday thermostats being classic examples of such controls). Finally, despite their homeostatic tendencies, systems can transform and change their properties.

From a systems theory perspective, disease results from the failure of an organism to maintain its internal equilibrium. Moreover, given the interdependence of system elements, general disorder can result from a change in one or a few elements. The disregulation theory of Schwartz (e.g., 1984) exemplifies this view. Schwartz emphasizes the inability of the brain to perform its many regulating functions when sensing or feedback systems fail.

Though a detailed analysis of systems theory is beyond the scope of this volume, we suspect that such an analysis would reveal some limits on the applicability of the theory to disease. The theory is without content in a sense. It tells one to look for interdependencies and regulatory processes but, being a metatheory, does not indicate what types should be found. It does not, for example, predict that the kidneys will secrete a blood pressure regulating hormone (renin).

There may also be problems with the ideas of definable system boundaries and hierarchical organization, with nature having "out-systemed" systems theory in a sense. It is not at all clear how well the subsystems of organisms can be differentiated, because particular organs, cells, and compounds can belong to multiple systems.

Finally, it is not clear how systems theory could be refuted. Because it is so general, it provides infinite opportunities for ad hoc theorizing and can lean toward saying merely, "Whatever does happen, can." Related to the difficulty of disconfirmation is a tendency for a systems theory view of disease to be tautological. To say that disease results from the failure of regulatory mechanisms can be to say that things go awry because they go awry.

In dealing with organisms and disease, systems theory is probably best taken as a broad but useful perspective—an admonition to expect complexity and interdependencies. The same could be said for holism in general.

To us, the need to adopt a holistic point of view comes from the data on the qualities of organisms, not from a metatheoretical preference. The internal processes of organisms and their relationships to their environments are characterized by *multifactorial, interactive, reciprocal* influences. By multifactorial, we mean simply that all processes are affected by numerous variables; there are no single causes but rather networks of influences. We mean interactive in the sense of a statistical interaction—a pattern of influence in which the effect of one factor is not constant but depends on the degree to which other factors are operating. The effects of classical chemical carcinogens and promoters offer a good example of interaction. Promoters alone do not induce cancers, but they can do so if given after an otherwise ineffective dose of a primary carcinogen.

In reciprocal causality, two elements or processes affect each other, and each can thereby affect itself. Reciprocal influence is ubiquitous in organismic function. As systems theory emphasizes, many processes are subject to negative feedbacks (e.g., the actions of suppresor cells to terminate immune responses, and most acts of coping with stress). Some reciprocal relationships involve positive feedback, however. In social interactions, for instance, people's responses to each other can result in escalating hostility or attraction rather than a return to a previous state. Stress may exacerbate pathology, the pathology and its consequences then serving as additional stressors.

When causation is multifactorial, interactive, and reciprocal, as it is in organisms, understanding any process thoroughly might require understanding many or all other processes—in other words the whole of the organism. Much of the content of the next three chapters will illustrate the interdependencies which presumably contribute to stress-disease relationships.

It is possible to get a sense of what holism really implies by thinking of a *biopsychosocial matrix* like that represented in Table 1. A sample of factors is listed in the rows of the matrix as independent variables (x's) and in the columns as dependent variables (y's). The question is, which x's are plausible influences on which y's? Does evidence or reasonable speculation from the evidence suggest, for example, that interleukin-1 can directly or indirectly affect itself (x_1, y_1) or caffeine intake (x_1, y_j)? As we shall see, those effects are plausible, and the same could be said for most relationships in a biopsychosocial matrix.

Table 1. A Biopsychosocial Matrix

		... y_i ...	y_j ...	y_k ...	y_l ...	y_m ...	y_p ...	y_q ...	y_r ...	y_s
Body Temperature	x_i ...	□	□	□	□	□	□	□	□	□
Caffeine Intake	x_j ...	□	□	□	□	□	□	□	□	□
Corticotropin	x_k ...	□	□	□	□	□	□	□	□	□
Interleukin-1	x_l ...	□	□	□	□	□	□	□	□	□
Job Performance	x_m ...	□	□	□	□	□	□	□	□	□
Minor Auto Accident	x_p ...	□	□	□	□	□	□	□	□	□
Pancreatic Oncogenesis	x_q ...	□	□	□	□	□	□	□	□	□
Receiving a Compliment	x_r ...	□	□	□	□	□	□	□	□	□
Trait Anxiety	x_s	□	□	□	□	□	□	□	□	□

THE ANTI-ANALYTIC ASPECT OF HOLISM

The fact that wholes appear to have emergent properties and need to be viewed as wholes seems to have led to the notion that the ordinary analytic methods of scientific inquiry are of no use in learning about them. This anti-analytic bias is not terribly salient, but it is there. Gordon (1980, p.11) characterized the holistic position as follows: "All things do appear seamlessly and wondrously interconnected, and all attempts to describe them are inadequate and, although heroic, are still somehow beside the point." Murphy (1947, p.988) defined holism as "the doctrine that the dynamics of a living whole permits of no differentiation of discrete elements." Scroggs (1985, p.240) represented holism in personality psychology as holding that, "If experience is analyzed and dissected, the result is something artificial and irrelevant."

This distrust of analysis appears to relate to the use of Gestalt-type perceptual analogies in explaining holism. Analyzing a newspaper photograph to learn that it consists of 150,000 or so black dots on a white ground would indeed tell one nothing about what had been photographed. Looking at the picture "as a whole" would.

However, such analogies are misleading when applied to understanding organisms. Photographs are static; the dots do not affect each other. Also, there is in most photographs a whole whose nature can be apprehended by sensory-perceptual systems specialized for that purpose. In contrast, organisms are dynamic; their parts continuously affect each other. And it is not possible to perceive a whole which sums up the biopsychosocial status of an organism in anything like the way that perceptions capture the essence of photographs.

As applied to stress and disease, or to other aspects of living things, holism is not non-analytic. It is *hyper*-analytic. It acknowledges that multitudes of functions must be analyzed in the process of building useful syntheses. We cannot conceive of understanding hypertension, for example, by trying to view hypertensives "as wholes" and ignoring the interacting processes which have produced the disorder.

In sum, our view of holism focuses on the idea that systems which involve multifactorial, interactive, reciprocal causation must be comprehended broadly—perhaps in their entirety—to guarantee an understanding of any of their functions. Further, we see an analytic understanding of specific subsystems (the parts of the whole) as necessary, though certainly not sufficient, for explaining the functions of the whole. At this stage of our knowledge the major implication of a holistic conceptualization of stress and disease is that we should expect complexity and should omit nothing from consideration. This may sound obvious and trivial, but in fact it is all too easy to forget how many variables probably contribute to stress and illness.

HOLISTIC MEDICINE

We would be remiss if we did not mention the holistic movement in medicine. Gordon (1980) has provided a good overview of this field's claims and purposes. Holistic medicine is in part a protest against a number of perceived overemphases in conventional medicine, among them the single cause-single effect view of pathology, the tendency to deal with disease outside the context of the rest of patients' lives, and the overuse of invasive methods.

Holistic medicine assumes that disease arises from the totality of circumstances in persons' lives, an assumption congenial to those interested in stress and disease. It also places substantial reliance on the organism's own healing resources and on persons' taking responsibility for their own health. It seeks to extend medicine from concern with disease alone to concern with all aspects of life quality.

To us, holistic medicine has one major problem. Things such as laying-on-of-hands, intuitive diagnosis, aromatherapy, herbs, interpersonal energies, and psychic healing are written about, and presumably used, as though they are known to work (e.g., Hastings et al., 1980; Read, 1983), although as far we know the data are scanty at the very best. Accepting interventions whose worth is poorly substantiated is particularly inappropriate from a holistic perspective. The more complicated a set of phenomena is, the larger the amount of data usually needed to establish generalizations about it.

The Concept of Stress

If one knows that two groups of individuals differ with regard to disease state and wants to decide whether stress contributed to that difference, one needs to be able to tell whether the two groups differ in stress. In this section we examine some of the major questions in defining and characterizing stress. We shall conclude that a wholly satisfactory definition probably cannot be given—that in at least some sense there is no such thing as stress.

It is almost a ritual for authors at least to mention that stress has not yet been adequately defined or to take some other notice of the problems with the concept. The Institute of Medicine Study Steering Committee (1982) lamented the fact that 35 years of trying had not produced a good definition. Many capable people have done stress research, have written on the topic, and have said that the term has not been defined satisfactorily. Why has a good definition been elusive?

One possibility that seems not to have occurred to too many—Ader (1980) and H. Weiner (1985) being among the exceptions—is that the term cannot be defined adequately because too many phenomena are involved to be represented by one word. Certainly a holistic view of living organisms and their transactions with their environments does not encourage the use of a single term for as broad a set of things as workers try to encompass under the rubric of stress. Wondering why stress has not been defined well is a bit like using one word (for instance, "furnishing") for every object in a house and then being surprised that it is difficult to cook on a hat rack or sleep in a dishwasher.

WORDS, SYMBOLS, AND DEFINITIONS

The problems with the term stress are similar to the problems with words and symbols in general. Words are arbitrary. Moreover, they often represent abstractions, and natural phenomena need not group themselves to correspond with our abstract distinctions.

In science at least, the meaning of terms is not in the symbols themselves or in their general usages, but rather in the theoretic and empirical relationships of the underlying constructs. Consider "charm" in referring to the properties of quarks in physics. It is doubtful that charmed quarks have winning smiles or have been put under a spell by fairies. If physics chose to substitute "happiness" for charm, no change in meaning would necessarily be implied. Similarly, "strain" or "zilsblat" could be substituted for stress with no change in meaning.

Since terms are arbitrary, those who study stress could have agreed to define it in any number of reasonable, or even unreasonable, ways. That they have not done so reflects, we believe, the issues of abstraction and of the boundaries of phenomena. Definitional questions are more easily resolved when the phenomena can be more easily specified. When objects are there in a naive, direct sense, it is a matter of agreeing on which symbols to use for which. Even useful scientific terms can be hard to define when they represent abstractions. Adrenal gland is more easily defined than anxiety partly because adrenals can be pointed to. Even if things are not immediately sensible they may be more easily defined when they are physical; it is probably no accident that "neutron" is better defined than stress.

Related to problems with physicalness and concreteness are problems of process and boundaries. Definitions can be hard to come by with living organisms because of organisms' complexities and because the interest is so often in processes rather than static entities. When concepts are abstracted from a flow of complicated interacting events then our abstractings need not reflect the way things are actually divided up in nature. There is the possibility, if not the certainty, that our concepts obscure things. And it is then that concepts, distinctions and definitions are most open to debates which can be stilled only by arbitrary agreements regarding which symbols shall stand for what.

What is clear is that environments, in combination with the characteristics of organisms, produce changes in organisms. Some try to use a word, "stress," for a subset of the phenomena that occur in organism-environment transactions. They have not agreed on what subset the word should apply to because there are no natural boundaries at the desired level of abstraction. Probably the only way to define stress is by arbitrary agreement, but such a definition would merely shuffle words or be too restrictive to capture the connotations that "stress" now has. The difficulties of conceptualizing stress will hopefully become more apparent as we go to some specific attempts.

DEFINITIONS OF STRESS

For our topic, one consequence of the arbitrariness of terms' uses concerns disagreements about whether stress is a stimulus condition, a response to stimulus conditions, or a relationship involving stimuli, organism characteristics and responses (e.g., Dohrenwend & Shrout, 1985; versus Lazarus et al., 1985). If the stimulus conditions, responses, or relationships can be specified, it matters not for which the term "stress" is reserved. It does not even matter whether the term stress is used at all. If the stimuli, responses, or relationships cannot be specified, the symbols used still do not matter much, for then one literally does not know what one is talking about. As we shall try to show, they probably cannot be specified.

Response Definitions

In a response definition, the term stress is used for changes which environmental conditions produce in organisms. The best known response definition is that of Selye (1976) in which stress is "the nonspecific response of the body to any demand" (p. 55). Central to Selye's viewpoint is that all demands will elicit a common core of stress responses. The eliciting situations are termed stressors.

Adrenal enlargement, reductions in the size of lymphoid organs and in blood lymphocytes, gastric lesions, loss of weight, and reduced inflammatory response were the general responses to demand in Selye's original studies. He also noted a nonspecific illness syndrome in human patients. It is important to note that in Selye's theory stressors also have specific effects that represent the organism's response to their particular characteristics. Examples of specific effects would be immunologic responses to infection and muscular changes with exercise.

The difficulties with response definitions such as Selye's have been noted frequently (e.g., Lazarus & Folkman, 1984; McGrath, 1970). The major problem is that responses do not covary consistently. Even if one restricts attention to responses widely thought to be at the physiologic core of stress, inconsistencies are easily found. The adrenocortical and sympathoadrenomedullary (SAM) responses are certainly among the most general components of stress taken as a response. To the extent that there is a unitary stress response, indices of these systems' activities should change together across situations, but they seem often not to do so.

It has long been recognized that the various psychophysiologic indices of SAM arousal correlate only poorly with each other (e.g., Lacey, 1967). Measures such as heart rate, blood pressure, and skin conductance are mediated by "clearly dissociable mechanisms" (Lacey, p. 36) even though they are not entirely unrelated. Studies of classic stress-responsive endocrine systems exhibit similar dissociations. Dominant mice in a colony have a dramatic adrenomedullary response, but subordinates have a strong adrenocortical response (Henry et al., 1975). Mason (1975) noted in humans and monkeys patterns of stress response that differ with regard to the catecholamines. In one pattern, norepinephrine is elevated but epinephrine (EP) is not; in the other, levels of both catecholamines increase. According to Mason, stressful situations involving amibguity and uncertainty are more likely to produce EP elevations.

Work on the endogenous opioids (enkephalins, endorphins) and stress-induced analgesia illustrates that stressor differences need not be large and obvious for different response patterns to occur. Three minutes of continuous footshock produces nonopioid analgesia in rats, whereas 20 minutes of exposure to 1 second shocks at 4 second intervals produces an analgesia mediated by opioids (Lewis, Sherman, & Liebeskind, 1981). The analgesia produced by shock to the forepaws of rats is opioid-mediated, but that produced by hind paw shock is not (Watkins & Mayer, 1982).

These findings confirm some of the present authors' worst fears about stress. Endogenous opioids and their responses to stressors have been implicated in things from pain perception to tumor growth. If small and a priori trivial differences in stressors can produce profound differences in such major components of stress response, what meaning can stress as a response have?

There is no shortage of other results showing that classic stress responses are not very coherent, sometimes simply fail to occur at all, or are bound up with individual differences in ways that seem to preclude a general definition of stress as a pattern of response. Some of these findings will come up later. A response definition of stress probably cannot be very precise. And even if, as in Selye, there were a constant core of responses to demanding situations, it would still be possible that influences on disease stem from specific responses to stressors rather than nonspecific ones.

Stimulus Definitions

In a stimulus-based view of stress, the focus is on the eliciting conditions rather than the organisms' responses to them. Therefore variability in the responses could supposedly be accepted and regarded as unimportant for purposes of definition.

With stimulus definitions, then, the difficulty is specifying the critical stimulus characteristics in a meaningful and coherent way without either being arbitrary or having recourse to the responses. As one example, consider some of Weitz's (1970) characteristics of stressful situations. Included are threat, in which the individual "perceives the situation as potentially dangerous"; blocking or frustration "which inhibits task completion"; "noxious" environmental stimuli; group pressure, which produces "fear of failure"; and speeded information processing, stressful because it results in "degradation of performance" (pp. 125-127). In each of these cases, the situation is considered stressful *because of the response*. Perception of danger, fear of failure, and quality of task performance are all clearly response variables. "Noxiousness" is also difficult to identify except in terms of the responses it elicits. When so-called stimulus definitions of stress require identifying stressful conditions by the responses to them, then they are really response definitions, and the problems of response definitions still apply.

Relational Definitions

If we cannot meaningfully define stress in response or stimulus terms, we are left with relational or interactive definitions. In these definitions stress refers to a particular relationship between the organism and the environment, or to the quality of the transaction between the organism and the environment.

We see a definition by Lazarus and Folkman as about as good as can be written. *"Psychological stress is a particular relationship between the person and the environment that is appraised by the person as taxing or exceeding his or her resources and endangering his or her well-being"* (Lazarus & Folkman, 1984, p. 19; italics in original).

Note, however, that this is really a response definition, one using internal psychologic responses. Only the person's responses—appraisals regarding resources and well being—are dealt with explicitly. If those appraisals are of a particular sort then a stress relationship exists regardless of the nature of the environment, and if they are not then a stress relationship does not exist. Nothing about the environment is specified except the association with a certain type of appraisal by the individual.

Responses may be central whether we like it or not. Perhaps there is no meaningful way to justify saying that a stimulus situation or an environment-organism relationship is stressful except on the basis of how the organism reacts. Perhaps the best attempts at defining stress must be limited by the low covariation among responses.

The problems with using responses to define stress may be worse when the defining responses are internal psychologic ones like appraisals. Psychologic responses are unlikely to relate to environmental conditions more simply than do physiologic responses, and they are more difficult to assess with precision. People may be unwilling or even unable to report internal states accurately (e.g., Nisbett & Wilson, 1977). We would be reluctant, in the case of someone in an objectively dangerous situation and demonstrating marked physiologic signs of stress, to declare non-stress merely because the person would not appraise the situation as threatening to his/her well being.

Another problem with the Lazarus and Folkman (1984) definition is that it seems to rule out findings from infrahuman animals. There is much that will be learned more slowly if data from lower animals are defined out of the field.

Despite the criticisms we have just made, we largely agree with the emphases in relational definitions. Stress most assuredly involves processes in which organism and environment variables interact. Appraisals are crucial to stress no matter how, or whether, one decides to define stress. The question in our minds is whether an adequate definition of stress—one that is precise and fits the connotations with which the term has been endowed—is possible. Because any definition seemingly must rest on responses and the responses are inconsistent, a good definition seem unlikely. One could argue that there is no such thing as stress.

Even if stress is undefinable, there is the practical issue of what variables to discuss when considering stress and disease. This issue can be addressed by looking at the types of variables which tend to be employed in the literature. It seems not unreasonable to speak in stress-like terms to the degree that (1) physically or normatively threatening or dangerous situations occur (when for example there is tissue damage, pain, or the objective threat of such things); (2) there is an objective/normative threat to such elements of psychologic integrity as acceptance, self-esteem, or the pursuit of important goals; (3) the individual believes that there is a threat to physical or psychologic integrity whether or not there is an objective threat; (4) the resources to meet threats are lacking or are believed to be lacking; (5) there occur physiologic changes associated with the term stress in the literature, regardless of whether threat is objectively present or is believed to be present.

Note that the stress idea is related to, and perhaps very difficult to distinguish from, many other phenomena. Terms like anxiety, worry, arousal, threat, dysphoria, and frustration have similar connotations. Frustration, implying as it does interference with goals and thus questionable resources for meeting demands, seems particularly like stress.

Under the proper conditions, nearly any stimulus situation can serve as a stressor. Even small stimulus changes—a raised eyebrow, an averted gaze, a swollen lymph node, a gauge reading—can signal an impending disaster or at least lead people to believe that disaster is imminent. Personality, life history, and the background situation combine with the stimulus in creating persons' interpretations of their situations (Lazarus & Folkman, 1984), and although some physical stressors may act independently of appraisals, it seems safe to say that the most numerous stressors facing the human inhabitants of developed nations are psychologic.

SEVERITY, TIME, AND RESPONSE TO STRESSORS

Before we leave the question of the meaning of stress, there are two other things which need to be addressed briefly. One is stress severity; the other is the time course of stress responses. Both of these issues relate to how stress is conceptualized and to how one might think about stress and disease. Each of these topics deserves more space than we can give it.

Severity of Stress

Stress is a matter of degree. Stressors are assumed to differ in their severity, with something like death of a spouse normatively considered very stressful and things like receiving traffic tickets much less so (Holmes & Rahe, 1967). Also, most measures of stress response, whether behavioral or physiologic, imply continua; the responses may be small or large depending on the stressor and the individual (Friedman et al., 1967; Keller et al., 1981; Mason, 1975).

In a conceptualization such as that of Lazarus and Folkman (1984) two general variables are involved, namely appraisal of demand (i.e., threat to well being) and appraisal of resources to meet the demand. Very broadly, stress responses should be smaller with lower demand and greater resources, but it is not clear exactly what form the function would have. Presumably, as long as resources comfortably exceed demand, stress response should remain low, increasing slowly if at all with increasing demand or decreasing resources. Only when demand level becomes close to resource level should stress response increase greatly.

We could also ask what happens if demand increases and resources keep pace. It is reasonable to suspect that when the stakes are high it takes a greater cushion of resource excess to keep stress responses low. It is one thing for a student to have barely enough time to study for a high school history quiz, but quite another for time to be precarious when a career-deciding professional examination is at issue. If this reasoning is correct, then demand and resources interact, and the function needs to be represented in three dimensions.

Stressor predictability and controllability are two related variables widely held to affect the severity of stress responses. There is evidence that uncontrollability and unpredictablility magnify responses to stressors. Current research and discussion particularly emphasize controllability (see Chapter 3).

Some of the most dramatic evidence for the effect of controllability comes from infrahuman studies in which stress effects utterly failed to occur in animals able to escape or avoid shock but did occur under yoked uncontrollable conditions (e.g., Laudenslager et al., 1983; MacLennan & Maier, 1983; Visintainer et al., 1982).

There is also a great deal of evidence on predictability from animal studies. Preference for predictable over unpredictable aversive stimulation has been found repeatedly as has greater physiological change with unpredictable stressors (e.g., Abbott et al., 1984; Seligman et al., 1971).

The fact that stress is quantitative adds to the difficulty of distinguishing stressfulness from other characteristics of situations. No two situations can be presumed identical in stressfulness. The study of stress becomes almost equivalent to the study of environmental conditions' effects upon organisms, and stress has rather little identity as a distinct phenomenon. Lazarus and Folkman (1984) and H. Weiner (1985) have noted this and have suggested that definitions be adopted which avoid the problem. The problem cannot be avoided, however. Whatever we mean by stress, it can occur in large or small amounts. If one reserves the term stress for large amounts, one must find other terms for lesser amounts, and the basic questions do not change at all.

Temporal Factors

The factor of time must always be kept in mind when considering stress and disease; it is critical in several ways and will come up several times in this monograph. At this point, we shall mention two aspects of the time course of stress responses—the temporal course of response to a single stressor encounter, and the changes in stress response that occur with continued encounters. These temporal effects have been studied most frequently with physiologic dependent variables.

Time Course of Response to Single Stressors —

The physiologic responses to a single brief stressor are frequently rather brief. In rats, shock produces an increase in corticosterone which begins within a few seconds and is usually over within 30-60 minutes (e.g., Friedman et al., 1967). A similar pattern of rapid increase followed by a relatively rapid decline occurs with prolactin and restraint (Krulich et al., 1974). In humans there is also a rather time-limited glucocorticoid increase to a brief stressor (e.g., Mason, 1975).

The time course is not necessarily the same with all stress responses. Krulich et al. (1974), for example, found that in rats moved to an unfamiliar room luteinizing hormone (LH) levels returned to baseline after 30-60 minutes, but growth hormone (GH) levels were still significantly elevated after four hours. With other stressors GH was depressed rather than elevated and remained depressed after LH levels had fallen to baseline.

A further complication is that some hormones can apparently have biphasic responses to stressors. We are not aware of a great deal of evidence for this, but its theoretical import requires that it be mentioned. Krulich et al. found in several of their experiments that plasma LH first rose above baseline and then fell significantly below baseline after an hour or two. They found the same pattern for FSH (follicle-stimulating hormone) in one experiment. Testosterone, which is often reduced by stress, may sometimes rebound above baseline after a stressful encounter (see Rose, 1980).

Adaptation —

We shall speak of adaptation to stress as the return of stress responses toward baseline with extended exposure to a stressor. The ability to adapt to aversive conditions is a major attribute of living things. Although stressors leave lasting marks, humans often restore their physiology more or less to normal, reduce their levels of distress, and rebuild their lives even after such disastrous events as the loss of a spouse, the destruction of a community, or brutal incarceration.

Adaptation is probably not a single phenomenon. There are at least two ways that it might occur. For one thing, experience with a demand provides the opportunity to learn to cope with it. Increased coping ability can reduce the demand's actual impact and its appraised danger when it recurs. If the stressor is a single event with long-term ramifications, the same thing applies. People can learn to cope with severe losses by developing new behavior patterns and by allowing distress to extinguish. In part, then, adaptation is closely allied to controllability, and some cases in which stress responses fail to occur are surely due to such adaptation. This means, of course, that the organism's learning history and the similarity of new stress situations to old ones are important determinants of stress responses.

Adaptation occurs even when learning to control the stressor is not possible. Learning may still be involved in that the organism can learn that stress episodes and their damage are limited (Burchfield, 1979). However, there may be simple biologic mechanisms of adaptation as well. For example, with repeated exposure to stressors neurons can increase both their capacity to synthesize neurotransmitters and the efficiency with which they utilize them (e.g., Anisman et al., 1985).

Adaptation to stressors is important in stress and disease. Since the biologic and behavioral responses to a stressor vary with amount of previous exposure to it, so should pathology. Opportunity for adaptation can eliminate or reverse stress enhancement of experimental tumor development (see Newberry et al., 1984). It has been hypothesized that failure to adapt to chronic stressors is responsible for stress exacerbation of human disease (Baum et al., 1981).

Dienstbier (1989) has marshalled evidence that physiologic "toughening" can follow repeated exposure to stressful conditions, particularly if coping is perceived to be possible. The toughened state is characterized by low baseline catecholamine levels, vigorous cate-

cholamine/SAM responses to stressors, and relatively low adrenocortical responses to stressors. One well known aspect of the toughening
process is the reduction in adult emotionality and stress hormone
response in rodents which are exposed in infancy to extra stimulation
(e.g., Denenberg, 1967).

If this sort of toughness extends to disease resistance, then a
relatively stressful existence may be healthy. However, the question of
when adaptation or toughening will and will not occur needs much
more attention, because it may be critical to understanding stress
effects on disease.

Notice how adaptation complicates the characterization of stress.
There is no natural point in the adaptation process at which to conclude that the organism is no longer under stress. Moreover, different
stress responses may not adapt at the same rate. Adrenorcortical responses may adapt more quickly than catecholamine responses for
example (Rose, 1980). Thus the pattern of stress response, as well as
the overall magnitude, varies over time.

What Is Disease?

The meaning of disease does not seem to us as tricky as that of
stress. There are some logical and semantic questions, however, and
there are also differences among pathologies which should produce
differences in their responses to stress.

DISEASE, ILLNESS, AND HEALTH

Disease can be defined as "an interruption or perversion of
function of any of the organs...[or] tissues or an abnormal state of the
body as a whole" (Stedman's Medical Dictionary, 1961). A straightforward extension treats "illness" as a synonym of disease and "health"
as the absence of disease, as in Stedman's.

However, some authors have pressed the terms health and illness
into service in making distinctions among disease-relevant variables.
Weiner (1977, p. xi) has separated disease and illness, suggesting that
an individual can have a disease without being ill and vice versa. He
seems to equate disease with actual physiologic disruptions and illness
with the experience of symptoms. Hypertension is often asymptomatic,
and hypertensives may thus be said to have a disease without being ill.
Those with somatization or conversion disorders (American Psychiatric
Association, 1980) might be examples of persons who are ill without
having (physical) diseases.

Schwartz (e.g., 1984) has distinguished between the current state of the organism and its *potential* to resist disease. In this terminology, "wellness" refers to the current state and "health" refers to the potential to be well. Thus people can be diseased (low wellness) yet be healthy if they are exhibiting resistance to the pathology and healing successfully. Conversely, they can be well (not diseased) but still be unhealthy. Putting Weiner's and Schwartz's usages together, one can be diseased and therefore unwell without being ill and while remaining healthy. On the other hand, one can be unhealthy, but neither diseased nor ill; or ill and healthy but unwell; or. . . .

Obviously, it does not matter which words are used for what as long as everyone agrees. The distinctions among actual biologic pathology, one's experience of and response to one's state of health, and one's potential to resist disease are important no matter what the terminology may be. We shall follow the old school, using disease and illness as synonyms and health as the absence of disease. Some refer to a sort of superhealth which implies not only the absence of disease (and of illness as in Weiner) but also unusual psychologic well being (Gordon, 1980). Superhealth is beyond the scope of this volume.

Weiner's contrast between disease and illness brings up the issue of behavior as an outcome variable in stress-disease studies. If people can feel ill without having diseases and can have diseases while feeling well, then what they *do* and *say* about their states of health is suspect as an indication of their actual biologic statuses (e.g., Costa & McCrae, 1985; Kellner, 1985; Mechanic, 1972; Wagner & Curran, 1984, Watson & Pennebaker, 1989). Terms such as *illness behavior* and *sick role* have been used to refer to responses to perceived illness (see Gatchel & Baum, 1983, pp.163-167). Persons will differ in how they interpret their symptoms, in the degree of distress needed for them to seek health care, and in the way they present their degree of perceived illness to others (including researchers). Variables such as utilization of health care services or reports of symptoms and diseases are illness behaviors and will not relate precisely to actual pathology. Even physician diagnoses might sometimes be suspect, although they represent a clear improvement over something like self-report of illness.

Unfortunately, direct measures of pathology are often difficult, expensive or unethical to obtain and so, despite their imperfections, questionable indirect measures might often need to be used. (We should point out that when the interest is in illness behavior per se, separating behavior from actual pathology is still a problem.)

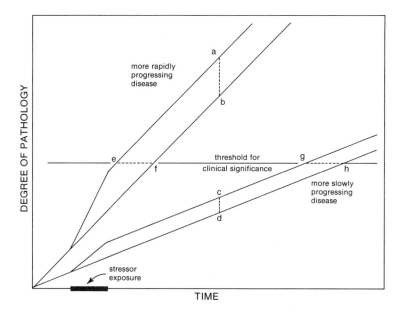

Figure 1. Illustration of possible effects of a stress episode on diseases that progress at different rates.

THE DYNAMICS AND DEVELOPMENT OF DISEASE

Even considering only direct measures of pathology, it is not always clear what it means to have a disease. When a disorder has developed far enough, there is ordinarily no problem in deciding that the individual is ill, but earlier in the progress of pathology the meaning of disease can be a bothersome issue. In many disorders, pathologic indices are on continua (e.g., blood pressure, degree of infection) and there need be no clear demarcation between health and disease. With some diseases (e.g., cancers), the earliest stages are not detectable.

Some general characteristics of diseases might affect their reaction to stress. All other things being equal, a disorder with a slow rate of progression should be affected differently by a stress episode than one which develops rapidly. Figure 1 depicts a hypothetical situation in which two diseases progress at different rates and in which the rate of pathologic change doubles during stress. The more rapid the underlying pathologic process, the greater will be the difference in

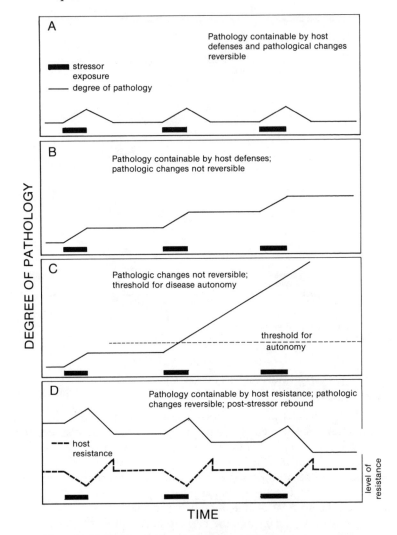

Figure 2. Examples of different possible relationships between stress and pathology which depend upon the dynamics of the pathologic processes and the ability of host resistance factors to contain the development of the pathology.

pathology as a function of stress (line segment a-b is longer than c-d in Figure 1). However, if there is a threshold for clinical significance (e.g., a degree of pathology that is likely to result in a diagnosis), the stress effect on when that threshold is reached does not depend upon how rapidly the disease progresses (line segments e-f and g-h are of equal length). Whether stress has unequal effects upon diseases which develop at different rates might depend on what outcome variable is examined.

The permanence of pathologic changes and the role of host resistance should also help to determine what effect stress will have. We can look at four simple examples (Figure 2) to illustrate some of the possibilities. When pathologic changes are reversible by host defenses, as in some infections for example, a stress episode may have no overall effect. Once the episode ends, host resistance forces can restore normality (Figure 2, panel A). When pathologic changes are not reversible, as may be the case with insulin-dependent diabetes or other disorders based on cell loss, then a series of stress episodes ought to have a cumulative effect (B of Figure 2). A third possibility is one in which pathologic processes can reach a threshold of autonomy at which host defenses, even if normal, can no longer check disease progression. When stress acts on such a disease by reducing host resistance rather than by enhancing pathologic processes directly, further stressor encounters would be irrelevant (Figure 2, C).

In the three preceding examples, there were no rebound effects at the termination of stress episodes or with adaptation. Panel D of Figure 2 illustrates a situation in which basal host resistance is sufficient to keep pathology from increasing and in which a post-stressor rebound increases host resistance above baseline. Under such circumstances, stress could diminish pathology even when the initial effect of stress is to exacerbate it.

These simple hypothetical situations cannot be taken as accurate reflections of relationships between particular diseases and particular stressors. Nor do they exhaust the possibilities (in none does the initial stressor exposure inhibit pathologic processes, for example). What we wish to illustrate is that different combinations of disease dynamics, host resistance, and stress response can plausibly produce a variety of outcomes. A holistic approach, sensitive to the operation of multiple variables in multiple patterns, does not suggest that stress should affect disease in only one manner.

SOME PROBLEMS OF METHODOLOGY

The difficulties in finding out whether, when, and how stress influences human disease contribute greatly to our belief that the context for stress-disease research findings is nearly as important as the findings themselves. If it were easy to answer these questions, it would not be quite so important to consider the conceptual problems with the term stress, to discuss stress effects on hormones, immune function, and behavior, or to know that there are many ways in which stress *might* affect disease.

There are logical, practical and ethical limits to what researchers can do to advance the understanding of any reasonably complicated relationship between people and their environments. (Is this why behavioral and social scientists do not worry that the success of their endeavors might make people's actions wholly predictable?) Such limits are hardly unique to the question of stress and disease, but this topic suffers from them as much as any.

The underlying problem is easily stated. *Science arrives at the conclusion that one factor (an independent variable) exerts a causal influence on a second factor (a dependent or outcome variable) by conducting research in which other possibilities are eliminated.* The greater the number of alternative possibilities ruled out, the more acceptable is the conclusion that the independent variable in question is actually an influence on the dependent variable.

There is no way to rule out all possibilities but one; scientific inquiry can never achieve total certainty. (Television commercials for headache remedies notwithstanding, the term "proof" should not be used where empirical questions are at issue.) However, even though infallibility is unattainable, there are crucial differences among methods in the degree of confidence they provide. The principal distinction in this regard is between experimental and non-experimental methods.

Experimental Versus Non-Experimental Research

If an experiment demonstrates an association between independent and dependent variable and if it is properly conducted (e.g., there is no systematic bias in the measurement of the dependent variable), then either the independent variable has in fact affected the dependent variable, or random error has produced an apparent influence. There are two easily recognized marks of an experiment. First, the researcher *manipulates* the independent variable. If the question is one of a stressor's influence on disease, the experimenter produces the stressor. Second, the experimenter can assign subjects randomly to levels of the independent variable. The experimenter can flip a coin to decide that Jones will be subjected to high stress and Smith to low stress. Replicated experiments (those which have been successfully repeated) set the standard of definitiveness for empirical cause-effect conclusions.

There may, of course, be serious questions about the *implications* of even well designed experiments. The independent variable may not be a pure manipulation of what the experimenter wanted, for example, or the dependent variable might not be the most relevant one for a particular question. But assuming routine precautions in the conduct of an experiment, an observed association must be due either to chance or to a real causal influence of the independent variable.

Non-experimental research may take many forms (e.g., Campbell & Stanley, 1966). All forms have in common a low degree of control by the researcher—too little to allow manipulation of the independent variable and random assignment of subjects. Thus there are an unknown number of possible reasons for observed associations between independent and dependent variables, genuine influence and random error being but two.

Suppose, for instance, that a researcher obtained a random sample of all U.S. adults who underwent marital separations during a particular two months and also a random sample of adults who did not undergo a separation. If significantly more of the separation subjects developed bacterial infections during the next 90 days, the researcher could not justifiably conclude that the marital separations (or the frictions that presumably preceded them) produced the high rate of infectious disorders. Even ignoring such obvious things as disparities between the groups in age and initial marital status, there are alternative explanations for the findings.

Perhaps the separated were, on average, consorting with more numerous acquaintances both before and after the separations, and those activities increased their exposure to bacteria. Perhaps susceptibility to disease is a factor in making spouses dissatisfied with one another. Perhaps the separated were, on average, more generally slovenly, that slovenliness making them both more likely to irritate their spouses and less likely to take simple hygienic precautions against infection. Perhaps more of the separated were in the early stages of some chronic disorder that both depressed their resistance to bacteria and altered their behavior in ways that made them difficult to live with. One perhaps follows another. As it is non-experimental, such research cannot distinguish separation as a causal factor from other possibilities.

Some types of research look experimental but are not, at least not completely. For instance, when time serves as an independent variable, results can be difficult to interpret because time is not really under the experimenter's control and can easily be confounded with other factors.

Another example is the very common paradigm in which a manipulated laboratory stressor is one independent variable and a personality factor is a second independent variable. Glass and colleagues (see Glass, 1985), for example, compared the responses of Type A and Type B men to defeat in a video game during which the superior opponent either did or did not harass them. The greatest physiologic changes occurred in the harassed Type A's, suggesting that antagonistic encounters are particularly important stressors for these individuals. Studies of this type are half experimental and half non-experimental. The stressor is manipulated by the researcher, but the personality variable is not. It may not have been the Type A-ness of the subjects which produced their higher physiologic responsiveness.

We emphasize the inconclusiveness of non-experimental investigations because it is easily overlooked. Researchers in the stress-disease area often use phrases such as "effect of" or "impact of" when their methods are not experimental. Another thing occasionally observed is the statement that if stressors occur before the period over which disease outcome is assesed then causation can be established (see, "Retrospective and Prospective Research", below).

Giving causal status to factors which have been shown only to be associated with disease may reflect the imperfections of human judgment. People (including researchers) tend among other things to use judgmental heuristics that bias decisions (e.g., Tversky & Kahneman, 1983). One aspect of this bias involves the influence of plausible causal scenarios. A readily available scenario linking two events is likely to be used in interpreting those events whether it is correct or not. Since "everybody knows" that stress is detrimental, an association between stress and pathology may be interpreted as causal without other, less cognitively available, possibilities being considered.

THE USES OF EXPERIMENTAL METHODS

The experimental approach has real limits. It is neither ethical nor feasible to randomly assign people to be stressed by researchers and followed until their disease outcomes are known. Experiments can be done only under circumstances which render them inconclusive as to whether stress participates in the etiology of human disease. Even when experiments can be done, there is the question of *external validity*, of whether the controlled and limited conditions of permissible experiments match the more complex conditions of real life.

Human Experiments

Experiments using human subjects cannot be used to ascertain whether stress affects the development of disease, but they can serve other purposes. Many, though hardly all, of the psychosocial and biologic processes that contribute to stress are subject to experimental investigation in humans. Experiments to determine whether stress management techniques can alter the post-diagnosis course of disease are also feasible. To the extent that the influences on disease after it is diagnosed parallel those on its original development, effects of stress management on post-diagnosis course provide evidence in favor of stress as a pre-diagnosis factor. It is also possible to study experimentally the effects of stress-reducing interventions on morbidity, particularly in high-risk groups where very large numbers of subjects would not be required. Work on techniqes such as relaxation is being done, and the initial results are relatively encouraging (e.g., Johnson, 1982).

Experiments With Infrahumans

Although research on animal models has become controversial, it is difficult to imagine great progress on the stress-disease question without it. Animal models have answered the question of whether stress *can* influence the development of disease. It can. They also provide crucial information on the mechanisms of those effects. Still further, they are the basis for much of what is known about pathologic processes. The early events in cancer, for instance, simply cannot be studied in humans. AIDS provides another timely example. The biology of retroviruses is very unusual, and it is terrifying to consider how little would now be known about this disease if researchers had not spent decades studying obscure retroviruses in mice and fowl.

The control which infrahuman models allow over disease initiation and environmental conditions permits studies of those models to detect subtleties in stress effects which would be much more difficult to detect in human research. Infrahuman research has shown clearly that stress can inhibit the development of disease as well as enhance it. Which occurs depends jointly upon the characteristics of the disease, of the host and of the stressor (e.g., Newberry et al., 1985; Plaut & Friedman, 1982).

Like all other approaches, animal models have weaknesses. Neither experimental diseases nor the responses of infrahumans to stressors parallel their human counterparts exactly. Experimental pathologies are often induced by artificial means. In no two species are basic biologic processes quite identical. Infrahumans almost surely lack the immense human capacity to worry about the future and interpret their own interpretations of imagined stressors. Just as it is easy to underestimate the importance of animal models and assume that they have no relevance, so it is easy to overgeneralize from them and assume that anything found in their study applies fully and automatically to humans.

In Vitro Experiments

The test tube and culture bath are indispensable. Things can be learned by isolating tissues and cells that cannot be learned from the study of whole organisms. Much of what is known about genes, the mechanisms by which chemical messengers act, and the biochemical basis of disease comes from the study of cells and tissues, not whole organisms.

The limitations of in vitro methods are as obvious as their advantages. When cells and tissues are studied away from the environment provided by the rest of the organism, some aspects of their functioning are certain to be unusual, even though it might be difficult to discover exactly which ones. One relevant example is provided by Keller et al. (1980). They studied the effects of hypothalamic lesions on the responses of lymphocytes (a variety of immune system cell to be discussed later) to activating agents called mitogens. The alterations of hypothalamic function suppressed the lymphocyte response, but only if the assay was carried out in whole blood. When lymphocytes were isolated before being tested, the effect did not occur.

THE USES OF NON-EXPERIMENTAL METHODS

Experimental and non-experimental methods complement each other. Non-experimental methods lack power to confirm cause-effect conclusions, but they often have greater external validity than experiments and can be employed where ethical and logistic considerations preclude experiments.

As we have implied, a most important thing to consider in evaluating a non-experimental study is the way the study controls for extraneous variables' effects. In stress-disease research, then, the larger the number of alternative possibilities eliminated, the more probable it is that stress actually has a causal role.

Retrospective and Prospective Research

The timing of the data collection is one aspect of a study that determines what alternatives can be eliminated. Temoshok and Heller (1984) provided one discussion of this topic in their review of psycho-social cancer research. In *retrospective* studies patients and controls are asked about stressors which occurred before the patients were diagnosed. The problem, of course, is that the biologic effects of the disease, the knowledge of having the disease, medical treatments, life-style changes, and other's reactions to patients having the disease can all alter the psychologic states of the patients and therefore alter their recall of previous stress. Retrospective studies can be strengthened if all stress-related reports in both the patients and the controls are susceptible to independent verification or disconfirmation, but that greatly increases the difficulty of the study.

Prospective stress studies attempt to assess stress before the disease is present. Thus, the disease and its concomitants should not affect the stress measures. Successful prospective studies identify *risk factors*—variables that predict the likelihood of a disorder in advance of morbidity.

Identifying risk factors is of major importance, but risk factors need not be causal factors. Other variables might be influencing both the risk factor and the disease. Depression may predict death from cancer (Shekelle et al., 1981), but the prediction might work because a genetic characteristic predisposes people to both depression and cancer, or because some people are depressed by their poor health behavior.

Moreover, even deciding whether stress is a risk factor can be a bit tricky. To know whether the stress assessment was made before the pathology began, the researcher must know when the pathology began, but that is often unknowable. The safe way out is to use a prospective delay so very long that the disease could hardly be having any effects at the beginning of the study. Unfortunately, long delays between stress assessment and disease outcome mean that stress effects occurring during the progression of the disease cannot be detected. The researchers are damned if they do and damned if they don't.

Long-term prospective research is often exceedingly expensive. One variation on the prospective study which is much less expensive is the *archival* study (Temoshok and Heller call this the retro-prospective study). In this approach, the researchers make use of data that were taken in the past for other purposes and retained. The archives of employers, educational institutions, prisons, and hospitals may contain records of stress-relevant variables that were obtained in the past. If later information on the health of those individuals can be obtained, the logic of a true prospective study holds.

Matching and Statistical Control

A prospective approach can control for the possibility that disease and the things that accompany it are affecting measures of stress. But there are many other things that it cannot control for— possibilities in which stress precedes disease in time but does not have a causal influence.

Most readers will know that there are ways to conduct and analyze non-experimental studies so as to improve the odds of being correct about causal hypotheses. These methods involve controlling for the effects of alternative possibilities either by matching high-stress with low-stress subjects on relevant variables or by assessing the possible alternatives and removing their effects statistically. Techniques such as partial correlation and multiple regression are used with the latter approach. These procedures should be employed whenever they are appropriate.

However, they are limited in what they can accomplish. Requirements for sample size, researchers' time, subjects' time, and money increase as the number of variables ruled out increases. Those requirements quickly become impractical to meet and do not in any case allow for controlling an indefinite number of variables. A logical limitation is that these control techniques can account only for alternative possibilities that occur to the researcher, whereas random assignment of subjects in an experiment can deal with possibilities that no one has yet considered.

We are left, then, with no clear way to demonstrate quickly and conclusively that stress influences the development of human disease. Non-experimental research cannot demonstrate causation even to the extent that the logic of inquiry allows. Experimental research cannot ethically be used to answer the basic question. It is the convergence of evidence from well conducted studies of all sorts which can convince a sometimes skeptical scientific community that stress effects on human disease are the best approximation to the truth. The present authors like Miller's (1981) idea of being adventurous in what we consider but cautious in what we claim.

The Question of Mediation

Understanding the mechanisms by which stress effects might occur is essential in developing practical methods for minimizing any illness burdens that come from too much or too little stress. More relevant to this book, information on mediating mechanisms is helpful in evaluating the hypothesis that stress affects disease. If stressors alter immune function, for example, it is more reasonable to think that they can alter susceptibility to infections or cancer.

Something must act on normal tissues to bring about the derangements that are called disease. Exogenous agents (e.g., drugs, bacteria, radiation) and endogenous factors (e.g., hormones, enzymes, other pathologies) would seem to exhaust the possibilities. Thus if stressors impact disease, they must act by altering effective exogenous agent exposure and/or altering the organism's internal economy. There are literally thousands of sequences of events that can connect a stressful situation to a change in pathologic processes. Determining which of these sequences act to affect which pathologies when which persons are exposed to which stressors is about as difficult a task as the present authors can imagine.

It involves understanding as much as possible about behavior, psychologic processes, biologic processes, and the characteristics of environments. It involves, in other words, the whole of organism-environment relations. All of the types of methodologic difficulties which come up in deciding *whether* stress affects disease remain, and they are multiplied because more steps need to be worked out.

To take a simple example, it is easy to show that the stressor of forced restraint inhibits the development of chemically induced rat mammary tumors (Newberry, 1978) but much more difficult to find out how this happens. Does it occur because of changes in food intake, immune function, circulating hormones, the metabolism of the carcinogen, blood lipids, or—the worst to contemplate—some very particular combination of those changes? As per the rule of establishing causation by eliminating alternatives, showing definitively that any one possible mediating factor is in fact operating requires research in which all of the other possibilities are ruled out.

Three types of evidence are usually used to evaluate the roles of putative mediators. The weakest of these is merely evidence that the putative mediator covaries with stress effects on the disease. Many variables change under stress. Showing that one does so does not mean that it is an operative mediator. Finding depressed immune function when a stressor produces sudden cardiac death would not mean that the immunodepression was responsible for the stressor's effects on the heart. The covariation approach can eliminate possible mediators from consideration, however. If some factor remains unchanged when stress affects pathology, it would be difficult to argue that that factor mediates the effect.

A second approach attempts to reproduce the stress effect by independent manipulation of the mediator. Assume that a stressor were known to exacerbate an infectious disease in mice (cf. Plaut & Friedman, 1982), and that a particular hormone, corticosterone, were known to increase in response to that stressor. The finding that direct administration of corticosterone also decreased resistance to the infection would then be important evidence favoring the hormone as a mediator of the stress effect. It would not be conclusive evidence, however. Under stress, with many factors changing at once, the infection-promoting effect of corticosterone might be offset by other hormones, perhaps by prolactin (see Berczi, 1986a). Moreover, it would be difficult to administer exogenous corticosterone so as to precisely mimic the pattern of its response to the stressor.

The strongest evidence for a particular mediator would be the observation that the stressor's effect on the pathology fails to occur when the stressor's effect on the proposed mediator is precluded. Continuing with our stress-corticosterone-infection example, suppose it were possible to block the corticosterone response to the stressor while leaving all other components of the stress response apparatus intact, and that under those conditions the stressor had no effect on susceptibility to infection. That finding would strongly implicate the hormone.

Unfortunately, it is often not possible to find a means of blocking only one element of the stress response. We know of no method which can do so for corticosterone; all of the possibilities which occur to us (adrenal decortication, aminoglutethimide, metyrapone, etc.) affect other systems rather directly. In addition, it might be possible to get false negatives with the blocking approach. Some process may actually be a mediator, but blocking it might produce compensating changes in other mediators and allow the stress effect to occur anyway.

It may be difficult to discover exactly how stress effects on health are mediated, but they have to be mediated in some fashion. Our next topic is the nature of the biologic stress responses which most experts believe carry much of the burden in linking stressful experiences to disease.

2:

Biologic Systems That Respond Under Stress

Understanding the spectrum of stressors' effects on organisms is necessary for understanding how and when stress might influence disease. For stressors to affect disease, they must have direct or indirect impacts upon psychologic and biologic processes, impacts which can carry their influences from the environment to pathology or from one pathologic process to another. In this chapter and the next we shall consider some of the ways in which stressors may change the functioning of organisms more or less directly. A very large amount of research has been done, but many things are still unexplored and there are seeming inconsistencies.

We hope to give the reader some sense of the diversity of stress responses and the intricacy with which internal systems influence each other. Psychologic stress responses will be considered in Chapter 3. The discussion in the present chapter will center on the neuroendocrine and immune systems. It should become clear as we proceed that these systems are very closely interrelated. The endocrine and nervous systems can sometimes hardly be distinguished from each other because they share organs and messenger substances. The endocrine system itself consists of more types of secreting tissues and hormones than most psychologists have considered. The immune system turns out to be an endocrine system in addition to, or as a part of, having a role in defense against disease.

NEUROENDOCRINE RESPONSES

Relations Between Nervous and Endocrine Systems

The nervous system is the major mediator of stress responses. The brain controls behavior and exerts great influence on peripheral physiology. Given what is being learned about the degree of influence the brain exerts on the periphery, there may be a tendency to underestimate the importance of other systems—to assume that the brain knows all and regulates all. Weiner (1977, p. 5) has characterized psychosomatics in this way: "This approach is formed by the implicit belief that all physiological processes in the body are ultimately regulated by the brain." If one takes this to mean a tight regulation, it is probably an overstatement (and Weiner notes that organs are self regulating as well). There are other control and response systems, some of which appear to have considerable autonomy even with today's knowledge. Moreover, on the principle of feedback, it might be about as correct to say that the periphery controls the brain as vice versa. But the brain is in the position of being able to respond both to the internal state of the organism and to the external environment. The adjustment of each of those to the other is largely a matter of brain function.

The endocrine system has been considered the second general means for intra-organism communication. However, nervous and endocrine function are so intimately related that it is difficult to take them as separate (Ganong, 1985). Even a brief exposition of their interrelationships can give a rather compelling sense of the degree to which organisms function as wholes.

Since the endocrine system is so basic to stress, and since we are organizing our discussion to emphasize interrelationships rather than to outline the endocrine system in the usual way, we provide Table 2. This table gives some (but by no means complete) information on many of the inter-cellular messengers which we mention, including abbreviations and alternative names, sources, and functions. Minor or less well known sources and functions are given in brackets. The reader should assume that some of this is not yet very well understood.

Table 2. Some Hormones, Some of Their Sources, and Some of Their Functions

Name(s) and Acronyms(s)	Source(s)	Functions
ADRENOCORTICOTROPIC HORMONE (ACTH, corticotropin, adrenocorticotropin)	Adenohypophysis [immunocytes]	Stimulation of adrenal cortical hormone synthesis. Learning & memory: increases motivation and retention. [antipyrogenic]
ALDOSTERONE	Adrenal cortex	Mineralocorticoid: increased sodium reabsorption by kidneys. [stimulates bradykinin production in kidneys and angiotensin production by increasing kallikrein production]
ATRIAL NATRIURETIC FACTOR (ANF)	Heart	Increase in sodium excretion. Vasodilation.
ANGIOTENSIN II	Lungs (and other tissues)	Vasoconstriction. Reduction of renal excretion of water and sodium. Stimulation of aldosterone secretion. [stimulation of vasopressin secretion; enhancement of norepinephrine release from sympathetic neurons]
ANGIOTENSINOGEN	Liver	Precursor to angiotensin II.
BETA-ENDORPHIN (ß-END)	Adenohypophysis (probably others as well)	Endogenous opioid. Possible systemic roles include pain modulation, immunomodulation, modulation of endocrine function. Behavior: activation, sedation, learning, memory.
CALCITONIN (CT)	Thyroid	Lowering of blood calcium by stimulating calcium uptake by bone. [reduces food intake]

Table 2 (continued)

CHOLECYSTOKININ (CCK, pancreozymin, PZ)	Gastrointestinal tract	Emptying of gallbladder. Release of digestive enzymes from pancreas. Stimulation of satiety and oxytocin secretion. [found in gastrointestinal neurons; stimulation of calcitonin secretion]
CORTICOSTERONE	Adrenal cortex	Glucocorticoid (rats & mice): Gluconeogenesis. Inhibition of glucose uptake. Synthesis of catecholamines. Behavior, learning, and memory. [reduction of thyroid hormone secretion; stimulation of growth hormone secretion; reduction of cells' sensitivity to insulin; impairment of low-density lipoprotein uptake by cells; stimulation of gastric acid secretion; inhibition of prostaglandin synthesis; maintenance or increase in arteriolar constriction and myocardial function; modulation of catecholamine receptor numbers]
CORTICOTROPIN-RELEASING FACTOR (CRF)	Hypothalamus	Hypophyseotropic: stimulation of ACTH secretion.
CORTISOL (hydrocortisone)	Adrenal cortex	Glucocorticoid: effects similar to corticosterone (above).
DEOXYCORTICOSTERONE (DOC)	Adrenal cortex	Mineralocorticoid (minor): effects similar to aldosterone (above). [precursor to brain GABA receptor ligand with anesthetic and hypnotic effects]
DOPAMINE (prolactin release-inhibiting factor, PRIF)	Hypothalamus	Hypophyseotropic: inhibition of prolactin secretion. (also brain neurotransmitter and precursor to epinephrine and norepinephrine)
ENKEPHALINS (met-ENK & leu-ENK)	Adrenal medulla, gut	Endogenous opioids: systemic effects probably similar to beta-endorphin. Brain and peripheral neurotransmitters.

Table 2   (continued)

EPINEPHRINE (EP, adrenalin)	Adrenal medulla	Catecholamine: vasodilation and vasoconstriction; bronchial dilation; relaxation of intestinal muscle; stimulation of platelet aggregation; increase in renin output; inhibition of insulin secretion; stimulation of glucagon secretion & glycogenolysis; stimulation of ACTH secretion; release of lipids from adipocytes.
EPIDERMAL GROWTH FACTOR (EGF)	Salivary glands (mice) (other tissues)	Stimulation of growth & healing of skin, lungs, etc. [sperm development (mice)]
ERYTHROPOIETIN (EPO)	Kidney (possibly only a controlling enzyme is secreted by the kidneys)	Stimulation of development of red blood cells (erythrocytes).
ESTRADIOL	Ovary	Oogenesis. Secondary sexual characteristics. Growth inhibition. Behavior. [stimulation of calcitonin secretion]
FOLLICLE-STIMULATING HORMONE (FSH)	Adenohypophysis	Stimulation of ovarian follicles and estradiol secretion. Spermatogenesis. Increase in testicular receptors for luteinizing hormone.
GASTRIC INHIBITORY PEPTIDE (GIP)	Gastrointestinal tract	Inhibition of gastric acid secretion. Stimulation of insulin secretion.
GASTRIN	Gastrointestinal tract (antrum)	Increase in gastric acid secretion. [stimulation of calcitonin secretion]
GLUCAGON	Pancreas	Glycogenolysis. Gluconeogenesis. Stimulation of insulin secretion.

Table 2 (continued)

GROWTH HORMONE (GH, somatotropic hormone, STH, somatotropin)	Adenohypophysis [immunocytes]	General promotion of growth, in large part due to stimulation of somatomedins. [impairment of motor performance; reduction in cells' sensitivity to insulin]
INHIBIN(s)	Gonads	Reduction of follicle-stimulating hormone secretion.
INSULIN	Pancreas	Increase in cellular uptake of glucose. Glycogen synthesis. Cellular uptake of potassium (K^+). Triglyceride formation.
INTERLEUKIN-1 (IL-1)	Macrophages (variety of other tissues)	Immunoregulation. [stimulation of ACTH secretion; promotion of fever; promotion of connective tissue and bone breakdown; promotion of coagulation; production of acute phase proteins; satiety; somnolence]
LUTEINIZING HORMONE (LH)	Adenohypophysis [immunocytes]	Stimulation of ovaries and testes.
LUTEINIZING HORMONE RELEASING HORMONE (LHRH, gonadotropin releasing hormone, GnRH)	Hypothalamus	Hypophyseotropic: stimulation of release of luteinizing hormone and follicle-stimulating hormone. [neuroregulator in sympathetic ganglia]
MACROPHAGE COLONY-STIMULATING FACTOR (M-CSF)	Vascular endothelium, immunocytes	Stimulation of proliferation and differentiation of monocytes/ macrophages and/or their precursors.
MACROPHAGE-GRANULOCYTE COLONY-STIMULATING FACTOR (MG-CSF)	Vascular endothelium, immunocytes	Functions similar to M-CSF (above) but for both monocytes/ macrophages and granulocytes.

Table 2 (continued)

MELATONIN	Pineal	Antigonadotropic effect: depresses gonadal function.
NERVE GROWTH FACTOR (NGF)	Salivary glands (mice) (and variety of other tissues)	Stimulation of neuron growth, particularly of peripheral sympathetic neurons. Best known as local substance released by innervated tissues; systemic role not well understood.
NOREPINEPHRINE (NE, noradrenalin)	Sympathetic NS, adrenal medulla. (Sympathetic and brain neurotransmitter)	Wide range of catecholamine effects, similar to those of epinephrine (above).
OXYTOCIN	Neurohypophysis	Milk release. Contraction of uterus. Contraction of umbilical blood vessels. [role in satiety & nausea]
PARATHYROID HORMONE (PTH, parathormone)	Parathyroids	Increases in blood calcium by bone demineralization, renal reabsorption, intestinal calcium absorption. Stimulation of vitamin D synthesis. Increased renal phosphate excretion.
PLATELET-DERIVED GROWTH FACTOR (PDGF)	Blood platelets	Promotes proliferation of smooth muscle, primarily in vessel walls. Probably mostly local action.
PROGESTERONE	Ovary (corpus luteum)	Preparation of reproductive organs for reproductive function. Sexual behavior. [precursor to brain GABA receptor ligand with anesthetic & hypnotic effects; increase in aldosterone secretion]
PROLACTIN (Prl)	Adenohypophysis	Mammary gland development. Lactation. [stimulation of adrenal androgen synthesis; maintenance of testicular receptors for luteinizing hormone; reduction in transcalciferin levels; stimulation of hair and sebaceous gland growth/development]

Table 2 (continued)

PROSTACYCLIN I$_2$ (PGI$_2$)	Vascular endothelium	Inhibits platelet aggregation. Member of prostaglandin family.
PROSTAGLANDIN-type compounds (PGE, PGF, TXA, LTE)	Many tissues. Synthesized in cell membranes.	Widespread effects via cAMP. E.g., smooth muscle contraction and relaxation, modulation of water excretion, stimulation of ovulation, platelet aggregation, inflammation, immune function. Perhaps mostly local effects and action as second messengers.
RENIN	Kidney	Converts angiotensinogen to angiotensin I.
SOMATOCRININ	Hypothalamus	Hypophyseotropic: stimulation of growth hormone secretion.
SOMATOMEDIN(s) (SMs, IGF-1)	Liver (and probably other tissues)	Growth. Responsible for many effects of growth hormone.
SOMATOSTATIN (somatotropin release inhibiting factor, SRIF)	Hypothalamus [GI tract, pancreas]	Hypophyseotropic: inhibition of growth hormone secretion. [regulation of gastrin secretion, nutrient absorption into blood; inhibition of glucagon and insulin secretion; inhibition of thyroid-stimulating hormone secretion; stimulation of ACTH secretion; neuroregulation in sympathetic ganglia]
TESTOSTERONE	Testes	Secondary sex characteristics and spermatogenesis. Behavior. Growth. [erythropoiesis; increased transcalciferin; stimulation of nerve growth factor and epidermal growth factor secretion by salivary glands (mice)]
THYROTROPIC HORMONE (thyroid-stimulating hormone, TSH, thyrotropin)	Adenohypophysis [immunocytes]	Stimulates T$_4$ and T$_3$ synthesis and secretion.

Table 2 (continued)

THYROTROPIN-RELEASING HORMONE (TRH)	Hypothalamus	Hypophyseotropic: stimulates secretion of thyrotropic hormone. [stimulation of prolactin and growth hormone secretion]
THYROXINE (T$_4$)	Thyroid	Permissive effects for many if not most other hormones. Growth. Metabolism increase. Multiple physiologic and behavioral effects of excess or deficiency. In part, precursor to triiodothyronine. [increased catecholamine receptor sensitivity; stimulation of growth hormone and prolactin secretion]
TRIIODOTHYRONINE (T$_3$)	Thyroid	Same as thyroxine.
VASOACTIVE INTESTINAL PEPTIDE (VIP)	Gastrointestinal tract [immunocytes]	Inhibition of gastric acid secretion. Vasodilation. (May have only local roles; found in GI neurons.) [stimulation of ACTH secretion; found in bone, genital, and nasal neurons]
VASOPRESSIN (arginine vasopressin, AVP, antidiuretic hormone, ADH)	Neurohypophysis	Increase in renal absorption of water. Vasoconstriction. [stimulation of secretion of ACTH and thyroid-stimulating hormone; role in learning and memory]
VITAMIN D (active form)	Kidney	Absorption of calcium from intestine. Bone growth and demineralization. [variety of possible roles in brain, mammary glands, pancreas]

Much of the information in Table 2 is taken from Hadley (1984) and Wilson & Foster (1985).

SOME ENDOCRINE AND NEUROENDOCRINE TERMINOLOGY

It may be helpful for readers unfamiliar with the biologic side of the stress-disease area to become acquainted with some terms and processes that will be used in subsequent discussions. One set of terms has to do with the degree to which inter-cell communication is focused and the distance over which it takes place. In *endocrine* communication, messenger molecules are secreted into the blood and carried by the blood to target tissues. The distance between the sending and receiving cell can be long or short, of course. Hormones are substances which carry endocrine messages. If an action is short range but still involves transport through the blood, it can be called a local hormone action. Hormones secreted by the hypothalamus to regulate pituitary function are termed *hypophyseotropic*.

In *paracrine* communication the messenger substance does not enter the circulation; it travels rather through the extracellular fluid. Paracrine communication is therefore short range almost by definition. If a cell secretes a substance which acts back upon that very cell, it is called an *autocrine* influence.

Classic neurotransmission may be considered a form of paracrine communication. It implies chemical transmission across a specialized synapse. Neurons are subject to other types of messenger influence as well, however. The term *neuromodulation* has been used for influences that do not meet the requirements for being called neurotransmission. Neuromodulators can be thought of as influencing the characteristics of the neurotransmission process. There are many ways in which this might occur: changes in the number or conformation of receptor molecules, the amount of neurotransmitter released, the rapidity of transmitter degradation or reuptake, the metabolic state of the receiving cell. A substance may serve as both a neurotransmitter and a neuromodulator. *Neuroregulation* encompasses both neurotransmission and neuromodulation (Ciaranello et al., 1982); it is a good term to use when the exact means by which a substance influences neural function is unknown. The terms *neuroendocrine* and *neurosecretion* are often used to refer to the secretion of hormones by neurons, something which occurs frequently. However, "neuroendocrine" may refer to the complex of related endocrine and neural systems when they are considered together—a usage which we adopt.

This is as good a point as any to discuss some of the means by which chemical messengers exert their effects on receiving cells. It is difficult to follow many stress-related literatures unless one has some familiarity with this terminology. Receiving cells possess specific receptors for specialized messenger molecules. The receptors are always or almost always protein molelcules. These receptor molecules may be in the cell membrane, in the cytoplasm, or in internal structures of the cell. The binding of a ligand to a protein receptor molecule may be thought of as changing the receptor's shape and thereby its function. The end result can be changes in almost any process in the receiving cell. The term *agonist* refers to a substance that has the effect of a natural messenger and often connotes an affinity for the natural messenger's receptors (the natural messenger itself is considered an agonist). The term *antagonist* refers to a substance that blocks the action of a natural messenger; antagonists often operate by occupying receptors without being able to activate them. We can give only highly simplified versions of these mechanisms, and we should also emphasize that much is still being learned in this very active area of research.

The most discussed modi operandi for cell membrane receptors involve the so-called *second messengers* (e.g., Roth & Grunfeld, 1985). The molecules that carry signals from one cell to another are sometimes called "first messengers," and the second messengers are then molecules that carry the message from the inside of the cell membrane to the interior of the cell. Peptide and catcecholamine first messengers often operate via the second messenger mechanisms that we now describe.

The best known second messengers are *cyclic nucleotides*—cyclic 3',5' adenosine monophosphate (cAMP) and cyclic 3',5' guanosine monophosphate (cGMP). The cAMP functions seem to be a bit more often discussed and we shall describe them. The basic sequence of events is one in which a series of protein molecules is activated one after another. Each activation results from the previous one.

Occupation of the receptor molecule's extracellular binding site activates (or in some cases which we shall not consider here, deac-tivates) a nucleotide cyclase—adenylate cyclase in the case of a cAMP system. The receptor molecule and the cyclase are linked by an inter-mediate regulatory protein, often called a G protein. The G protein transmits the message from the receptor to the cyclase after the G protein binds guanosine triphosphate. In its active form the adenylate cyclase catelyzes the conversion of adenosine triphosphate (ATP; also the major carrier of energy in the cell) to cAMP.

The role of cAMP is then to activate one of a class of enzymes called *protein kinases*. Protein kinases function to phosphorylate (add phosphate groups to) other proteins, and thus to change their activities. In a cAMP second messenger system, then, the result of a first messenger's binding to its cell membrane receptor is a change in the activity of proteins in the cytoplasm of the cell. A messenger acting via cGMP triggers a similar sequence of events.

The chemical deactivation of cyclic nucleotides is an important way in which these second messenger systems are modulated. Enzymes called cyclic nucleotide phosphodiesterases (PDE's) perform this function.

A more recently discovered type of second messenger system involves cell membrane phospholipids (e.g., Majerus et al., 1986; Marx, 1987; Roth & Grunfeld, 1985). In this system (Figure 3), the activation of a cell membrane receptor by an extracellular first messenger activates, via a G protein, a membrane enzyme called a phospholipase (phospholipase C; PLC). PLC acts to split one or more types of phosphatidylinositide, forming *diacylglycerol* (DG) and *inositol triphosphate* (ITP). DG and ITP both act as second messengers. ITP releases calcium ion (Ca^{2+}) from stores within the cell. DG acts with the Ca^{2+} and another phospholipid such as phosphatidyl serine to activate a protein kinase called kinase C (PKC). Protein phosphorylation can then alter cellular function as it does in the cAMP system. PKC activation and ITP may also act to open calcium channels in the cell membrane (not illustrated in Figure 3). Norepinephrine (NE), acetylcholine, ACTH, and vasopressin are among the many messengers which can act via this phospholipid mechanism in at least some cases. We should also mention that arachidonic acid and its metabolites are linked to this phospholipid second messenger system.

Steroid hormones operate in a very different manner than peptide and catecholamine messengers (Clark et al., 1985). Steroids are lipid soluble and can therefore diffuse through the lipid membranes of cells. Steroid receptors, therefore, are usually not on the cell membrane but in the cytoplasm or the nucleus of the cell. When steroids bind to their

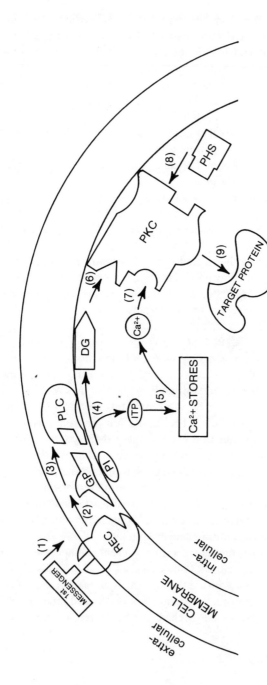

Figure 3. Some general aspects of membrane phospholipid second messenger systems. (DG, diacylglycerol; GP, G protein; ITP, inositol triphosphate; PHS, phosphatidyl serine; PI, phosphatidyl inositide; PKC, protein kinase C; PLC, phospholipase C; REC, cell membrane receptor.) Binding of a first messenger to REC (1) activates GP (2), resulting in the activation of PLC (3). PLC catalyzes the conversion of PI to DG and ITP (4). ITP in turn acts to release stored calcium ion (5). PKC is activated by DG (6), calcium (7), and PHS (8), and phosphorylates a target protein (9), thus changing that protein's function.

receptors, the steroid-receptor complexes act in the nucleus to regulate gene expression. The transcription of particular DNA regions into messenger RNA is enhanced or inhibited when the steroid-receptor complex attaches to the DNA or nuclear proteins.

The types of messenger action that we have described are not the only ones. There are other second messenger systems and other classes of mechanisms by which first messengers can affect protein kinase activity and cell membrane channels. Also, one first messenger can act in multiple ways. Thyroid hormones, for example, function in part like steroids, but they also have effects upon the cell membrane and mitochondria that do not depend upon the transcription of DNA (Hadley, 1984).

NEURAL ENDOCRINE ORGANS

Some major circulating hormones are secreted by neural or nearly neural structures (see, e.g., Hadley, 1984; Reichlin, 1985). The pituitary has long been called the master gland because of its control over peripheral endocrine glands, but in fact the brain is the master gland. The hypothalamus "is" the neurohypophysis (posterior pituitary) and controls the adenohypophysis (anterior pituitary). Oxytocin and vasopressin (arginine vasopressin or AVP, also known as antidiuretic hormone, ADH) are synthesized and secreted by magnocellular neurosecretory neurons. The cell bodies of these neurons are in the hypothalamus, and their axons terminate in the neurohypophysis. They respond to presynaptic influences with the release of their hormones much as other neurons respond by releasing neurotransmitters. The hypothalamus also secretes hormones that regulate anterior pituitary output. These releasing and release-inhibiting hormones (sometimes called "factors," particularly before they are completely characterized) are synthesized in the parvocellular secretory neurons of the hypothalamus, released into hypophyseal portal vessels in the median eminence, and carried by portal blood to the anterior pituitary. Some of these hypophyseotropic hormones must reach the general circulation. However, their concentrations are likely to be quite low, and they may have no physiologic functions beyond the pituitary.

The pineal is another brain structure with secretory functions. Actually, it is a brain structure embryologically and geographically, but has little direct neural connection to the rest of the brain. It is innervated by the peripheral sympathetic nervous system, oddly enough.

The function of the pineal in mammals has been obscure for quite some time. It now appears that its major secretion, melatonin, has an antigonadotropic effect and that the pineal plays a role in seasonal changes in reproduction. Numerous other functions have been suggested for the pineal (Hadley, 1984).

There are neural endocrine structures in the periphery as well. The adrenal medulla is developmentally neural, and its chromaffin cells function somewhat like typical post-ganglionic sympathetic neurons. They respond to preganglionic cholinergic fibers and release primarily catecholamines. Their major product is epinephrine (EP). Although the adrenal medulla secretes some NE, most circulating NE derives from sympathetic nerve endings (Landsberg & Young, 1985), and the peripheral sympathetic nervous system could thus be said to be a diffuse endocrine organ. Landsberg and Young doubt that circulating NE has significant effects. However, its levels are usually higher than those of EP (basal levels perhaps five times as high in humans), and we find it difficult to believe that that much catecholamine would have no effect.

THE BRAIN AS AN ENDOCRINE TARGET ORGAN

The brain is a target of hormones as well as a source of hormones. Pituitary and peripheral hormones feed back to the brain, most obviously to the hypothalamus, to regulate pituitary secretions (e.g., Reichlin, 1985). These are usually negative feedbacks in which pituitary or peripheral hormones act to reduce their own outputs. However, estrogens promote pituitary luteinizing hormone (LH) secretion in the middle of the ovarian cycle, and this positive feedback effect may be partly on hypothalamic gonadotropin releasing hormone (GnRH; also called luteinizing hormone releasing hormone, LHRH). In many cases peripheral hormones feed back to the anterior pituitary as well as to the hypothalamus.

Hormones' actions on the brain subserve more than just endocrine regulation. They also affect basic neural processes and behavior. Among the best known psychoneural/behavioral effects of hormones are those of the gonadal steroids (e.g., Hines, 1982; Rose, 1985). Prenatal or early postnatal androgens "masculinize" both the pattern of GnRH secretion and certain aspects of behavior (e.g., rough play in monkeys). Gonadal hormones have activational influences on sexual behavior in later life, influences which depend in part on the earlier brain-organizational influences of those same hormones. There is some evidence that low androgen levels reduce aggressiveness in humans (see Hadley, 1984). The etiology of premenstrual syndrome, the symptoms of which may include depression, anxiety and fatigue, is at least partly endocrine (Reid & Yen, 1981).

Adrenocortical steroids also have significant psychoneural actions. They increase the reuptake of NE in brain (Maas & Medneicks, 1971). Deoxycorticosterone has anesthetic and hypnotic properties. These are apparently produced by metabolites that function as natural ligands for GABA (gamma aminobutyric acid) receptors. At least one of these metabolites, 3α,5α-tetrahydrodeoxycorticosterone, is increased by adrenocorticotropic hormone (ACTH) and may have a role in brain response under stress (Majewska et al., 1986). A metabolite of progesterone has the same GABA receptor effect. Corticosterone elicits submissiveness in male mice if it has been paired with defeat (Leshner et al., 1980). A variety of psychoneural manifestations can accompany excessive corticosteroid secretion and corticosteroid therapy. Among those reported are fatigue, depression, mania, and social withdrawal (Rose, 1985).

ACTH and related peptides are also known for their effects on brain and behavior. Like many peptides, ACTH is cleaved from a larger precursor, in this case called *pro-opiomelanocortin* (POMC). POMC contains the sequences for several hormones and neuroregulators, including three melanocyte-stimulating hormones (MSH's), ß-endorphin (ß-END), met-enkephalin, and ß-lipotropic hormone (ß-LPH, a possible prohormone for ß-END and met-enkephalin). ACTH appears to facilitate learning and retention in both animals and humans (De Wied, 1980; Richardson et al., 1984). It may act by increasing the motivational value of environmental cues. A number of other pituitary peptides appear to affect learning and memory processes as well. It appears that such effects result at least in part from hypophyseal hormone secretion rather than synthesis of the peptides in the brain, since systemic administration of the hormones can be effective.

Opioid peptides are secreted by the pituitary (ß-END, dynorphin and ß-LPH), the adrenal medulla (met- and leu-enkephalin) and possibly cells of the gut (enkephalins) (see, e.g., Landsburg & Young, 1985; Reichlin, 1985; Rose, 1985). These compounds clearly have psychoneural effects (J.L. Henry, 1982; Kalin & Loevinger, 1983). Their role in analgesia is best known (Watkins & Mayer, 1982). They can also produce behavioral activation, sedation, and euphoria, and can affect learning, memory, and the secretion of pituitary hormones. Opioids have important functions as neuroregulators synthesized in brain as well as putative hormonal functions.

The effects of thyroid hormones on psychoneural function are obvious in cretinism. Both hypothyroid and hyperthyroid conditions have effects in adults as well (Rose, 1985). Depression-like symptoms and reduced cognitive functioning tend to characterize adult-onset hypothyroidism. Anxiety, irritability, difficulties in focusing attention, and psychotic symptoms can occur in hyperthyroidism. Within normal ranges, thyroid hormone levels correlate with cognitive performance (Tucker et al., 1984). Rose (1985) cites evidence that thyroid hormones increase the sensitivity of catecholamine receptors and notes that this could account for many of the behavioral characteristics that accompany differences in thyroid function.

There are hormonal effects on psychoneural function that are rather less well known than most of those we have just discussed. Among those are the reduction in fever by ACTH and α-MSH (Murphy et al., 1983), the stimulation of oxytocin secretion and the reduction of food intake (possibly related to mechanisms of nausea) by cholecystokinin (CCK) (Verbalis et al., 1986), and the inhibition of motor performance by growth hormone (Kelly, 1983). The point is that hormones have widespread effects upon the function of the nervous system and thus upon behavior and psychologic characteristics.

SUBSTANCES SHARED BY THE NERVOUS AND ENDOCRINE SYSTEMS

Still another link between the nervous system and the endocrine system is that some of the same molecules serve as circulating hormones and also as neuroregulators synthesized in the nervous system. EP and NE have long been known to have both roles (Ganong, 1985). Krieger (1983) has provided an excellent overview of some of the others.

At least in retrospect it is not surprising that the compounds synthesized by the hypothalamus and released as hormones have other functions within the brain itself. Among the hypothalamic hormones found in other parts of the brain are LHRH, thyrotropin releasing hormone (TRH), somatostatin (somatotropin release-inhibiting factor, SRIF), corticotropin releasing factor (CRF; Koob, 1985), oxytocin, and vasopressin. The neurotransmitter dopamine serves as the prolactin release-inhibiting hormone (PRIF).

There is evidence that many substances best known as pituitary or peripheral hormones are synthesized in (non-neurosecretory) neurons or perform neural functions (e.g., Hadley, 1984; Krieger, 1983; Reichlin, 1985). CCK, vasoactive intestinal peptide (VIP), and insulin are among those that appear to act in the brain. Some of these hormones appear to function in the peripheral nervous system as well. Somatostatin, CCK, VIP, and enkephalins have been found in gastrointestinal neurons. LHRH apparently serves as a neurotransmitter in sympathetic ganglia (Krieger, 1983). VIP is found in neurons which innervate bone (Hohmann et al., 1986), the genitals and the nose (Reichlin, 1985).

In other words, a large number of substances have roles in different "systems" of the organism. Somatostatin is a prime example (Hadley, 1984). It is best known as a hypophyseotropic hormone secreted by the hypothalamus to inhibit pituitary growth hormone (GH) output. It is also present in other brain neurons and serves as a neuroregulator of some sort. In the periphery, it serves as a local hormone in the gut to regulate the secretion of gastrin. In the pancreas, it acts in a presumably paracrine fashion to reduce the secretion of insulin and glucagon. Its blood levels increase after meals, and it may act as a peripheral hormone to regulate the rate at which nutrients move from the digestive tract to the blood. It is most unlikely that somatostatin is unique in the variety of roles it plays.

CAUTIONS IN INTERPRETING NEURAL-ENDOCRINE RELATIONSHIPS

Although it is clear that the nervous and endocrine systems are very intimately related, it can be difficult to decide exactly what type of neural-endocrine connection is described by any particular piece of research. There are several reasons for this difficulty in interpretation. Since many substances function as hormones and are also synthesized in the nervous system for discrete neuroregulatory functions, there can be a problem in telling whether a particular effect reflects hormonal impacts on the nervous system or changes in the nervous system's intrinsic synthesis of neuroregulators. CRF injected into the brain produces sympathetic arousal (Koob, 1985). But that finding does not tell us whether in real life it reaches the brain by transport in the blood, or exerts this effect as a result of intrinsic neural release, or both. Peripheral hormones may have psychoneural influences by acting directly on the brain, but they might also act via afferent neural impulses, as for example by altering gut motility. Clinical hypo- and hyperendocrine syndromes provide useful indications of the possible effects of hormones on psychoneural processes, but they often represent multiple dysfunctions. The behavioral changes that accompany Cushing's disease, for example, might reflect an effect upon the brain of ACTH, cortisol, altered peripheral energy metabolism, changes in the signals sent by immune system cells, or all of those.

Finally, it should be noted that studies which use exogenous hormones, while essential, need not mimic endogenous hormone actions faithfully. Pharmacologic doses are often used in order to gather basic information. Moreover, most hormones are secreted intermittently, and exogenous administration will usually not follow the natural patterns.

Brain Neurochemistry and Stress

Most of the work on brain activity under stress has involved the levels and turnover of neurotransmitters. NE has been the most studied (e.g., Anisman et al., 1985). The initial exposure to a stressor typically reduces the levels of NE in many areas of the brain. This reduction appears to be due to an increase in the utilization of the neurotransmitter. Noradrenergic neurons increase their activity, and the biosynthesis of NE cannot keep up with its use. With repeated exposure to the stressor a type of adaptation occurs. The NE depletion which was originally observed diminishes or disappears; NE levels in the brain are at or near normal. Adaptation in this case may not mean reduced neural activity, however. Neuronal capacity to synthesize NE increases, and the efficiency of NE reuptake probably increases as well, meaning that high levels of noradrenergic activity need no longer result in reductions in the overall level of NE.

Interestingly, brain levels of gamma-aminobutyric acid (GABA) seem to increase under stress, and its breakdown is retarded (Andreev et al., 1983). GABA is an inhibitory neurotransmitter, and its buildup may indicate a damping of inhibitory processes under stress.

There has been some research on brain cyclic nucleotides and stress. Meyerhoff et al. (1985) have cited some of the relevant research in the context of their own work. Stressful stimulation has been shown to elevate both cAMP and cGMP levels in rodent brain. The data of Meyerhoff et al. indicate, however, that the cGMP increases are probably due to the motor activity elicited by many stressors.

Endocrine Interrelationships

As we have indicated, circulating hormone levels have long been taken as major indices of stress. They are also important means by which stress might affect disease. In attempting to understand stress and stress-disease relationships from a holistic perspective, it is helpful to recognize that the endocrine system involves more tissues than one might think, and that hormones relate to each other in multiple ways. There are within the endocrine system the same types of interconnectedness that one finds between neural and endocrine functions.

THE EXTENT OF THE ENDOCRINE SYSTEM

Behavioral scientists may be used to thinking of the endocrine part of the neuro-endocrine complex as consisting of a few glands whose hormonal outputs either represent their major functions or have been known for decades. The pituitary, gonads, adrenals, thyroid, parathyroids, endocrine pancreas, and probably the gastrointestinal tract would be the organs most frequently recognized as endocrine.

However, hormones are also produced by a variety of other tissues (see Hadley, 1984; Wilson & Foster, 1985). The kidneys secrete erythropoetin, which stimulates red blood cell precursors in bone marrow to proliferate when increased oxygen carrying capacity is needed. They also secrete the active form of vitamin D—1α, $25(OH)_2$-cholecalciferol—which they convert from a precursor produced by the liver. The liver secretes somatomedins in response to GH. Salivary glands, at least in mice, release significant amounts of nerve growth factor (NGF) and epidermal growth factor (EGF) into the general circulation. EGF stimulates sperm development in male mice, and its production is in turn stimulated by androgens and progesterone (Tsutsumi et al., 1986).

Several types of endocrine functions are performed in or by the cardiovascular system. As its name suggests, platelet-derived growth factor (PDGF) is produced by blood platelets. PDGF's most important function is probably as a local hormone, being released at sites of vascular damage to promote smooth muscle proliferation. It may be important in the development of atherosclerosis and hence ischemic heart disease. Blood vessel endothelium (the innermost cell layer) secretes prostacyclin I_2 (PGI_2). PGI_2 is one of the arachidonic acid metabolites (others being prostaglandins, leukotrienes, and thromboxane A_2). PGI_2 is an extremely potent inhibitor of platelet aggregation and, like PDGF, is probably most important as a local hormone. The endothelium also secretes a macrophage colony-stimulating factor and a macrophage-granulocyte colony-stimulating factor (Clark & Kamen, 1987) (see "The Immune System," below). The heart also has an endocrine role. Atrial natriuretic factor (ANF) is released from secretory cells of the atria (Debold, 1985). It functions to increase the excretion of sodium in the urine and as a vasodilator, and can be secreted in response to stressors (Eskay et al., 1986).

There are cases in which some steps in messenger biosynthesis occur in the blood, and in which it is therefore not clear exactly what should be called a hormone in the strict sense. The bradykinin system is one example (Guyton, 1986; Hadley, 1984). Kininogens are circulating proteins that are cleaved by enzymes called kallikreins to form bradykinin(s). Bradykinin is a powerful vasodilator that can apparently be produced in many tissues. In the lungs, bradykinin participates in the edema that accompanies asthma. It may also participate in the skin vasodilation that accompanies sweating.

The renin-angiotensin system also relates to vascular tone and involves kallikrein (Guyton, 1986; Hadley, 1984). Renin is secreted by the juxtaglomerular cells of the kidneys; it is, if you will, another renal hormone. It is produced from a prorenin by the action of kallikrein. Renin is itself an enzyme that converts a plasma protein, angiotensinogen, to angiotensin I. Angiotensin I is in turn converted to angiotensin II. This step occurs largely in the lungs, and the lungs could therefore be considered endocrine organs. Angiotensin II is a potent vasoconstrictor; it also reduces renal excretion of water and salt, and stimulates the secretion of the mineralocorticoid aldosterone by the adrenal cortex. There is an angiotensin III, produced from angiotensin II, which has many of the same properties as angiotensin II. We should point out that the renin-angiotensin system factors are present in the brain and are probably involved in the CNS regulation of blood pressure (Krieger, 1983). Also, a renin precursor has been found in ovarian follicles (Glorioso et al., 1986).

As angiotensin II stimulates aldosterone production, so does aldosterone stimulate the production of kallikrein, possibly creating a positive feedback between aldosterone and renin/angiotensin. Hadley (1984, p. 359) suggests that bradykinin may also contribute to renin release by stimulating prostaglandins in the kidneys. ACTH can increase aldosterone secretion, and catecholamines can increase renin output. Thus the renin-angiotensin system (and possibly the kallikrein-bradykinin system) are potential links between stress and hypertension (e.g., Herd, 1981).

MULTIPLE ENDOCRINE INFLUENCES ON PERIPHERAL PROCESSES

One manifestation of the holistic nature of organisms and the intricacies of the endocrine system is the fact that very many peripheral physiologic events are regulated by multiple hormones. We have just mentioned some of the factors that contribute to blood pressure regulation, and we shall mention a few other relevant cases at this point.

Blood glucose level serves as a very good example (Cryer, 1985; Hadley, 1984). A dozen or so gastrointestinal hormones are involved in digestion and thus in the appearance of glucose in the blood. Insulin promotes the uptake of glucose, most importantly by liver, muscle, and adipose cells. Glucagon is the pancreatic anti-insulin hormone; its basic functions are to stimulate glycogenolysis (the breakdown of glycogen stores into glucose) and to promote gluconeogenesis (the synthesis of glucose from protein and lipids).

The release of insulin and glucagon appears in turn to be under multiple controls. Glucose itself stimulates insulin secretion, but several endocrine factors are relevant as well. The gastrointestinal hormones gastric inhibitory peptide (GIP) and enteroglucagon stimulate insulin release. Pancreatic glucagon increases the secretion of insulin (seemingly paradoxically), and somatostatin reduces the output of both insulin and glucagon—influences that are probably paracrine. Sympathomedullary activation tends to inhibit insulin secretion and stimulate glucagon secretion (e.g., Schuit & Pipeleers, 1986). Catecholamines also promote glycogenolysis. Adrenal glucocorticoids promote gluconeogenesis. Growth hormone has the initial effect of lowering blood glucose, but in the long term it inhibits glucose uptake by cells and reduces their sensitivity to insulin.

"Growth" is hardly a single process (neither is carbohydrate metabolism, of course). Hadley (1984, p. 289) lists 20 factors that have growth promoting or *mitogenic* (cell division-stimulating) properties. Many of these are largely limited to one or a few types of tissue (e.g., prolactin and mammary gland development, thymus hormones and lymphocyte proliferation, platelet-derived growth factor [PDGF] and vascular endothelium proliferation). However, even if one considers only such gross measures as bone and muscle mass, growth provides another excellent example of something that requires multiple hormones.

Pituitary GH is by far the best known hormone with regard to the broad, general stimulation of growth. Even here, though, there are complexities. For one thing, many GH effects are indirect, produced by a class of factors called somatomedins (SM's). SM's are grouped with the insulin-like growth factors (IGF's); SM-C and IGF-I are identical or highly similar molecules. At least some SM's are secreted by the liver in response to GH stimulation. GH can act to promote the differentiation of cells to a state in which they are responsive to the mitogenic influences of SM's (Zezulak & Green, 1986).

General growth also requires insulin and thyroid hormones. Insulin probably exerts part of its effect through making glucose available in cells for protein synthesis, but it also promotes amino acid uptake by cells. The thyroid hormones thyroxine (T_4) and triiodothyronine (T_3) provide the classic example of hormones' permissive effects; almost nothing, including growth, proceeds normally in their absence. Steroid hormones are also involved. Glucocorticoids are inhibitory to growth, at least at high concentrations. Estrogens also inhibit growth, possibly by reducing liver response to GH. Androgens stimulate growth by stimulating protein synthesis (their anabolic effect) but tend also to limit bone growth because they induce epiphyses to ossify.

MULTIPLE EFFECTS OF SINGLE HORMONES

The foregoing has included several instances in which particular hormones influence rather disparate processes. We shall mention a few additional instances involving hormones that we shall not discuss extensively later. Androgens act on bone marrow to promote erythropoesis, affect liver enzymes such as those that metabolize drugs, and alter mitochondrial function in the kidneys (e.g., Clark et al., 1985).

Parenthetically, it is worth noting that many effects of testosterone occur when it is metabolized to dihydrotestosterone or estradiol.

Prolactin also illustrates the fact that a single hormone can have a variety of effects (Hadley, 1984). In addition to its well known functions in lactation, prolactin stimulates the development of hair and sebaceous glands—reasonable because, like the mammary glands, these are integumental structures. It also influences adrenal androgen synthesis (Bondy, 1985), maintains the testes' receptors for LH and reduces the level of transcalciferin (a binding protein that transports cholecalciferol from the skin into the circulation for eventual conversion to active vitamin D by the kidneys [Hadley, 1984]).

HORMONES' INFLUENCES ON EACH OTHERS' SYNTHESIS AND SECRETION

Just as hormones act jointly to influence other functions, they act jointly in influencing endocrine outputs themselves. A common series of steps in controlling the outputs of classic endocrine glands is for hypothalamic releasing and/or release-inhibiting hormones to regulate pituitary hormones, and, in the case of peripheral glands, for the hypophyseal hormones in turn to regulate outputs of the final hormones. Thus, for example, hypothalamic thyrotropin releasing hormone (TRH) stimulates the production of thyrotropin (thyroid stimulating hormone, TSH), and TSH stimulates the production and secretion of T_3 and T_4. Even when this hypothalamic-hypophyseal-peripheral sequence is not the major control, we tend to think of a single influence determining the level of each individual hormone (blood calcium and parathyroid hormone [PTH], neural impulses and EP, etc). It is indeed the case that there is usually one major influence on a given hormone, but there is also much evidence for secondary influences (e.g., Bondy, 1985; Hadley, 1984; Reichlin, 1985).

Multiple influences on insulin secretion have already been mentioned, as has the fact that prolactin affects testicular LH receptors. Another example of a peripheral hormone that is influenced by several others is calcitonin; its secretion is stimulated by androgens, estrogens, gastrin, and cholecystokinin. Glucocorticoids tend to reduce thyroid hormone secretion.

With regard to pituitary hormones, both the idea of single feedbacks from the periphery and the idea of single-purpose release or release-inhibiting hormones are oversimplified (Hadley, 1984). Pituitary gonadotropins are affected not only by feedback from gonadal steroids but also by gonadal peptides called inhibins which reduce follicle-stimulating hormone (FSH) output, by glucocorticoids, and by melatonin from the pineal. GH and prolactin secretion are stimulated by thyroid hormones, and GH particularly by the combination of thyroid hormones and adrenal glucocorticoids. AVP/ADH secretion is thought to be stimulated by angiotensin II as well as by blood pressure, volume, and osmolality receptors. In turn, ADH can serve as a releasing hormone in the anterior pituitary; it stimulates the secretion of ACTH and TSH (Lumpkin et al., 1987). Thyrotropin releasing hormone (TRH) stimulates the secretion of prolactin and GH (Caroff et al., 1984) as well as TSH. Somatostatin inhibits TSH output in addition to GH output. Dopamine, the prolactin release-inhibiting hormone, also reduces the secretion of TSH and gonadotropins (Reichlin, 1985).

A WELTER OF MESSAGES

The internal communications of living organisms are astounding—constant neural traffic, a multitude of messengers liberated from many tissues, and intricate links within and between the endocrine and nervous systems. We shall see later that the immune system, long thought to operate independently, also participates in the organized complexity of internal messages. Every tissue (every cell?) seems to be communicating. Nearly every process is subject to multifactorial, reciprocal, interactive influences. The interdependence of peripheral physiologic functions and their relationships to the brain make an a priori case for stress influences on disease and for the usefulness of a holistic viewpoint.

The Pituitary-Adrenocortical System and Stress

The emphasis placed on the pituitary-adrenocortical axis by Selye, the relative consistency of its response to stressors, and the broad range of its peripheral influences have made this system one of the most frequently cited candidates for mediating stress effects upon disease. There are in fact a wide variety of means by which adrenal corticosteroids might affect pathology. In some cases, one would expect an exacerbation of pathology by these steroids, and in others protection against disease would be expected.

CHARACTERISTICS OF THE PITUITARY-ADRENOCORTICAL SYSTEM

Effects of Glucocorticoids

The adrenal cortex can synthesize all major classes of steroids—glucocorticoids, mineralocorticoids, estrogens, progestogens, and androgens (see Bondy, 1985, from which our treatment of this system is largely taken). Our primary concern is glucocorticoids. The major glucocorticoid of primates, dogs and guinea pigs is cortisol (hydrocortisone); that of rats and mice is corticosterone. It is sometimes not appreciated that these compounds are not equivalent. Cortisol is approximately three times as potent as corticosterone in standard assays of glucocorticoid effects (Haynes & Larner, 1975). This means that studies in which cortisol is administered to rats or mice may produce results that are not physiologically meaningful unless doses are low. The synthetic glucocorticoids can be even more potent; dexamethasone is about 70 times as powerful as corticosterone (Haynes & Larner, 1975).

As their name implies, glucocorticoids have major influences on carbohydrate metabolism. They promote gluconeogenesis and the storage of glycogen in the liver. They also reduce the entry of glucose into cells. The secretion of insulin may be increased by glucocorticoids (possibly as a result of blood glucose elevation), but glucocorticoids can reduce cells' responsiveness to insulin. The secretion of glucagon is stimulated by glucocorticoids. It can reasonably be said that glucocorticoids have a net diabetogenic effect.

Glucocorticoids are also involved in lipid metabolism, but Bondy (1985) notes that their effects are difficult to separate from other influences. Glucocorticoids can increase food intake, augment release of stored lipids by catecholamines, and impair the uptake of low density lipoproteins (LDL) by cells.

Glucocorticoids' effects extend beyond basic metabolism. In the gastrointestinal tract, glucocorticoids stimulate gastric acid secretion (and might thereby exacerbate gastric ulcer symptoms), increase the blood supply to the gastric mucosa, and participate in regulating electrolyte absorption. We shall discuss the effects of glucocorticoids on immune function when we consider stress and the immune system.

Glucocorticoids have complex effects on the cardiovascular system. Myocardial function and arteriolar tone are reduced if glucocorticoid levels are extremely low. Glucocorticoids inhibit the synthesis of several prostaglandin-type compounds, and excess PGI_2 may contribute to vasodilation under hypo-glucocorticoid conditions. These types of effects suggest that excess glucocorticoids might contribute to hypertension. Corticosteroids can reduce the number of catecholamine receptors on heart muscle cells. This might reduce cardiac output under stress, but Williams (1984) has indicated that they also prevent the reduction in catecholamine receptors that ordinarily accompanies excessive sympathomedullary activation.

Control of Adrenocortical Output

The major control over glucocorticoid secretion is, of course, the hypothalamus-pituitary axis. Corticotropin-releasing factor (CRF) stimulates pituitary ACTH secretion, and ACTH increases the glucocorticoid output of the adrenals. The somata of CRF secretory neurons are in the paraventricular nucleus of the hypothalamus. They receive excitatory input from the suprachiasmatic nucleus, amygdala, and raphe nuclei, and inhibitory input from the hippocampus and locus ceruleus (Reichlin, 1985).

There are several negative feedback effects in the hypothalamic-hypophyseal-adrenocortical system. Glucocorticoids act upon the hypothalamus to reduce CRF output and on the pituitary to reduce ACTH output. In addition, ACTH feeds back to suppress CRF secretion.

There are two salient aspects of temporal variation in glucocorticoid levels. First, there is an overall circadian pattern. Shortly before and during the early part of sleep, levels are quite low; they begin to increase during the last half of the sleep period. Second, during the period of wakefulness, secretion seems to be episodic since levels can vary as much as 10-fold. The active-period episodic variations do not result from feedback. Surprisingly, there appears to be a direct neural influence on the responsiveness of the adrenal cortex to ACTH. This may contribute to the circadian pattern. Another possibly minor contributor to glucocorticoid levels may be prolactin. Prolactin can reduce steroid inactivation by reducing the level of 5-α reductase in the adrenal (Ogle & Kitay, 1979).

ACTH secretion is itself subject to more influences than just CRF and feedback. Axelrod & Reisine (1984) have reviewed evidence

ACTH release is stimulated by ADH, circulating EP and NE, somato-statin, and vasoactive intestinal peptide. As with so many other things thought critical to stress-disease relationships, glucocorticoid levels seem to be affected by a large number of variables.

The major mineralocorticoid is aldosterone. It acts to enhance the reabsorption of sodium by the kidneys and the excretion of other ions, particularly potassium. Angiotensin II and III are the most important hormonal stimulants of aldosterone secretion, although ACTH does have an effect. Potassium seems to have a direct stim-ulatory effect on the aldosterone-secreting cells. Progesterone and pregnancy increase aldosterone levels. It should be noted that the glucocorticoids corticosterone and cortisol have some mineralocorticoid activity. (Corticosterone is about 15 times as potent as cortisol in this regard; this is another reason for care in interpreting studies in which cortisol is administered to rats and mice.)

The adrenal cortex secretes testosterone and such weak andro-gens as androstenedione and dehydroepiandrosterone. It is not clear (to us at least) that adrenal androgens have much physiologic signif-icance under normal circumstances, although if they have, it should be greater in females because the ovaries secrete only very small amounts of androgens. The patterns of adrenal androgen secretion tend to parallel those of glucocorticoids. Pituitary gonadotropins do not affect adrenal androgen output; control is vested in ACTH and prolactin.

GLUCOCORTICOID RESPONSE TO STRESSORS

Stressors can overcome the feedback and circadian inhibitions of glucorticoid secretion. A wide variety of taxing and demanding con-ditions have been shown to increase glucocorticoid levels (see, e.g., Asterita, 1985; Mason, 1975; Rose, 1980, 1985), and the fact that they do so is quite well known. The exceptions and limitations to this generalization are therefore of greatest interest, but there are not many well confirmed principles which predict when a presumably stressful situation will fail to produce pituitary-adrenocortical activation.

Perhaps the clearest thing is that adaptation or something similar to it often dampens the adrenocortical response rather rapidly with continued exposure to a stressful situation. This has been found in lower animals (e.g., Murison, 1983) and in humans (e.g., Levine, 1978). Rose (1985) has said something of this sort in emphasizing novelty as an elicitor of glucocorticoid secretion. Ciaranello et al. (1982) put it in terms of unpredictability and the failure of expectancies to be met. They noted that in rats the elimination of food reward increases corticosterone levels and even the anticipation of food becoming available can decrease them (see Coe et al., 1983; Coover et al., 1977).

It is probably not enough to say that predictability or novelty or disconfirmed expectancy produces the adrenocortical response. For one thing, situations are seldom wholly novel or unpredictable, particularly for humans. Some aspects of a situation may be predictable and others not, and the effects of various proportions of predictability and unpredictability have not been much studied. Moreover, expectancies have contents as well as degrees of veridicality; accurate expectancies may be quite unpleasant. Tennes and Kreye (1985) found that the cortisol levels of schoolchildren were higher on achievement test days than on more ordinary days, and that on test days children of higher intelligence tended to have higher cortisol levels than did those of low intelligence. The achievement tests were presumably neither novel nor unexpected. But they were important, in that there was a demand with significant stakes and there was a chance of failure to meet the demand. The less capable children may have been under lower demand because others expected little of them.

It may be better to say that glucocorticoid increases are produced by the expectancy that a significant failure is possible than to say that they are produced by novelty or the disconfirmation of expectancies per se. Unexpected events may elicit a response because, in signalling that the individual did not fully comprehend the situation, they signal that a threat may be more likely than had been anticipated. This view of the role of novelty and unpredictability brings one back to stressors as threats to well-being (Lazarus & Folkman, 1984).

Partly consistent with stress as threat is J.P. Henry's (e.g., 1982) view that "dejection," implying loss of control, is the key to pituitary-adrenocortical response. This theory might predict adaptation—return of glucocorticoid levels toward baseline—if experience teaches that a potentially adverse situation can be mastered or that its adverse consequences are not as severe as might have been feared (cf. Burchfield, 1979; Dienstbier, 1989).

Williams (1985) has proposed that mental work, as opposed particularly to passive sensory intake, is a critical factor in glucocorticoid output. Williams and colleagues found that doing mental subtraction for a small positive incentive increased cortisol levels significantly whereas a simple reaction time task with no incentive did not. Williams related this finding to other literature on neuroendocrine responses in drawing the mental work conclusion. This is an interesting theory, but tasks that require mental work may also engender evaluation apprehension, even in the laboratory setting and even if the evaluation is the subject's own. It will be important in evaluating the Williams view to design tasks that require mental work but do not tap threat of poor performance. It is also worth remarking that Hyyppa et al. (1983) found that cortisol levels fell in response to demanding mental work.

Even when the theoretical generalizations just discussed are taken into account, there remain occasional findings in which glucocorticoids do not respond as expected. To us, one of the most striking of these is in a study reported by Natelson et al. (1976). They found that the introduction of uncontrollable shocks for rhesus monkeys performing shock avoidance failed to increase cortisol levels. This was the case both early and late in the series of eight daily sessions. Here, the critical events were novel, painful, uncontrollable, in violation of expectancies, and likely to provoke some sort of mental work. Moreover, behavioral signs of distress did increase at the introduction of the uncontrollable shocks, indicating that the animals perceived the novelty of these stimuli and were in some sense disturbed by them. There are human studies indicating that such things as increased workload and exposure to a phobic object need not increase cortisol. In fact, cortisol levels are occasionally depressed under seemingly stressful conditions (see Rose, 1980).

There are also cases in which adaptation seems to occur slowly if at all. In rats, the corticosterone response to electric shock adapts but that to cold swim does not, or at least does so considerably more slowly (Weiss et al., 1976). Baum et al. (1985) found that persons living near the site of the nuclear plant accident at Three Mile Island had higher cortisol levels 15 months after the event than did controls in a demographically similar community 80 miles from Three Mile Island. It is difficult to know how much these elevated cortisol levels reflected a failure of adaptation to the initial accident. They may have been due instead to discrete events related to but later than the original accident (later newspaper or television stories, etc.). However that may be, the Baum et al. data suggest that it is possible for very a chronic pituitary-adrenocortical activation to occur in response to ongoing uncertainty and threat.

The Sympathoadrenomedullary (SAM) System and Stress

CHARACTERISTICS OF THE SAM SYSTEM

The SAM system consists of the sympathetic nervous system (SNS) and the adrenal medulla, the latter being embryologically and functionally related to the SNS. As a possible mediator of stress effects on pathology, the SAM response to stress receives at least as much attention as the adrenocortical response. Our treatment of the SAM system's basic features is taken from Landsberg and Young (1985) unless otherwise indicated.

The autonomic nervous system's two divisions, the sympathetic and parasympathetic, innervate most tissues, although they are best known for their innervation of smooth muscles and glands. It is the SNS which has received the most attention as a stress response system but, since the two autonomic divisions often have opposing effects, sympathetic-parasympathetic balance is probably as important to disease as is SNS activity taken alone. SNS outflow from the spinal cord to target organs basically involves one relay in either paravertebral ganglia or in more peripheral ganglia. The preganglionic SNS neurons are cholinergic; that is, acetylcholine is their neurotransmitter. Nearly all postganglionic SNS neurons utilize NE as their neurotransmitter. The adrenal medulla is in a sense part of the SNS; it might be thought of as a greatly modified sympathetic ganglion.

Several messenger substances are involved in the peripheral SAM system in one way or another. We have already mentioned endogenous opioids (e.g., Landsberg & Young, 1985). Somatostatin and substance P (SP) are neuroregulators in sympathetic ganglia; among other things, they act to increase levels of tyrosine hydroxylase (Kessler et al., 1983). (SP is a neuroregulator found in brain and gut and well known as a possible transmitter of pain impulses in the spinal cord; Hadley, 1984.) As another example, sympathetic neurons containing vasoactive intestinal peptide (VIP) innervate bone (Hohmann et al., 1986) and may play a role in the balance of bone deposition and resorption—something related to osteoporosis, normal growth, and general calcium metabolism. Dopamine appears to have a peripheral neurotransmitter role connected with the SAM system (Landsberg & Young, 1985). However, the catecholamines EP and NE are the chief substances released during SAM activation, and we shall concentrate upon them. The chromaffin cells of the adrenal medulla release primarily EP. Nearly all postganglionic sympathetic neurons release NE.

The catecholamines are synthesized from the amino acid tyrosine in a series of steps. The enzymes responsible for the synthesis are frequently referred to in the literature. The three most often mentioned are tyrosine hydroxylase (which converts tyrosine to dopa and is the rate-limiting enzyme), dopamine ß-hydroxylase (which converts dopamine to NE), and phenylethanolamine N-methyltransferase (PNMT, which converts NE to EP). The adrenal medulla receives a blood supply from the adrenal cortex, and adrenal glucocorticoids increase the levels of PNMT in adrenomedullary chromaffin cells. Thus the pituitary-adrenocortical system influences the ratio of EP to NE in the medulla.

There are at least four types of adrenergic (NE- and/or EP-sensitive) receptors on cell membranes. They are designated α_1, α_2, β_1, and β_2. The distribution of these receptors across types of cells is complex. Basically, vasoconstriction and relaxation of intestinal smooth muscle are mediated by α_1 receptors. Receptors of the α_2 type occur at the axon terminals of many neurons, including postganglionic SNS neurons. Their activation reduces NE release by SNS neurons. Blood platelet aggregation is also mediated by α_2 receptors. β_1 adrenoceptors are responsible for catecholamine-induced lipolysis (release of lipids from fat cells) and for stimulation of the heart by the SAM system. β_2 receptors produce vasodilation and dilation of bronchial passages. They also potentiate NE release by SNS neurons and in that regard act in a fashion opposite to α_2 receptors.

EP and NE are not equally potent as agonists for the different types of receptors. EP is somewhat more potent for the α receptors. EP and NE are approximately equal as β_1 agonists. EP is considerably more potent for β_2 receptors.

Although central nervous system influences on preganglionic sympathetic neurons are obviously the critical factors regulating SAM effects on target tissues, there are subtleties. For one thing, sympathetic ganglia are more than mere relay stations. As we have already pointed out, substance P, somatostatin, and GnRH are all apparently active in sympathetic ganglia. Dopaminergic interneurons serve to inhibit activation of postganglionic neurons.

At the final neuroeffector junctions, numerous factors can affect the release of NE. NE is itself one of these. NE released at the junction can stimulate the α_2 and β_2 receptors on the releasing axon terminal and therefore reduce or increase subsequent NE release (an autocrine effect). Landsberg and Young (1985) note that NE released by one axon terminal could affect neighboring terminals as well (a paracrine effect). Circulating EP from the adrenal medulla might also augment NE release by stimulating the β_2 receptors at axon terminals. Acetylcholine has a net inhibitory effect on NE release at SNS neuroeffector junctions, as do histamine, E-type prostaglandins, and adenosine. Angiotensin II has an enhancing effect. Thyroid hormones either reduce or fail to affect SNS activity, but they increase tissue sensitivity to catecholamines.

SAM effects are also modulated by changes in the number of adrenoceptors present on target cells. The most general effect is probably the reduction in receptor numbers in the continuing presence of agonists. This "down-regulation" serves to moderate the effect of intense adrenergic activity. At least some of the receptors are internalized as part of this process. Steroids are among the other influences on adrenergic receptor numbers. Estrogens, for example, act to decrease the number of α receptors on platelets. Glucocorticoids can prevent the down-regulation that occurs with exposure to catecholamines (see, e.g., Foldes et al., 1982). This may be a means by which the adrenocortical response to a stressor can potentiate the SAM effects of that stressor. Thus the net effect of SAM activation on any tissue will vary with the types and numbers of adrenergic receptors its cells possess as well as with the amounts of EP and NE present.

EFFECTS OF SAM ACTIVATION

Catecholamines influence a bewildering variety of tissues and functions. We merely mention a few of them (Landsberg & Young, 1985).

Catecholamines can affect the secretion of other hormones either alone or by altering endocrine cells' responsiveness to other factors. Not infrequently, α-receptor and β-receptor activation have opposing effects (e.g., on calcitonin, parathyroid hormone, progesterone, pancreatic hormones). Catecholamines are thought to increase secretion of gastrin, testosterone, and erythropoetin. The net effect on insulin seems to be inhibitory; that upon pancreatic somatostatin, thyroid hormones, progesterone and melatonin may be stimulatory. Circulating catecholamines are thought to stimulate ACTH release (Axelrod & Reisine, 1984).

The SNS stimulates body heat production in cold and trauma. Catecholamines liberate metabolic fuels, stimulating gluconeogenesis, glycogenolysis, and the release of free fatty acids by lipolysis. They stimulate cholesterol biosynthesis and can increase the levels of low- and high-density lipoproteins.

SAM RESPONSE TO STRESSORS

As with glucocorticoids, plasma catecholamine levels usually increase under stress. This reflects both SNS activation and adrenal medullary activation. As is true of other components of the stress response, there are some limits on the idea of a general, inevitable catecholamine increase, however.

Landsberg and Young (1985) discussed several more-or-less physical stressors. Exercise stimulates both SNS activity and adrenomedullary secretion. Starvation reduces SNS arousal but stimulates the adrenal medulla. Hypoglycemia (as induced by insulin administration) strongly stimulates the adrenal medulla and pushes plasma EP to very high levels. Interestingly, eating also stimulates the SAM system. Exposure to cold increases sympathetic stimulation of some organs but not others and has relatively little effect on the adrenal medulla. With injury, the initial SAM response is adrenomedullary, accompanied in some cases by an actual decrease in SNS activity; but with time, the medullary response diminishes and SNS activation increases. It is clear that physical stressors generally enhance SAM activation, but it seems clear as well that this enhancement can be selective.

There is also diversity in SAM response to more psychologic stressors. Brady (1975) presented data collected by him and his colleagues showing that in monkeys, stress can produce an increase in circulating NE without provoking an EP increase. This occurred, for example, in response to an audible signal that had been paired with shock and also during shock avoidance. The increase in NE without an increase in EP suggests that SNS activation was occurring without adrenomedullary activation. In humans, blood pressure and skin conductance responses to a laboratory stressor have been found not to co-vary well, suggesting that SAM effects on the cardiovascular system can be decoupled from other effects (Fredrikson & Engel, 1985). As we mentioned when we considered the concept of stress, it has long been known that different elements of the SAM stress response can be dissociated (Lacey, 1967).

There does not appear to be solid agreement on when NE and EP will respond differently to a psychologic stressor. Mason (1975) has suggested that when uncertainty and unpredictability are added to aversiveness, an EP response will be added to the NE response (his Pattern II). According to this view, then, NE will increase to a wider range of stressors than will EP. On the other hand, Frankenhaeuser (1975) has suggested that EP will be more responsive than NE. J.P. Henry's (1982) theory associates increased EP output with dejection and pituitary-adrenocortical activation (consistent with Mason's Pattern II), and associates NE output with anger and more active coping.

Whatever the critical conditions are for stressors to elicit different patterns of catecholamine response, it is reasonable to suspect that different response patterns might have different effects on pathologic processes. Stressors that elicit both EP and NE increases may have greater effects simply because more catecholamine is in circulation. Also, the addition of EP to a stress response should mean relatively intense activation of β_2 receptors. We can speculate that this might mean greater bronchodilation and vasodilation, and conceivably less likelihood that the stress response would potentiate hypertension and asthma attack. When physical stressors are involved, the well documented differences in catecholamine response patterns and the selectivity of SNS activation might mean differential effects on different pathologies.

As is true of the glucocorticoid response, the SAM response to stressors can undergo adaptation. Hansen et al. (1978) reported that initial tower jumps for military parachute trainees were associated with significant increases in both EP and NE, as compared to a baseline day before jump training began. These increases were observed both before and after the morning jumps took place. With repeated jumps, the levels of both catecholamines declined. Pre-jump EP was actually significantly below baseline on the last two jumps assessed.

Frankenhaeuser (1975) and Rose (1980) have cited evidence that catecholamine adaptation may not occur as readily as glucocorticoid adaptation, particularly if the stressful stimulus retains its ability to elicit psychologic distress. One instance of chronic change in the SAM system was reported by Henry et al. (1975). They found that adrenal tyrosine hydroxylase remained elevated for at least 40 days in the dominant males of a stabilizing mouse colony. Baum et al. (1985) found in their Three Mile Island (TMI) study that residents of that area had higher urinary NE than controls at 15 months after the nuclear plant accident. TMI subjects' EP levels were not significantly above those of controls but were nearly so.

Pardine and Napoli (1983) studied the relationship of self-reported life stress to students' heart rate (HR) and blood pressure (BP) responses to the laboratory stressor of a bogus intelligence test. High and low life stress subjects did not differ in baseline HR or BP; nor did they differ in their initial responses to the IQ test. However, the high life stress subjects did show slower HR and systolic BP recovery from the IQ stressor. Slow recovery from daily stressors could chronically elevate measured stress responses in studies such as that of Baum et al.

To summarize, SNS outflow and circulating catecholamines very frequently increase in response to stressors. However, there are some instances in which the EP and NE responses are dissociated, with EP increases seemingly being less frequent. Adaptation of SAM responses occurs but can occur more slowly or less often than glucocorticoid adaptation.

Other Hormonal Responses in Stress

Although glucocorticoids and catecholamines are by far the most studied and discussed components of the endocrine stress response, the interdependence of physiologic processes would lead one to expect that the levels of other hormones would also vary with exposure to stressful conditions, and so they do. Many hormones have been shown to respond under stress, and in this section we mention a sample of them. Asterita (1985), Curtis (1979), and Rose (1980, 1985) provide much of the basis for our brief discussion.

Prolactin (Prl) levels are frequently elevated under stress. A wide variety of conditions have been observed to elicit this response in humans, among them surgery and other medical procedures, parachute jumping, the laboratory stressor of mirror drawing (see Curtis, 1979;

Rose, 1980, 1985), exercise (e.g., Loucks & Horvath, 1984), and jumping into deep water (Vaernes et al., 1982). In one study, the cold pressor test did not significantly alter Prl levels (Bullinger et al., 1984).

Animal experiments have also shown Prl to increase under stressful conditions. There is some evidence, however, that when a stress episode is prolonged (one or more hours) or is repeated chronically, prolactin levels can be significantly depressed (Jobin et al., 1975; Taché et al., 1978). There is also evidence that ovarian and adrenal hormones may be required for a full Prl response to stressors (Milenković et al., 1986).

There is agreement that growth hormone (GH) levels often increase in response to stressors. Individual differences have been emphasized with this hormone, however. Some persons seem to respond to stress with GH increases and others do not (Curtis, 1979; Rose, 1980, 1985), it being thought that those high on anxiety-relevant traits are more likely to respond. Kosten et al. (1984) have reported one of the relevant investigations. They studied GH during interviews about the deaths of subjects' severely ill spouses. Those who gave a GH response were relatively high in assessed anxiety, and the combination of high anxiety and high defensiveness was even more strongly associated with GH response. The idea that this sort of preexisting psychologic disequilibrium increases the chances of a GH response is consistent with Rose's (1980, 1985) suggestion that a stronger stressor is needed to provoke a GH increase than, say, a cortisol increase.

The frequent finding of stressor-induced GH increase seems to contradict the suggestion of GH hyposecretion in psychosocial dwarfism and maternal deprivation syndrome. In these disorders, growth retardation (with behavioral abnormalities) occurs in a setting of social neglect and/or psychologic distress for children (see Reichlin, 1985; Underwood & Van Wyk, 1985). There are possible reconciliations of the stress literature with the fact of retarded growth under stressful conditions. It may be that chronic psychologic stress reduces GH output at least in some children; that sleep deprivation occurs in these cases and prevents the normal nighttime GH surge; that the deficit is in somatomedin production; or that nutritional deficits accompany psychosocial deprivations and can produce some or all of the growth failure.

Of the pituitary-gonadal axis hormones, testosterone seems to have been the most studied in relation to stress. Perhaps this is because the female cycle makes pituitary-ovarian responses more difficult to investigate. Testosterone levels are usually found to fall in response to stressors (Asterita, 1985; Curtis, 1979; Rose, 1980, 1985). It is unclear how often this decline results from a reduction in gonadotropin output, because gonadotropin levels do not necessarily fall with stress-induced testosterone declines (Rose, 1980, 1985).

There are instances in which testosterone levels have been shown to increase under presumably stressful conditions. In rats, testosterone increased after 30 minutes of exposure to ether or ether plus laparotomy (incision through the body wall) (Frankel & Ryan, 1981). Rose (1980) mentioned testosterone increases in monkeys who won aggressive encounters. In individuals classified as displaying the Type A behavior pattern, testosterone levels increased during a reaction time task (Williams, 1985)—a mild stressor which Williams considers a sensory intake task rather than a mental work task. Urinary testosterone levels rebounded above baseline following a 72 hour avoidance conditioning session in monkeys (Mason et al., 1968) or exposure to heat stress in boars (Larsson et al., 1983). Davidson et al. (1978) found that in comparison to a baseline day, parachute trainees had reduced plasma testosterone both immediately before and immediately after their first tower jumps. However, with increasing experience, the prejump testosterone levels climbed significantly above baseline. Findings such as those we have just mentioned indicate that in some manner adaptation to or relief from stress can increase levels of testosterone.

Luteinizing hormone (LH) has also been the subject of some stress research. However the reported responses of this gonadotropin under stress have been quite diverse. In female rats, brief stressor exposure has been found to increase (Du Ruisseau et al., 1978; Euker et al., 1975) and more protracted exposure to decrease (Du Ruisseau et al, 1978; Taché et al., 1976) circulating LH. However, Hulse and Coleman (1983) reported that shock at the time of the preovulatory LH surge reduced LH release. In males, Du Ruisseau et al. found no effect, and Taché et al. (1978) found LH depression followed by return to baseline with repeated exposure to forced exercise or immobilization. In humans, LH has been shown to increase in response to exercise, gastroscopy, and surgery (Monden et al., 1972; Sowers et al., 1977). Pontiroli et al. (1982) reported that in males, but not females, LH values increased after cholecystectomy (gall bladder removal). Other investigators (Nakashima et al., 1975) found serum LH levels to increase during surgery and then fall to levels significantly lower than presurgery values two days post-operatively. Johansson et al. (1988) compared LH levels immediately before and after medical school examinations to levels in earlier baseline blood samples. Males' LH levels were reported as significantly lower immediately before the examination and immediately after it than at baseline. However this was not true of females. (Testosterone levels did not change in either sex as a function of the examination.) It seems clear, then, that LH is stress-responsive, but the pattern of its response is unclear and may be complex.

Since endogenous opioids are secreted by the pituitary along with ACTH and also by the adrenal medullae, their levels would be expected to increase as part of the stress response. ß-endorphin (ß-END) has been the most studied. Its levels have been shown to increase with a variety of stressors, among them examinations, surgery, exercise, and electric shock (Asterita, 1985; Cohen et al., 1983; Rose, 1985). Although Cohen et al. mention two studies in which ß-END failed to increase under stress, ß-END may be about as common a part of the hormonal stress response as glucocorticoids or catecholamines.

THE IMMUNE SYSTEM

The immune system constitutes a major defense against infectious organisms and, possibly to a lesser extent, against cancer. Broadly construed, it includes specialized *lymphoid* and *reticuloendothelial* cells, which we shall refer to in the aggregate as lymphoreticular (LR) cells or immunocytes. These cells and the substances they produce can respond in complex ways to molecules which they detect as foreign. The immune system does not contribute to pathology only by failing to contain pathogens, however. Its responses to pathogens may be damaging to the organism, and it can attack self tissues. It is clear as well that the immune system has functions beyond the traditional ones of direct defense against foreign material. The details of immune function are the subject of massive amounts of research.

It is now beyond dispute that the immune system is affected by neuroendocrine factors and stress-relevant psychologic variables. For this reason, and because of its role in host resistance to numerous disorders, the immune system has received a great deal of attention as a possible mediator of stress-disease relationships. Behavioral scientists are probably less familiar with the immune system than with neuroendocrine systems, and we shall present an overview of immune function before discussing stress effects.

The Basic Functions of the Immune System

Our discussion of the elements of immune function is drawn from Barrett (1983), Borysenko (1987), and Kimball (1986) unless otherwise indicated.

The immune system is usually able to discriminate self from non-self (foreign) molecules. It responds to foreign molecules and to cells or particles which carry those molecules on their surfaces. A molecule which can trigger a classic acquired immune response is referred to as an *antigen*. Antigens may be associated with infectious agents or transplants. They may also be novel molecules produced by the organism itself, as may happen in cancer. Only large molecules such as proteins, nucleic acids, and polysaccharides are generally antigenic. The immune system does not recognize and respond to whole antigen molecules, however. It reacts to discrete regions called *antigenic determinants*, and an antigen may have many determinants. It can respond to small molecules only if they are presented attached to large ones (the small molecules then being called haptens).

Immune systems' exquisite molecular recognition abilities are used in non-immunologic research to assay a variety of substances, and the term antigen is often used for any molecule, pathogenic or not, that is being studied via immunologic assays. This can be particularly confusing when marker molecules on the surfaces of LR cells are assessed by immunologic methods and called antigens, as they often are.

EFFECTOR FUNCTIONS OF THE IMMUNE SYSTEM

Immunologic attacks on foreign materials employ four types of final effector functions. These are not independent, however; some cells and cell products participate in most of them.

Antibodies or *immunoglobulins* (Ig's) are proteins released into the general circulation and secreted in certain tissues. There are several classes of Ig's—IgA, IgD, IgE, IgG, and IgM. They differ in their functions, the tissues in which they are most concentrated, and the number of basic Ig units which comprise them. Put simply, the basic Ig unit can be thought of as a Y-shaped molecule having two antigen-binding regions and, as the stem of the Y, what is termed the Fc region. The Fc region interacts with other molecules of the immune system, particularly Fc receptors on LR cells, and it thus participates in the ultimate disposition of antigens bound to the antigen-binding regions. Hundreds of thousands of different antigen-binding sites can be synthesized, and the immune system can respond to an almost limitless variety of antigens.

The mere binding of antibodies to antigens can be effective against some types of pathogens. Ig's can neutralize toxins and link pathogens together to block their actions. To a considerable extent, however, the role of Ig's is to facilitate other effector functions.

Phagocytosis is the ingestion of material by cells. Macrophages, neutrophils and eosinophils are major phagocytic cells. *Opsonization* is a process in which substances attach to pathogens and thereby promote phagocytosis. Some Ig's are potent opsonins, holding targets close to phagocytes and, in some cases, neutralizing target electrical charges which would otherwise keep them separated from the phagocytes.

Activation of the *complement* system provides a third effector pathway. Complement is a series of circulating proteins, termed C1 through C9. The binding of Ig to antigen triggers a complex series of complement reactions. In this cascade, complement proteins are joined and cleaved in a variety of ways (cleavage products are indicated by lower case letters; e.g., C3a); some 20 or so molecules play active roles.

A major result of complement activation is lysis of target cells by the complex (C1s,C4b,C2a,C3b,C5b,C6,C7,C8,C9) in combination with antigen-antibody complex. This attack unit produces pores in target cell membranes. Other products of the complement reactions act as chemotaxins to attract leukocytes (e.g., C5a), as anaphlatoxins which stimulate histamine release by basophils and mast cells (e.g., C3a, C5a), and as opsonins (C3b).

In *cell-mediated cytotoxicity*, immune system effector cells contact (or nearly contact) target cells and release toxins which kill the targets. Some mechanisms of cell-mediated cytotoxicity involve perforation of target membranes in a manner similar to complement-mediated lysis. The substances released by cytotoxic cells include active oxidizing molecules, proteolytic enzymes, and lipolytic enzymes. Cytotoxicity can require the presence of specific antibody or can be antibody-independent.

Convention distinguishes *humoral* from *cell-mediated* immunity. Humoral immunity centers on circulating molecules. Its defining characteristic is that cell-free serum from immunized organisms is effective against pathogens. In cell-mediated immunity, then, serum is not sufficient; intact cells are required. This distinction can seem a bit confusing since cells must produce the humoral factors and humoral factors are involved in activating the cells. Humoral and cell-mediated immune function are in fact closely connected, even though the distinction is important.

CELLS OF THE IMMUNE SYSTEM

Lymphocytes and Related Cells

Like all cells of the immune system, lymphocytes develop from precursors in the bone marrow. The two broad classes of lymphocytes differ in the locations at which they mature and in their functions.

B lymphocytes (B-cells) mature in the bursa of Fabricius of birds and in (possibly several) "bursal equivalent" locations in mammals. When activated by antigen and by chemical stimulants from other LR cells, mature B-cells differentiate into *plasma cells* and secrete antibodies. Each plasma cell secretes immunoglobulin with one specific type of antigen binding site. The B-cells express their Ig's on their cell surfaces, and the surface Ig's act as antigen receptors. Thus a B-cell will respond only to antigens against which its antibody will be effective. It appears that B-cells can also process antigens and present them to T lymphocytes (see "Macrophages", below; Unanue & Allen, 1987).

T lymphocytes (T-cells) make up the second group of lymphocytes. These mature in the thymus. They perform a wider variety of functions than do B-cells, some serving as effector cells and others acting to regulate the immune response. Like B-cells, individual T-cells are responsive only to particular antigens; they have antigen receptors on their surfaces, but those receptors are not Ig molecules. There are several subsets of T-cells.

Cytotoxic T-lymphocytes (also known as CTL's, T_c-cells, or killer T-cells) are contact cytotoxicity effectors. In addition to being antigen-specific, CTL's will attack only targets which express certain molecules of the *major histocompatibility complex* (MHC). The target must usually express the same MHC antigen as the CTL. (The MHC molecules on cell surfaces are diverse and are different from one individual to another. They were originally discovered as antigens responsible for rejection of grafts and transplants but are now known to be important in regulating immune responses.) The MHC restriction on CTL action means that CTL's should generally attack only deranged or infected cells of the organism itself. However, they are quite active against foreign transplants and in this case they seem to be directed primarily against the foreign MHC antigens.

Helper (T_h) and *suppressor* (T_s) T-cells are regulators. When activated by exposure to their specific antigens, T_h-cells secrete substances (types of lymphokines; see below) which stimulate B-cells and other T-cells. A most important factor in AIDS immunosuppression is the destruction of T_h-cells by the human immunodeficiency virus (HIV). T_s-cells have the opposite function; their signals act to dampen the immune response.

There are more lymphocyte subsets than we have mentioned. Different groups of B-cells differ in their need for, or the necessary type of, T_h help. There are also additional subclasses of T-cells.

Lymphocytes are responsible for *immunologic memory*. If the immune system has once responded to a particular antigen, it can often respond more rapidly and strongly if it re-encounters that antigen. Some lymphocytes stimulated by antigen in the first exposure become *memory cells*, ready to respond quickly to subsequent exposures. This memory function and the relative strength of the resulting *secondary immune response* are the bases for vaccination.

Some immunocytes are lymphocytes morphologically but do not express the surface molecules that would identify them as either T- or B-cells. Of these, *natural killer cells* (NK cells) (e.g., Herberman & Ortaldo, 1981) are the most often discussed in the context of stress and disease. Microscopically, NK cells look like large granular lymphocytes (LGL's). They are contact cytotoxic, particularly to tumor cells and virally infected cells. In contrast to CTL's, NK cells do not require the sequence of antigen processing and clonal expansion (to be discussed below) for their activity; rather, they are part of what is called *natural immunity* (see, e.g., Chirigos et al., 1981).

Another type of lymphocyte-like cell is the *null cell* or K cell. Null cells are also cytotoxicity effectors. Their action requires the presence of antibody; they are one of the cell types participating in *antibody-dependent cell-mediated cytotoxicity* (ADCC).

Macrophages

Macrophages develop from blood *monocytes* when monocytes migrate into tissues. Monocytes and the various types of macrophages are often referred to in the aggregate as *mononuclear phagocytes*. Macrophages were once thought to be merely phagocytes, but are now known to have numerous roles, more perhaps than any other cells of the immune system (see, e.g., Unanue & Allen, 1987). One function of macrophages is in *antigen processing*. Lymphocytes do not respond well to most antigens in isolation. This is particularly true of T-cells. Macrophages partially digest antigens and present portions of them (roughly, the antigenic determinants) on their surfaces. When lymphocytes with the appropriate receptors encounter those determinants on macrophages (or other *antigen-presenting cells*), they can respond. The presentation of antigens to lymphocytes must also involve the MHC molecules on the accessory cell. This restriction prevents uncontrolled lymphocyte responses.

Another way in which macrophages participate in immune function is through substances which they secrete. Macrophages produce a number of compounds which have diverse effects (see below), but the most important for immune function is *interleukin-1* (IL-1). IL-1 activates T- and B-cells. Some IL-1 effects may occur via a membrane-bound form of the molecule rather than the secreted form (Unanue & Allen, 1987). Macrophages also secrete interferon, some of the complement proteins, and numerous other substances.

The direct effector functions of macrophages extend beyond phagocytosis. When activated by certain immunoregulatory substances, macrophages can become cytotoxic effectors, seemingly able to function in ways similar to NK and null cells. This activation also increases macrophages' mobility and phagocytic activity.

Granulocytes

There are three types of granulocytes (polymorphonuclear leukocytes). *Neutrophils* are best known as phagocytes, but they may also act as cytotoxic effectors (Weiss et al., 1983). *Eosinophils* are also phagocytic. *Basophils* release histamine, and other compounds such as heparin, from their granules, thus participating in inflammation and allergic reactions. Basophils have receptors for IgE, and the binding of antigen to this IgE is the major stimulus for the basophil response. Tissue *mast cells* function much like basophils.

Table 3 lists some of the cell types of the immune system, along with their functions and secretions. Like the earlier table of hormones, it is representative rather than complete.

EVENTS IN ACQUIRED IMMUNITY

At this point, we can describe in general terms what occurs in the most classic type of immune response, namely actively acquired immunity which results from a first encounter with an antigen. This description will be helpful in following the subsequent discussion of immunoregulation.

Table 3. Some Immunocytes, Some of Their Functions, and Some of Their Secretions

Cell Type	Functions	Secretions
LYMPHOCYTES B-cells/plasma cells	Antibody (Ig) produc-. tion. Antigen process- ing.	Immunoglobulins.
Suppressor T- cells	Inhibition of activity of other immunocytes.	Soluble immune response suppressor & other inhibitory cytokines.
Helper T-cells	Stimulation of other lym- phocytes & NK cells.	Interleukin-2, B-cell differentia- tion factor, interferon(s).
Cytotoxic T-cells	Cell-mediated contact cytotoxicity.	Lymphotoxins (oxidizing molecules, lipolytic & proteolytic enzymes)
Delayed hypersen- sitivity T-cells.	Stimulation of antigen- specific inflammation.	Macrophage chemotaxin, macrophage migration inhibition factor.
NATURAL KILLER CELLS	Cell-mediated contact cytotoxicity.	Cytotoxins, presumably similar to lymphotoxins.
MACROPHAGES	Antigen processing & presentation. Stimula- tion of other immuno- cytes. Phagocytosis. Cytotoxicity. Systemic endocrine role.	Interleukin-1, prostaglandins, inter- feron(s), complement molecules, tumor necrosis factor, cytotoxins.
GRANULOCYTES Neutrophils	Phacocytosis. Contact cytotoxicity.	Cytotoxins, presumably similar to lymphotoxins. Elastase.
Eosinophils	Phacocytosis. Activity against parasites.	Cytotoxins.
Basophils	Promotion of inflamma- tion and allergies.	Histamine. Heparin.

In this sort of specific or acquired immunity, the organism's defense against a pathogen results from a series of events triggered by the appearance of antigen (Figure 4). Antigenic material will typically encounter the immune system in the *secondary lymphoid organs*—the spleen, lymph nodes, tonsils, gut-associated lymphoid tissue. Here macrophages or other antigen-processing cells present the antigen to lymphocytes. Helper T-cells (T_h) are particularly important at this stage. A complex set of interactions involving cell-cell contacts and secreted stimulatory substances results in the activation of the relatively few lymphocytes specific for the antigen. The activation process produces both *clonal expansion* (the proliferation of the antigen-specific lymphocytes) and any final *differentiation* needed to convert lymphocytes to fully functioning effector cells (e.g., B-cells to plasma cells) or to memory cells.

A considerable amount of time (up to about 10 days) may elapse between the appearance of antigen and the full development of the specific immune response. After this, the immune response will weaken as the effects of suppressor cells and other inhibitory regulatory processes come to dominate the stimulatory processes.

Note that in natural immunity, this extended sequence of events is not necessary. Natural effector cells such as NK cells and activated macrophages can act without clonal expansion. They are pre-primed against certain types of pathogens. Natural effector cells do become more active in response to signals from other LR cells, however.

INTRINSIC REGULATION OF IMMUNE FUNCTION

Although the immune system is affected by a variety of other organismic systems, it possesses many intrinsic controls which act to maintain defenses which are vigorous but not excessive. We have mentioned MHC restriction in macrophage-lymphocyte interactions and in CTL-target interactions, but there are several other mechanisms as well.

The term *cytokine* applies to numerous substances secreted by LR cells. A particular compound is more likely to be considered a cytokine to the degree that its secretion is limited to immune system cells and its function is limited to immunomodulation. Cytokines are called *lymphokines* when secreted by lymphocytes and *monokines* when secreted by monocytes/macrophages.

The nomenclature of cytokines can be confusing. These substances have often had more than one name, either because they were discovered more than once or because of attempts to develop tidier naming systems. Readers should also be aware that some cytokine designations may represent different functions carried out by single compounds. Conversely, some designated by a single name are really families of compounds.

We shall mention only a few well known cytokines here. Three major types are stimulatory—*interleukin-1* (IL-1), *interleukin-2* (IL-2),

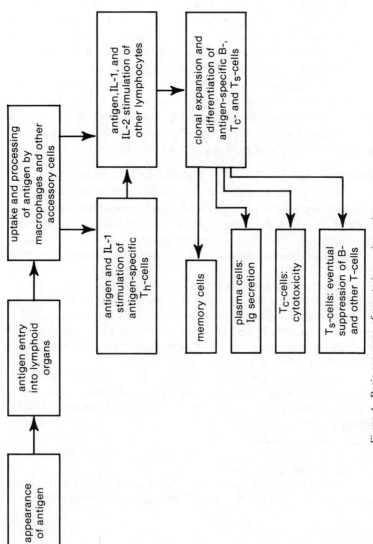

Figure 4. Basic sequence of events in a primary immune response.

and *B-cell differentiation factor* (BCDF). IL-1 is secreted primarily by macrophages, although it may also be secreted by other types of cells, including stimulated B-cells (see Durum et al., 1985). Various stimuli can provoke IL-1 secretion by macrophages, including antigen-antibody complexes, complement component C5a, bacterial toxins, and signals from activated T-cells. The immunologic functions of IL-1 are also diverse. Most often mentioned is probably the stimulation of T-cells. However, B-cells, neutrophils, NK cells, and macrophages themselves are thought to be stimulated as well.

IL-2 acts in the activation and growth of lymphocytes, and appears to be a crucial stimulus for their function (Smith, 1984). They are also its major source. Antigen and IL-1 can produce expression of T-cell receptors for IL-2 and also the secretion of IL-2 by T-cells (e.g., Waldmann, 1986). The results of IL-2 action on the receptors are the T-cell activation and multiplication necessary for an effective immune response. IL-2 secretion by T_h-cells is important in stimulating B-cells to proliferate.

BCDF is, at its name implies, a stimulator of B-cell maturation. It is secreted by T-cells (presumably T_h-cells) and acts upon B-cells which have been stimulated by antigen, IL-1, and IL-2 to move them toward differentiation into Ig-secreting plasma cells.

Interferons (IFN's) are a group of related proteins produced by LR cells and by many other types of cells as well. Their effects are too many and complex for us to detail. IFN's were discovered as inhibitors of viral infections. In this role, IFN's disrupt viral protein synthesis and thereby prevent viral replication. Gamma-IFN (a.k.a. immune IFN) is also an immunoregulator. It is secreted by lymphocytes and macrophages, and serves to activate those cells and NK cells. It appears that gamma-IFN is the same as a cytokine known as macrophage activation factor (MAF).

Colony-stimulating factors (CSF's) act to advance the differentiation of blood cell precursors toward their final forms and functions, and also to activate differentiated forms (Clark & Kamen, 1987). Granulocyte CSF, macrophage CSF, and granulocyte-macrophage CSF act on the cell lineages that their names imply. Another CSF, called interleukin-3, seems to play a role with all types of blood cells except lymphocytes.

Numerous other cytokine activities have been described, among them attraction of macrophages (macrophage chemotaxin), reduction of macrophage motility (macrophage migration inhibiting factor, MIF), inhibition of granulocyte migration (leukocyte inhibitory factor), inhibition of lymphocyte function by suppressor T-cells (soluble immune response suppressor), and the destruction of targets by killer T-cells (lymphotoxins).

The thymus produces immunoregulatory substances which promote the maturation of T-cells and almost certainly circulate to stimulate the activities of mature T-cells. Barrett (1983, p. 86) lists five of these hormones, but he notes that they have not been well characterized and consist of families of compounds.   The names thymosin and thymopoetin are those most encountered in the literature.

We have mentioned the role of T_s-cells in terminating the immune response.   Suppressor activity develops later than helper activity and may reflect delayed proliferation of the suppressor cells. Interestingly, NK cells (Abruzzo & Rowley, 1983) and macrophages may play suppressor roles. Interference with suppressor functions may contribute to autoimmune disease or other immune system-induced pathologies.

Another process that regulates immune function is the production of *anti-idiotypic antibodies* (i.e., antibodies to antibodies). When Ig's are produced in response to an antigen, the antigen-binding sites on those molecules will constitute protein regions (called *idiotypes*) that are plentiful for the first time. The immune system can produce antibodies to the idiotypic regions of the first antibodies, thus interfering with their function and reducing their production.

Relations between the Immune System and the Rest of the Organism

Even considered alone, the immune system embodies a complex, interactive set of relationships. However, the immune system does not exist in isolation.   Even beyond its traditional role in dealing with pathogens, it is influenced by and in turn influences the rest of the organism (Ader, 1981; Janković et al., 1987).

NEUROENDOCRINE INFLUENCES ON IMMUNE FUNCTION

Befitting the diversity of endocrine influences in general, many hormones affect the immune system (see, e.g., Alqvist, 1981; Berczi, 1986a; Plaut, 1987 for reviews). It is believed that endocrine influences are an integral part of the normal regulation of immune function (Besedovsky et al., 1986). LR cells have receptors for a wide variety of neuroendocrine substances, and their function can be both depressed and enhanced by activation of those receptors. Unfortunately, but not unexpectedly, endocrine effects on the immune system are variable. They depend upon the hormone, of course, but also upon the measure of immune function studied, the maturity and activation of the LR cells, the timing and dose of hormone, and whether the experiment is carried out in vivo or in vitro. We can give only the sketchiest description of this morass and urge interested readers to consult reviews for details.

Glucocorticoids and Catecholamines

The fact that glucocorticoids often diminish immune function is as clear as anything in this area. Indeed, these compounds are frequently used medically to reduce inflammation and control organ transplant rejection. We summarize some of the points made by Alqvist (1981), Berczi (1986b), and Plaut (1987).

Glucocorticoids reduce the numbers of blood lymphocytes. In highly sensitive species such as mice, lymphocytes can be killed by exogenous glucocorticoids. In less sensitive species, including humans, much of the reduction in blood levels is due instead to changes in circulation patterns; lymphocytes tend to sequester in bone marrow.

LR cell function is often inhibited even if the cells remain viable, however. Thus Ig production, lymphocyte proliferation in response to *mitogens* (substances which, unlike antigens, stimulate large proportions of lymphocytes), antigen processing, phagocytosis and cytotoxicity by macrophages, the release of histamine by basophils, and NK cell activity have all been shown to be inhibited by glucorticoids. In at least some cases, the effects of exogenous glucocorticoids have been shown with physiologic doses—an important point because many studies use pharmacologic doses. ACTH administration tends to mimic the effects of glucocorticoids, and adrenalectomy tends to produce opposite effects. Plaut (1987) has suggested that many of the effects of glucorticoids on lymphocytes result from the inhibition of IL-1 and IL-2 production, and administration of these cytokines can often prevent glucocorticoid-induced immunodepression.

There are exceptions to the general impairment of immune function by glucocorticoids. However, these have not yet been shown to fit a general pattern, the problem being that the number of relevant parameters is so great that no experiment can vary them all simultaneously. There is some evidence for the following. Blood granulocyte levels increase in response to glucocorticoids, probably due to an increase in the release of neutrophils from the bone marrow. Lymphocytes and macrophages may be more resistant to glucocorticoids when they are mature and activated than when they are immature or unstimulated. In response to glucocorticoids, T-cells can elaborate a cytokine which, when present along with glucocorticoids, augments production of Ig's. NK activity can be enhanced by glucocorticoids as well as inhibited, and there may be a biphasic effect in which an initial increase in NK activity is followed by a decrease. Low levels of glucocorticoids are probably necessary for optimal immune functioning.

There has been less research on the immune system's response to catecholamines than on glucocorticoid effects. However the situation with catecholamines is seemingly much the same as with glucocorticoids (Alqvist, 1981; Berczi, 1986b; Plaut, 1987). The stimulation of adrenergic receptors on LR cells frequently hampers their functions, but there are apparent exceptions.

There is evidence that catecholamines inhibit mitogen-induced lymphocyte proliferation, immediate hypersensitivity, and CTL activity. On the other hand, catecholamines can produce leukocytosis (increase in circulating leukocyte numbers). The production of Ig's can be either increased or decreased, with increases being more likely from catecholamine stimulation early in maturation and/or activation. NK cell cytotoxicity can be either increased or decreased. Inhibition of immune function by catecholamines (and probably by many other non-steroids) is thought to result largely from increases in cyclic AMP levels in LR cells. Alqvist (1981) has suggested that stimulation of α-adrenergic receptors may enhance immune function by stimulating the degradation of cAMP, but there are instances of inhibitory effects from α-receptor activation (Berczi, 1986b).

Other Hormones and Peptides

It is known that gonadal hormones affect immune function (Berczi, 1986c; Grossman, 1984). The findings seem to us too diverse to support many generalizations, although Berczi (1986d) ventured to conclude that estrogens generally enhance immune functions and androgens usually inhibit. Studies indicating that females have stronger immune responses (and often greater susceptibility to autoimmune disorders) are rather abundant. On the other hand, the removal of both ovaries and testes has been shown to strengthen immune function. Grossman (1984) cites several studies in which estrogens inhibited various measures of immune function (e.g., lymphocyte proliferation, NK activity). Grossman also noted evidence for inhibition of thymus function by gonadal hormones.

Berczi (1986b) and Plaut (1987) have cited several findings in which endogenous opioids influenced immune function. ß-endorphin has increased (rats) and reduced (humans) lymphocyte response to mitogens, increased NK activity, and acted as a chemotaxin. Enkephalins have been found to enhance mitogen response but also to reduce antibody production as indexed by the plaque-forming cell (PFC) assay. Data from Rowland et al. (1987) indicate that met-enkephalin may be able to enhance or depress immune responses, depending upon antigen dose and the strength of the immune response it elicits. Shavit and colleagues (e.g., Shavit & Martin, 1987) have suggested that endogenous opioids play a key role in stress-induced immunodepression.

Berczi (1986d, 1986e; Berczi & Nagy, 1986) has argued that growth hormone (GH) and prolactin (Prl) have general and basically identical immunostimulatory effects. That their effects should be similar is not surprising because they are similar chemically (Hadley, 1984). These hormones can significantly relieve the immunodepression which occurs in hypophysectomized animals and can antagonize the inhibitory effects of ACTH. Ig production, NK activity and delayed (T-cell mediated) hypersensitivity are among the functions that have been potentiated by GH and Prl.

As a final example, E-type prostaglandins have repeatedly been shown to affect immune function (Plaut, 1987). Indeed, Plaut suggests PGE_2 as the hormone or autacoid (a term sometimes used for certain local hormones) most likely to have genuine endogenous immunoregulatory functions. PGE_2 is secreted by monocytes and macrophages, and could be considered a monokine. PGE_2 has a variety of inhibitory actions on lymphocytes. Among other things, it inhibits their proliferation, their production of IL-2, and their cytotoxicity. It can either inhibit or enhance NK cytotoxicity, enhancement occurring if the cells are exposed to it before their activity is assessed. Under certain circumstances it can enhance Ig production. PGE_2 may act in part by stimulating a subset of suppressor T-cells.

PGE_2 illustrates the delicacy of intrinsic immunoregulatory processes. It is secreted by macrophages but acts to reduce the production of IL-1 by macrophages, therefore serving a possible autocrine negative feedback function. Moreover, glucocorticoids reduce PGE_2 production and thus have the potential to moderate the suppression of IL-1 by PGE_2 while they are themselves inhibiting IL-1 and other aspects of immune function.

Some other factors for which there are data suggesting an influence on the immune system are progesterone, vasopressin, oxytocin, thyroid hormones and thyrotropin (TSH), parathyroid hormone, somatostatin, substance P, insulin, angiotensin-II, acetylcholine, histamine, and vasoactive intestinal peptide (Berczi, 1986a; Plaut, 1987). In many of these cases, there are receptors for the substance on immunocytes, suggesting that the effects are at least partly direct. There are, of course, many opportunities for indirect effects as well.

EFFECTS OF THE IMMUNE SYSTEM
ON OTHER FUNCTIONS

A holistic approach, implying as it does that everything might affect everything else, would suggest that the immune system might influence other organismic processes. Evidence for such influences is now rather plentiful. The spleen and thymus are innervated, seemingly by sympathetic neurons, and activity in those neurons may depress immune function. However, the effect is bidirectional. Activation of the immune system by exposure to antigen reduces the levels of NE in secondary lymphoid organs, suggesting that sympathetic outflow to those organs is diminished during immune responses (Besedovsky et al., 1986). The means by which the immune system affects sympathetic function has not been determined, but there are many possibilities.

A variety of organs and tissues are sensitive to substances whose chief functions have been thought to be immunoregulatory. The effects of IL-1 are perhaps the best known. IL-1 stimulates the production of ACTH by the pituitary and therefore the production of glucocorticoids. (Besedovsky et al., 1986; Wolosky et al., 1985). It has an extraordinary variety of other functions as well (Dinarello, 1985). IL-1 promotes fever (it is an endogenous pyrogen, acting on brain to increase body temperature set point), the breakdown of collagen and cartilage, bone resorption, somnolence and sleep, blood coagulation, the proliferation of glial cells, production of "acute phase" proteins by the liver (proteins produced in response to injury and inflammation), and satiety. It participates in the regulation of blood iron, zinc, and copper levels. It is, in other words, a broad-based regulator of organism function, including brain function.

Other cytokines also have multiple functions. PGE's produced by macrophages can stimulate the development of new blood vessels (angiogenesis), something helpful in wound healing but also necessary for the development of solid tumors (Folkman & Klagsbrun, 1987). Tumor necrosis factors (TNF's, also known as cachectin) are secreted by macrophages and lymphocytes. They were originally known for their ability to antagonize the growth of certain cancer cells (Sugarman et al., 1985). They are now known to stimulate the growth of some normal cells (Sugarman et al., 1985) and to be responsible for much of the toxicity of certain bacterial infections (Tracey et al., 1986). Factors produced by T-cells have been found to stimulate the growth of neurons (Gurney et al., 1986) and glial cells (Merrill et al., 1984).

We have already noted that gonadal hormones may affect the function of the thymus. Grossman (1984) also summarized evidence suggesting that the thymus affects the pituitary-gonadal axis. Athymic mice have low gonadotropin levels, and various thymosin subtypes are able to increase or decrease the release of luteinizing hormone and hypothalamic gonadotropin-releasing hormone. It seems, in other words, that the thymus is a part of the normal network of factors regulating reproductive function.

Still another way in which the immune system may influence the rest of the organism is through LR cells' production of "traditional" hormones. Some of these findings have been reviewed by Blalock et al. (1985). When activated, LR cells can seemingly secrete ACTH, endogenous opioids, thyrotropin (TSH), vasoactive intestinal peptide (VIP), growth hormone (GH) and luteinizing hormone (LH).

Neutrophils secrete an enzyme (an elastase) which promotes blood coagulation. The elastase degrades antithrombin (AT-III) and may be responsible for hypercoagulability in some infections. Heparin enhances the destruction of AT-III by neutrophil elastase, despite the fact that heparin also functions *with* AT-III in preventing clots from forming (Jordan et al., 1987).

Whatever else it is, the immune system is part of the overall neuroendocrine regulatory system of the organism. Just as neural and endocrine functions influence each other to the point that they become difficult to distinguish, so the immune system, through its secretions, is part of the endocrine system and contributes to the network of internal communications through which organisms adapt to internal and to externally-produced perturbations.

THE IMMUNE SYSTEM AND PATHOLOGY

Immune function can contribute to pathology in at least three ways. The most obvious occurs, of course, when it fails to control pathogens. A variety of immunodeficiency syndromes are commonly described (Robbins et al., 1984). However, the immune system's participation in disease is not limited to its function in defense against pathogens. Immunologic attack can be trained on self antigens, and pathology can be a byproduct of otherwise normal immune function (e.g., Robbins et al., 1984, pp. 163-205).

In *autoimmune disease*, the normal *immunologic tolerance* for self antigens is compromised, and the organism attacks itself through the very mechanisms by which it defends itself against foreign pathogens. There are probably several ways in which the immune system can be induced to undertake such assaults. For example, an antigenic determinant of a self molecule could be combined with a drug or pathogen molecule and in the process of responding to the novel complex, antibodies might be made to the self determinant. Another possibility is that loss of suppressor cell function could in some fashion allow autoimmunity to develop. Viral infections have been implicated in the genesis of autoimmune reactions but the details of their roles remain unclear.

Systemic lupus erythematosus and scleroderma are among the disorders considered to have a clear autoimmune origin. There are many others, notably multiple sclerosis, rheumatoid arthritis and diabetes mellitus, which appear to have autoimmune aspects but in which the etiologic primacy of autoimmunity is still uncertain.

Another form of immune system-induced pathology need not involve autoimmunity in the strict sense. Rather, the vigor of more or less normal immune system reactions have pathologic consequences. *Hypersensitivities* provide examples (Robbins et al., 1984). Immediate hypersensitivity is illustrated by allergies. IgE specific for some antigen (allergen) stimulates the release of histamine and cytokines by basophils and mast cells when the allergen is encountered. The most severe form of this reaction is *systemic anaphylaxis*, in which contraction of bronchioles, pulmonary edema and shock develop rapidly. Other types of hypersensitivity can be damaging via the formation of excess antigen-antibody complexes in blood or tissues, via complement-mediated cytotoxicity, or through macrophage-induced damage in the course of inflammation. (When these hypersensitivity reactions develop to self antigens rather than foreign antigens, they would be autoimmune.)

Cytokines may participate rather directly in pathology. IFN and IL-1 can stimulate fibrosis (the deposition of collagen) in the lungs (Immune Interferon, 1987). Some evidence indicates that IL-1 is toxic to the endocrine cells of the pancreas (Bendtzen et al., 1986) and might therefore play a role in diabetes. Cachectin/TNF can produce a wide variety of disturbances—including renal necrosis, internal hemorrhage, hypotension and respiratory arrest—when its production is stimulated by bacterial endotoxin (lipopolysaccharide components of gram-negative bacterial cell walls) (Tracey et al., 1986).

Stress and Immune Function

Since stress affects neuroendocrine function broadly and the immune system is linked to neuroendocrine processes, it is not surprising to find stress associated with changes in immune function. This topic has been discused extensively (e.g., Ader & Cohen, 1984; Borysenko & Borysenko, 1982; Jemmott & Locke, 1984; Kiecolt-Glaser & Glaser, 1987; Lloyd, 1984; Monjan, 1981; Palmblad, 1981; Shavit & Martin, 1987). The clearest and most frequent finding is of immuno-depression under stressful conditions. This result has been reported with a wide variety of immune function measures and stressors. Gluco-corticoids and catecholamines have most often been considered as the mediators of stress-induced immunodepression.

There are some exceptions to the general finding of immunode-pression under stress and to the notion that glucocorticoids and cate-cholamines are the only mediators. We shall cite a few studies which illustrate both the association of stress with impaired immune function and the existence of exceptions to the common hypotheses.

INFRAHUMAN STUDIES

We have previously noted that neuroendocrine responses can adapt and occasionally rebound with continued exposure to stressors. There is some evidence that this occurs with immune function as well. Monjan and Collector (1977) reported that mouse lymphocyte prolif-eration to the mitogens concanavalin A (con A) and lipopolysaccharide (LPS) was depressed by 4 to 20 days of exposure to intense sound but enhanced by 35 days of exposure. A similar function was found for cytotoxicity to P815 mastocytoma cells. Monjan (1981) indicated that this finding had been replicated. Greenberg et al. (1984) found that NK cell clearance of lymphoma cells was inhibited by 15 minutes of intermittent electric shock but augmented by 60 minutes of shock. Three days of confinement to the shock apparatus prior to a shock session also enhanced clearance of the tumor cells, as did four admin-istrations of ACTH over two days. The importance of recovery from stress has been suggested by Steplewski et al. (1986; see below).

A change from immunodepression to immunoenhancement with longer stressor exposures does not always occur, however. Shavit and colleagues (Shavit & Martin, 1987) found NK activity in rats to be reduced by 14 and 30 days of shock sessions. Another pattern was reported by Teshima and Kubo (1984). In their data, macrophage phagocytic activity was enhanced by up to eight hours of restraint stress and thereafter declined below baseline.

The type of stressor may also be important. Monjan (1981) reported that the procedure of taking blood samples from the orbital sinuses of mice enhances lymphocyte response to mitogens, particularly in animals exposed to sound stress for three days. Thus adding the retroorbital bleeding procedure reversed the pattern found with sound stress alone. Laudenslager et al. (1983) demonstrated that escapable shock did not depress lymphocyte mitogen response to con A and PHA though inescapable shock did. In fact, the escapable shock enhanced response to con A.

The Laudenslager et al. study suggests that various measures of immune system status may respond differently to stress manipulations. Another example is a study by Steplewski and Vogel (1986). They compared animals restrained for 11 days (3 hrs. per day) with controls and with animals which were restrained but were allowed to recover for 12 days. The initial restraint appeared to reduce T_h-and T_s-cell numbers, to increase the numbers of neutrophils and large granular lymphocytes (LGL's; probably NK cells), and not to affect NK cytotoxic activity. The status of the stress-recovery animals was rather different in comparison to controls: T_h and T_s numbers were above control levels, while neutrophil levels were lower than in controls. NK activity was enhanced. The fact that immune system parameters tended to rebound following the cessation of the stress regimen is another indication of the importance of temporal parameters.

Animal studies also provide evidence that the mediation of stress-induced immunodepression involves more than merely glucocorticoids and catecholamines. (We are aware of no truly compelling evidence *for* glucocorticoid or catecholamine mediation.) Keller et al. (1983) found that electric shock inhibited lymphocyte response to PHA in adrenalectomized (AdX) rats, including those given replacement corticosterone. In the AdX animals, presumably neither glucocorticoids nor epinephrine could have mediated the stress effect, although sympathetic norepinephrine could have. Interestingly, both AdX and AdX-plus-corticosterone acted to lower the responsiveness of lymphocytes in non-shocked animals, a finding which suggests that the relationship between immune function and adrenal hormones is not yet thoroughly understood.

Another report calls the role of glucocorticoids into question rather indirectly. Pavlidis and Chirigos (1980) found that 18 and 22 hours of restraint inhibited the cytotoxicity of interferon-activated mouse macrophages to MBL-2 leukemia cells. They also studied the effects of 10 mg/kg dexamethasone, prednisone and cortisol, finding that prednisone and cortisol inhibited macrophage cytotoxicity by about 50% and the more potent dexamethasone inhibited it by about 95%. The very high steroid doses used by Pavlidis and Chirigos allow one to speculate that macrophage activity in their assay is quite resistant to glucocorticoids. In attempts to prevent transplant rejection in humans, 1-2 mg/kg of prednisone is given per day. Pavlidis and Chirigos thus used *5-10 times a high pharmacologic dose* of a steroid over 10 times as potent as the natural corticosterone of the mouse. That only a 50% reduction in macrophage cytotoxicity occurred suggests that this aspect of immune function might be impervious to any level of glucocorticoids that stress could stimulate.

Shavit and associates (Shavit & Martin, 1987) have emphasized endogenous opioids as mediators of stress-induced immunodepression. One of their initial experiments (Shavit et al., 1984) demonstrated that a footshock schedule producing opioid-mediated analgesia also reduced NK cytotoxicity against YAC-1 lymphoma cells. This did not occur in animals given the opioid antagonist naltrexone. Later findings (see Shavit & Martin, 1987) suggested that opioid effects on the brain may be responsible for the effect of footshock which they observe and that the adrenal cortex may be the link between brain and immunocytes in their experiments. Taking the Keller et al. (1983), Pavlidis and Chirigos (1980) and Shavit et al. (1987) results together, it appears that there is more than one mediating sequence connecting stress with immunodepression and that which operates depends upon the specific characteristics of the situation.

HUMAN STUDIES

Jemmott and Locke (1984) reviewed studies associating stress-related variables and immune function in humans. Their review makes it clear that a variety of immune response measures (e.g., lymphocyte response to mitogens, phagocytosis, NK activity) and a variety of stress-related variables (e.g., bereavement, stressful life events, examinations, sleep deprivation) are involved in stress-immunodepression relationships. We shall mention a few findings published after that review.

Locke et al. (1984) studied NK cytotoxicity as a function of stressful life events and self-reported psychiatric symptoms (the latter used as an index of coping ability) in a sample of college students. Life stress was not related to NK function, but higher self-reported psychiatric symptoms were associated with lower NK activity. In addition, life stress and symptoms interacted. Subjects with the combination of high stress and low symptoms had the highest NK activity, significantly higher than those with high symptoms, regardless of the latters' stress levels. Were the Locke et al. data to be interpreted causally, the pattern would indicate that life stress *increases* NK activity in persons little subject to psychiatric symptomatology (i.e., presumably persons with good coping skills) and may (but less clearly from the data) reduce NK activity in those more likely to report symptoms. It is also of interest to note that Locke et al. found no relationship between NK function and reported illnesses.

Unemployment has been associated with reduced lymphocyte response to the mitogen PHA and the antigen PPD (purified protein derivative of tuberculin) (Arnetz et al., 1987). Subjects were two groups of Swedish women assessed at varying times ofter being laid off from factories and a control group continuously employed during the study. PHA and PPD responses were reduced after 12 months as compared to 4 or 9 months of unemployment. Cortisol levels did not vary significantly, however, suggesting that some other factor may have been responsible for the reduced lymphocyte responses.

There have been several studies of stress-related variables and salivary IgA (see, e.g., McClelland, 1989). This class of antibody is secreted at mucous membranes as an initial line of defense against pathogens. Stone et al. (1987) related IgA response to mood. Twenty-five times over eight weeks, dental students were assessed for mood and levels of salivary IgA against orally administered rabbit albumin. The levels of specific IgA were significantly lower when mood was more negative and higher when mood was more positive. Total IgA protein did not relate to mood in this study and Stone et al. questioned the value of that measure.

Kiecolt-Glaser, Glaser and their associates have reported a series of studies relating stress to human immune function (see Kiecolt-Glaser & Glaser, 1987 for an overview). One line of research by this group has dealt with changes in immunologic parameters in medical students undergoing examinations. Several aspects of immune function were shown to be impaired during examinations as compared to presumably less stressful periods. Among them were NK activity, number of T_h-cells, and lymphocyte responses to mitogens.

Marital status was related to immune system variables by Kiecolt-Glaser et al. (1987). Compared to married women, women recently separated from their husbands had fewer T_h-cells, fewer NK cells, and lower lymphocyte responses to the mitogens con A and PHA. Among the married women, poor marital quality was associated with lower lymphocyte PHA response. Among separated or divorced women, higher levels of attachment to the (ex)husband—and presumably therefore greater distress at the marital disruption—were related to lower T_h-cell percentages and reduced lymphocyte responses to mitogens.

Studies which experimentally manipulate stress-relevant variables in humans are particularly important. Kiecolt-Glaser, Glaser et al. (1985) demonstrated that relaxation training significantly improved NK activity in institutionalized but well functioning elderly individuals. Increased social contact without relaxation was also tried but had no effect. Pennebaker et al. (1988) attempted to use a different type of "therapeutic" intervention, written disclosure of psychologic traumas, to improve mitogen responses in undergraduate subjects. This manipulation did reduce health care utilization, but its effect on lymphocyte function was unclear because the relevant statistical tests were either nonsignificant or not completely reported.

The number of immunologic measures studied by the Kiecolt-Glaser and Glaser group allows an evaluation of the consistency of stress-associated immunodepression across indices of immune function. The generality is impressive, but there have been exceptions. As an example, stressful life events did not predict NK activity and mitogen response in nonpsychotic psychiatric admissions; loneliness did and interacted with life stress such that low-loneliness/high-stress individuals had high lymphocyte responses to pokeweed mitogen (Kiecolt-Glaser, Ricker et al., 1984). Plasma IgA levels were higher during medical school examinations than during a baseline period (Kiecolt-Glaser, Garner et al., 1984). In some cases there have been measures for which no relationships have been found. Thus attachment to an (ex)husband did not predict NK cell percentage even though it predicted T_h-cell percentage (Kiecolt-Glaser et al., 1987).

In sum, there is good evidence for immunodepression by stress. Many experimental studies are clear in this regard, and many nonexperimental studies are consistent with them. One broad question which remains is whether the occasional exceptions to immunodepression with stress are meaningful. There are just enough exceptions to the general finding to argue against blanket generalizations, but is there a pattern in the situations in which stress enhances immune function or fails to exert an effect? The complexity of the immune system and of stressors' influences on physiologic functions in general suggests that there may be, but there are not enough replication attempts on the exceptions to allow any conclusions.

Another issue is the clinical significance of stress-associated immunodepression. By and large, the effects appear not to be drastic. (One exception is a 96% reduction in leukocyte interferon production during medical school examinations [Glaser, Rice et al., 1986]). Effects which appear numerically minor may be clinically significant, however. Determining how important stress-induced immunomodulation actually is requires precisely duplicating stress effects by other means or blocking the stress effects, and both of those are often difficult to do.

It is worth noting that, if immunodepression by stress is clinically important, one would expect that pathology produced by a misdirected or overactive immune system could be ameliorated by stress, at least under some conditions. Such effects have in fact been found (e.g., Levine & Saltzman, 1987). On the other hand, if stress can stimulate immune function, it might thereby promote immune-system-induced pathology. The latter of these two possibilities seems to have been implied in the discussion by Lehman et al. (1991), who found that long-term stress increased the incidence of insulin-dependent diabetes in genetically susceptible rats.

Psychologic Factors and Stress

Stress involves a person's psychologic state and behavior in numerous ways. For one thing, stressors will affect behavior, cognition, and emotions—which is to say that psychologic, social, and behavioral changes are parts of the stress response. Stressors can alter the way memory functions, make one depressed, euphoric, or angry, and temporarily or permanently alter one's motives and life goals.

However, the same types of psychologic factors also help to determine how stressful a situation is. How one responds to a demand depends upon who one is—upon one's memories, skills, personality, values, and self-concept. Moreover, behavior and other personal characteristics can be stressors in themselves; just knowing (or believing) that one has undesirable characteristics can be distressing.

Not surprisingly, many of the variables that are both contributors to and responses to stress enter into reciprocal relationships with each other. Stress may, for example, result in failure at some task (reduced performance as a response to stress), and that failure can serve as an additional stressor. Stress-induced alterations in the way a person behaves toward others will probably produce changes in others' responses to the person.

We shall introduce the topics of this chapter by outlining some of them in the terminology of Lazarus and associates (Lazarus & Folkman, 1984) and then addressing the general roles of judgmental processes and individual differences. Following those discussions, we shall deal in somewhat more detail with psychologic factors as components of stress responses and psychologic factors that help to determine how stressful particular situations are for particular persons. One consequence of the multiple roles played by psychologic variables is that certain topics will come up more than once in the chapter.

AN APPRAISAL-COPING VIEWPOINT

The Lazarus group's approach centers on appraisal and coping. As we noted in Chapter 1, for Lazarus and Folkman (1984) psychologic stress occurs to the degree that individuals interpret (appraise) their situations as threatening to their well-being and judge their resources for meeting (coping with) demands as inadequate or questionable.

Primary appraisal in this scheme is appraisal of the degree of possible harm and/or benefit presented by a situation. A stress appraisal is a judgment that harm has occurred or is threatened, or that there is a challenge whose mastery will bring benefits. A situation may, of course, be judged to present multiple threats of harm and possibilities of advantage.

The term *secondary appraisal* refers to the process of evaluating what can be done to maximize well-being in dealing with a stressful situation. The individual evaluates the probable success of various actions and the likelihood that she/he can successfully carry them out. In other words, secondary appraisal involves assessing one's *resources* for coping with a threat or challenge.

We think of resources as personal, material, or social. Personal resources are characteristics of the individual, be they biologic or psychologic. Such things as intelligence, appearance, strength, psychologic defenses and biologic resistance to disease may contribute to coping with stressors. Material resources are basically money and the things it buys. Social resources are those carried by members of the person's social network. Friends, coworkers and family members may apply their personal and material resources to one's problems, and can provide emotional comfort (see "Social Support," below). Hobfoll (1988) actually defines stress in terms of resources—as the threat or perceived threat of a net loss of resources or of an insufficient return from the investment of resources. Hobfoll's model defines resources broadly and can thus accomodate a wide variety of stressor types.

Coping processes follow appraisals. Lazarus and Folkman distinguish *problem-focused* and *emotion-focused* forms of coping. Roughly, problem-focused strategies are directed at the source of threat—at the stressor and its demands. Their purpose is to reduce the demand placed on the individual by satisfying it or inducing those making the demand to alter it. Emotion-focused coping aims at reducing the impact of the demand upon the individual without altering or satisfying the demand—that is, at reducing the stress response rather than altering the stressor. Classic defense reactions such as denial are obvious examples of emotion-focused coping, but emotion-focused coping need not be defensive. Relaxation, for instance, can allow persons to reduce their emotional and physiologic responses to stressors without distorting their appraisals.

Lazarus and Folkman make it clear that problem-focused and emotion-focused coping are necessarily linked to each other and to appraisal. Emotion-focused coping can reduce arousal and thereby permit problem-focused coping to be carried out more effectively (though if arousal is reduced too drastically, the individual may no longer be bothered enough to act). Problem-focused coping may reduce affect when it portends success in dealing with stressors or increase affect by concentrating attention on stressors. Appraisals are obviously important influences on the choice of coping strategies, and they also change as a function of coping success or failure. Moreover, appraisals are themselves coping strategies. Reappraising a situation, as by accentuating its positive aspects and downplaying its negative aspects, is a form of emotion-focused coping.

Some, but hardly all, of the events which occur in a stress episode according to our interpretation of Lazarus and Folkman (1984) are illustrated in Figure 5. The basic sequence of events is from appraisal through coping attempts to outcomes. Primary appraisal depends partly upon the objective character of the stressor. Secondary appraisal occurs if primary appraisals signify that action is required. We presume that, in addition to depending upon information about resources, secondary appraisal requires additional information from the environment to determine precisely how to utilize resources. The appraisals affect the psychophysiologic status of the individual (e.g., emotions, hormone outputs), which, in order to simplify matters, we take in this diagram to be an endpoint. Coping attempts can begin as soon as primary and secondary appraisal processes have generated evaluations. The coping processes in turn will produce some sort of results (outcomes).

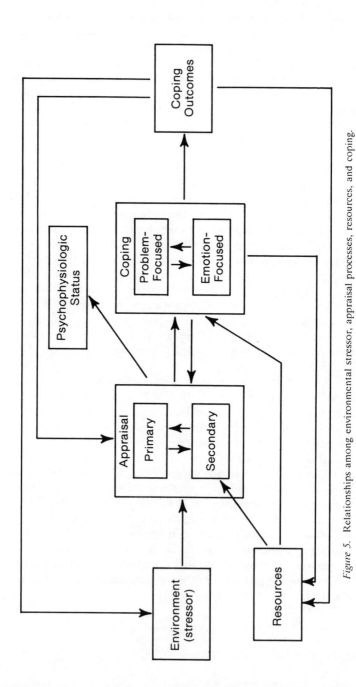

Figure 5. Relationships among environmental stressor, appraisal processes, resources, and coping.

When outcome information becomes available, it can feed back to both the primary and secondary appraisal processes and, if problem-focused coping has been used, can also alter the stressor. To the extent that outcomes are successful, then, primary appraisals of threat may be reduced, secondary appraisals may consequently report increased adequacy of resources, and the environment may signal reduced demand. Presumably, the pattern of psychophysiologic variables will then be one of reduced stressfulness. Outcomes and coping processes may deplete or augment resources.

Stress processes at the psychosocial and behavioral levels are clearly dynamic. There can be constant flux. Stressors and resources can change as the result of coping or external conditions not connected to coping attempts. One stressor can replace or add to another. The search for resources in the environment or in memory can at any time turn up something new, either good news or bad. The individual is continually learning from the environment and her/his own actions; that learning both modifies reactions to current circumstances and adds to the information available for reacting to future situations.

INTERPRETIVE PROCESSES AND INDIVIDUAL DIFFERENCES

The Lazarus group's approach embodies two important features of current views of stress—emphases on cognitive/interpretive processes and on individual differences. Appraisals are interpretations; often, situations are stressful only because they are so interpreted. (If you are about to be mugged but do not think you are about to be mugged, you will not respond as though you were about to be mugged. Psychology has discovered the importance of meaning several times.) Individual differences in interpretations imply differences in responses to presumably stressful conditions. Before we describe some of the psychologic responses to stressors and psychologic variables which help to determine how stressful a situation is, we need to elaborate a bit on the general roles played by cognitive factors and individual differences.

Interpretive Processes

Basic cognitive processes such as perception, attention, encoding and retrieval from memory are involved in all psychologic phenomena. In contemporary stress theories, interpretations of events seem to be the most discussed aspects of cognitive functioning, and we shall concentrate on them. Interpretations can be thought of as outcomes of more basic operations, and their relevance can be taken as evidence for the relevance of basic information processing functions. Almost automatically, humans interpret their environments, their behavior, and themselves (e.g., Jones, 1986). They even interpret their interpretations (Ellis, 1978). (Lower animals are presumably as cognitively active as their capacities allow.) *Any* factor which contributes to or reflects interpretive processes is relevant to stress.

Attributions and *expectancies* are two basic and closely related types of interpretations. Attributions are judgments about causes. One may attribute an event to one's own characteristics or actions (e.g., ability or effort), to others, to physical nature, or to luck or fate. There are several theories as to what induces a particular source of influence to be singled out as a "cause" for an event. Hilton and Slugoski (1986) discussed these in presenting their model, one which emphasizes conditions "abnormal" for the general circumstances of the target event or unlikely to be assumed on the basis of background knowledge.

The consequences of an attribution vary with a cause's judged stability and controllability, with the range of things that it is judged to be capable of influencing, and, in the case of causal attributions for a person's behavior, with the locus of attributed causation (person or environment) (e.g., B. Weiner, 1985). If someone attributes a pleasant happening to a stable, controllable, global influence, he/she is likely to react very differently than if the attribution is to a temporary, uncontrollable factor having a narrow judged range of influence. In the latter case, there would be few ways to assure that the pleasant event would recur. Causal attributions thus affect behavior and expectancies.

Expectancies are subjective predictions. They derive from personal experiences with situations and from such indirect sources as observations of others and didactics. Expectancies can be about nearly anything. When they concern the causes of future events, they are much like attributions. Mischel (1973) discussed "behavior-outcome" expectancies (predictions about the effects of one's own actions) and "stimulus-outcome" expectancies (which concern the sequelae of signals from the environment). Behavior-outcome expectancies are related to *self-efficacy* (Bandura, 1982). Self-efficacy concerns personal resources for performing a task, and perceived self-efficacy is basically the degree of expectation that, if one attempted the task, one would succeed.

Generality is an important characteristic of expectancies. Some expectancies refer to single situations (my local market will have fresh artichokes Wednesday afternoon). Others may be so broad as to be virtually independent of situations and can be seen as personality traits (if anything can go wrong, it will). Perhaps the best known generalized expectancy to be hypothesized is internal-external *locus of control* (Rotter, 1966). Locus of control is the degree of expectancy that one's life outcomes are due to one's own ability and effort (internal) or to luck and environmental forces (external). Since it deals with causation, locus of control can be considered an attributional style. (There may not actually be one single, highly generalized locus of control expectancy [Coombs & Schroeder, 1988]).

It is difficult to generate a framework to incorporate all of the types of interpretations humans can generate. We can only suggest a few generalizations and give some examples. We have already noted the general idea that people interpret nearly everything that touches them. Another broad principle is that interpretations need not reflect reality very accurately. Terms such as "cognitive myopia" (Hogarth, 1981) and "mindlessness" (Langer & Piper, 1987) have been used to denote broad human tendencies toward inadequate judgment.

Inherent limitations in the information processing apparatus can be one reason for interpretive errors. This is obvious when the sheer quantity of relevant information exceeds the individual's capacity to process it, but there are other limitations as well. We have alluded (Chapter 1) to logical errors such as overdependence on easily available information (e.g., Tversky & Kahneman, 1983). Probably related to the availability bias is the finding that imagining events can increase the frequency with which they are judged to occur in real life (Slusher & Anderson, 1987). There may also be limits on the amount of information reaching consciousness. Nisbett and Wilson (1977) discussed many studies in which subjects apparently could not report the effects of significant stimuli and internal psychologic processes upon their behavior.

Motivation influences the accuracy of interpretations. Attitudes and beliefs often conform to the dictates of *cognitive consistency*. By the consistency principle, we are motivated to hold congruent ideas, and if we have contradictory cognitions we will tend to change or reject some of them. Any belief, motive, or behavior can provide cognitions to which other cognitions will be adjusted. Cognitive consistency might predict, for example, that someone who firmly believes a situation to be benign would downplay contrary information. Information about the self can be treated very much like information about the environment (Higgins, 1987). Hypochondriacs, for instance, reject the idea that they are well. The self-consistency idea also predicts that individuals with strongly held low self-esteem may resist positive information (see, e.g., Swann et al., 1987).

Another important motive is a general need to view oneself positively. People often interpret their circumstances in ways which make them look good to themselves and others. The *self-enhancement* motive may be separate from and potentially in conflict with the tendency to self-consistency (Swann et al., 1987); it may also set core cognitions around which consistency is organized.

Biasing influences can be seen in a number of stress-relevant interpretive tendencies that have been described in the research literature. There is, for example, a tendency to be self-serving in attributions (Pettigrew, 1979; Pyszczynski et al., 1985; Weary-Bradley, 1978), as by attributing one's successes to personal qualities and one's failures to circumstances. Self-serving biases also occur in judgments about dividing rewards (O'Malley & Becker, 1984). The "just world" effect is a tendency to believe that people get what they deserve and therefore to blame misfortunes on the victims (Lerner & Miller, 1978). "False consensus" is a tendency to believe that one's opinions and behaviors are more widely shared than they actually are.

Though they obviously can be harmful, judgmental biases often have beneficial effects. Crocker and Major (1989) reviewed literature on self-esteem in stigmatized groups such as women, racial minorities, the disabled and the physically handicapped. They argued that such individuals may protect their self-concepts by explaining negative events as due to prejudice, by viewing their limitations as relatively unimportant, or by judging themselves relative to others in their own disadvantaged group rather than in relation to the more advantaged.

Self-protective interpretive biases extend to judgments about disease risks. Adolescent smokers overestimate the proportion of people who smoke (Sherman et al., 1983). Weinstein (1984) found undue optimism in persons' assessments of the health risks attending a variety of their behaviors. Ditto et al. (1988) found self-protective appraisals in subjects who took a bogus saliva test purportedly indicating increased risk for pancreatic disease. Subjects who tested positively for the "risk factor" tended to downplay the seriousness of their situations. For example, their estimates that the risk factor did in fact portend pancreatic disease were lower, and so were their estimates of the seriousness of the disease.

The idea that people's judgments can reflect self-enhancing and self-protective strategies is closely related to the psychodynamic notion of defense. In theories such as psychoanalysis, people engage in defensive processes such as repression and denial to protect themselves from anxiety, just as in newer theories people operate with such processes as cognitive consistency and self-serving attributions.

Whatever the theoretical language, defensiveness complicates attempts to understand psychologic and psychobiologic processes. On the psychologic level, the existence of defensiveness makes us question the meanings of our measures. What people report about their feelings and experiences can be incorrect. Defensive individuals' responses to psychologic tests may indicate that they are happy and content when they are actually quite dysphoric.

An even thornier problem is partly conceptual. What should defense imply for psychobiologic processes? If someone has seemingly "defended" against a threat, is he then biologically calm because he no longer perceives a threat; is he perhaps still biologically aroused because he is still "unconsciously" threatened; or is he in fact still consciously threatened but just unwilling to acknowledge his feelings to others? If the first of these possibilities obtains, we would not expect the person to show strong biologic signs of stress, but in the latter two cases we might.

Unfortunately, the research data are equivocal. Cook (1985), for instance, reported that persons classified as "true repressors," selected on the basis of a repression-sensitization scale and a consistently avoidant coping style, showed high skin conductance responses when giving a talk about themselves. On the other hand, a number of studies have suggested that strong defenses as assessed clinically are associated with low cortisol responses under stressful conditions (Vickers, 1988).

In sum, many data, and common experience, indicate that people need not judge their situations or themselves objectively. Therefore, the stressfulness of situations can be misappraised; people can underestimate or overestimate either the threats they face or the resources available to manage them. This means that putative stressors' effects should vary from situation to situation. It also means that assessing stress accurately can be a messy business.

Individual Differences

Differences among individuals derive from genetic variation in combination with environmental history variation. The resulting personal characteristics interact in complex ways with situational variables to determine psychologic processes (e.g., Endler & Magnusson, 1976). Given that cognitive processes and the information on which they operate differ from individual to individual, people should react differently to potential stressors. It is in this sense that stress theories such as that of Lazarus and Folkman (1984) are interactive. The characteristics of the situation and of the organism interact in determining responses to stressors. Differences in the interpretive processes we have just discussed represent a major type of stress-relevant person variable, but it is difficult to imagine a psychologic or social individual difference factor that would be utterly irrelevant to stress.

It is useful to recognize that since individual differences derive in part from experience, the study of individual differences and of experiential effects often cannot be separated clearly. If research focuses on individual differences—as assessed, say, by personality inventories— experience (including stressful experience) is part of what is being investigated. On the other hand, experiences have effects largely because they produce changes in persons.

Individual difference variables can operate at any stage in the stress sequence outlined in Figure 5. Among other things, differences in motives and behavior patterns affect the situations to which people subject themselves and therefore the stressors which they encounter. Individuals high on "sensation seeking," for example, tend to choose activities which involve physical risk. They may also have high levels of gonadal hormones and low levels of monoamine oxidase, an enzyme which degrades catecholamines (Zuckerman et al., 1980). Persons with the Type A behavior pattern seem to select or create demanding situations (Byrne & Rosenman, 1986). Field dependent individuals are sensitive to social cues and and tend to seek more social contact (Witkin & Goodenough, 1977). In a study by Aldwin et al. (1989), emotionality as assessed by the Eysenck neuroticism scale predicted both major life events and daily hassles ten years later.

Individual differences also influence how organisms respond to situations. We have already mentioned some variables which might be considered personal resources. Differences in abilities and cognitive style will influence appraisals and the quality of coping. Persons characterized as more "reflective" as opposed to more "impulsive" tend to be cognitively thorough, to have greater anxiety about performance, and to have less anxiety about their basic competence (Messer, 1976). One would expect reflectives and impulsives to find different situations stressful. There appears also to be a general tendency toward *negative affectivity*—a predisposition to respond to a variety of situations with a variety of negative emotions (Watson & Clark, 1984; Watson & Pennebaker, 1989). Physiologic differences (e.g., in biosynthetic enzymes) will affect the pattern of hormonal response to stressors.

Individual differences do not imply complete idiosyncracy in responses to stress. However, aside from extreme circumstances which would be appraised as challenging or threatening by most people (H. Weiner, 1985), we should expect considerable variation, with some individuals reacting strongly to situations which others take with relative equanimity. One implication of individual difference effects is that we cannot expect supposedly stressful conditions to influence disease in a simple, uniform way.

PSYCHOLOGIC COMPONENTS OF STRESS RESPONSE

The behavioral and psychologic consequences of stressful conditions are probably quite important to health. They affect physiologic responses and also affect subsequent stressor exposure. Many behaviors, such as nutritional choices, exercise, and adherence to medical regimens are directly health-relevant (Matarazzo, 1980).

Stressors influence emotions, cognitive and behavioral performance, and social relationships. Thus almost regardless of how it is conceptualized, stress relates to every facet of psychologic functioning, and understanding stress requires understanding psychologic processes in general.

Affective Responses to Stressors

Although emotion has proved difficult to conceptualize (e.g., Mandler, 1975; Zajonc, 1984), the very notion of stress as a threat to well-being and the traditional emphasis on sympathoadrenomedullary responses (e.g., Lacey, 1967) imply that emotions have to be involved in stress.

If stress affects emotion, it almost has to affect motivation. It is difficult to think of goal-directed (motivated) behavior as not involving some emotional responses to the goal and the quest for it; it could also be said that motivated behavior has the control of emotions as a general aim. Stressors' demands must impinge upon the urgency and salience of goals. Often, goals directly related to the stressor will become more salient and strongly desired. Thus, although we will couch this discussion in terms of emotion, it should be recognized that we are in some sense discussing motivation as well.

EMOTIONS IN THE SERVICE OF COPING

It is not too unreasonable to divide the affective responses to stressors into (1) those which more clearly represent coping attempts and (2) those which seem to be elicited more or less independently of coping and/or to be elicited when coping fails (i.e., emotions as outcomes, below). Authors who theorize about coping often set up taxonomies which differentiate in one way or another between attempts to deal with distress directly and attempts to moderate it by satisfying or reducing demands. Lazarus and Folkman's (1984) distinction between emotion-focused and problem-focused coping is just one of these.

Wilson's (1985) contrast between "fear control" and "danger control" is rather similar to the Lazarus and Folkman distinction. Suls and Fletcher (1985a) focused on cognitive aspects of coping in distinguishing between "avoidant" and "attention" strategies. Avoidant strategies direct attention away from distress or its source, and attention stategies involve focusing upon them. The avoidant strategies in this scheme are particularly directed at moderating emotional responses; attention strategies might be seen as problem-focused in that they can be preparations for instrumental action. Billings and Moos (1981) discussed three types of coping. Their "active-cognitive" coping includes both attempts to reinterpret stressful situations in a positive way and the cognitive generation of solutions to the problem; "active-behavioral" coping involves instrumental actions to gather information and influence demands; "avoidance" includes a variety of maneuvers which would neither prevent unpleasant outcomes nor stimulate emotionally positive appraisals.

Though they are hardly identical, each of these taxonomies includes strategies which aim at altering affect without altering demand. We should note that in nearly any theory of coping, strategies can be conceptualized and investigated both as individual difference variables (e.g., persons with strong or weak tendencies to deny the existence of threat) or as situationally determined (e.g., problem-focused coping in controllable situations and emotion-focused coping in uncontrollable situations).

Several more or less specific emotional coping tendencies have been discussed. Some of this work indicates that one's interpretations of others are significant in managing emotional components of stress. A review by Sherwood (1981) concluded that *attributive projection* reduces stress responses. In attributive projection, the individual does not deny possessing an undesirable characteristic, but she/he believes that others also possess it. Thus one may respond to one's poor performance at work by telling oneself (and others) that nearly everyone does this job poorly. Perhaps thinking that the negative trait is common reduces the sense of threat or unworthiness by letting one believe that others could not be highly condemnatory. Attributive projection is obviously similar to the false consensus effect.

Another process which involves interpreting other people is what Wills (1981) has called *downward comparison* (see also Taylor et al., 1990). Two of Wills' basic hypotheses are that comparing oneself with those who are worse off can enhance one's sense of well-being, and that these comparisons are elicited by reductions in the sense of well-being (i.e., under stress). Wills argued cogently that downward comparisons contribute to a wide variety of social phenomena including prejudice, hostile aggression, and social attraction. His analysis thus implies that all of those phenomena derive from stress to some extent.

A rather different type of emotion-focused coping involves *distraction*. Since information processing capacity is limited, attending to something other than a stressor should reduce the emotional response to the stressor. There is evidence that distraction is effective—in dealing with pain, for example (McCaul & Malott, 1984). Perhaps even more than other emotion-oriented coping responses, distraction has the potential to be either adaptive or maladaptive. Distraction from a stressor about which little can realistically be done allows resources to be directed at other goals, but distraction from a manageable threat can have harmful consequences. Matthews and Carra (1982) found that, compared to those of Type B's, Type A women's reports of menstrual symptoms suggested a tendency to ignore them. Matthews and Carra noted that this finding was consistent with other evidence that Type A individuals disregard events that interfere with goal-directed tasks.

Although it might seem at first glance to be important only in problem-focused or instrumental coping, learning is relevant to managing emotional responses. We alluded in Chapter 1 to Burchfield's (1979) treatment of adaptation in terms of learning. In her view, organisms learn the limits of the damage that stressors can do and also learn to make stress responses in advance of the actual appearance of the stressor. Similarly, Foa and Kozak (1986) argued that the exposure to feared situations reduces clinically significant fear.

The type of coping that will be used will depend upon both the nature of the stressor and individual differences in coping style. Regarding the type of stressor, Folkman et al. (1986a) studied eight types of coping and several classes of (appraised) stressors. The qualities of the stressors related in complex ways to the coping strategies employed.

With threats to self-esteem, subjects were relatively unlikely to report seeking help from others and relatively likely to report using confrontation (e.g, anger, standing their ground) and escape-avoidance (e.g., hoping for a miracle, wishing that the situation would go away). With stressors related to work goals, self-control (e.g., keeping feelings to oneself, trying not to act too hastily) and planful problem-solving (e.g., drawing on past experiences, increasing effort) tended to be reported. When the threats were to physical health, escape-avoidance and seeking help were most used.

With regard to individual differences, a study by Folkman and Lazarus (1985) suggested a great deal of variation among subjects in their coping with an examination. Wishful thinking and seeking support were associated with a feeling of threat in anticipation of the exam. Subjects who saw the test as a challenge tended to use problem-focused coping and to avoid self-isolation. Strube (1985) found that Type A individuals were more likely than Type B's to attribute success to personal qualities and failure to external factors.

EMOTIONS AS OUTCOMES

We now look at a somewhat different involvement of emotions, namely as outcomes in themselves—whether as elicited following initial appraisals or, after coping attempts, as consequences of coping outcome. Stressors should be able to stimulate a wide variety of affective responses. It is not very difficult to imagine positive emotions resulting from the identification of a stressful challenge or from learning that failure to cope is less damaging than anticipated. However, negative affect is much more often discussed. Higgins (1987), for example, argued that a variety of negative emotions can result from inconsistencies between self-representations.

Obviously, *fear* (or anxiety) will often be part of the stress response. Threat to well-being and doubt about ability to cope almost define the conditions for fear. It is possible for stress to rearouse old fears as well. Clinical fears such as phobias can emerge under mild or seemingly irrelevant threats; the hormonal responses to stress arouse fearful associations but disrupt the neural systems which would otherwise restrict an old fear to its former context (Jacobs & Nadel, 1985). Some of the evidence for fear rearousal comes from animal models of fear-motivated behavior (Richardson et al., 1984).

Depression has received much attention as a stress outcome. (As a psychiatric diagnosis, the term denotes more than sadness, melancholy or hopeless mood, but those affective features are major criteria

[American Psychiatric Association, 1980.]) One influential view of depression emphasizes attributions about stressful events (e.g., Peterson & Seligman, 1984). From this perspective, depression and loss of self-esteem tend to occur when a person's attributions for aversive events are internal, stable, and global. Thus, attributing a failure to one's genetically limited intelligence creates a risk for depression. Genetically determined intelligence is personal, cannot be changed, and is likely to affect a wide variety of future outcomes. Such ideas about one's relations to one's world can hardly fail to diminish self-esteem and hope.

The status of the stress-attribution-depression theory is not yet clear. Brewin (1985) contrasted several possible models for those relationships. He noted that the evidence supports some more than others but that the research has been too simple to provide good tests of the models. We would add that none of Brewin's models involves reciprocal causation and therefore all are likely to be oversimple. It is reasonable to speculate, for instance, that depression results in part from, but also tends to produce, internal, stable, global attributions for bad events.

Our final example of a stress-induced affect is *anger*. Stress is much like frustration in implying interference with goal attainment. If "goal" encompasses such ongoing desiderata as maintaining self-esteem and reputation, then most stressful situations will involve frustration in some form. Although anger and aggression are influenced by many factors, such as observing others model hostility and the prospect of reward for aggressive behavior, frustration has long been considered a major determinant (e.g., Berkowitz, 1962). A review by Rule and Nesdale (1976) concluded that provocation and frustration do indeed engender anger and aggression. More recent thinking by Berkowitz (e.g., 1990) involves the idea that aversive experiences *in general* elicit anger and other aggression-related internal processes.

Overall self-esteem and variability in self-esteem from situation to situation predicted the experience of anger in a study by Kernis et al. (1989). Persons with high but variable self-esteem were particularly prone to anger. These individuals may be especially sensitive to such threats as negative evaluations from others.

PERSONALITY AND INDIVIDUAL DIFFERENCES
IN AFFECTIVE RESPONSE

Psychologic individual differences, whether in coping style or in other factors, have repeatedly been shown to influence emotional stress responses. Folkman et al. (1986a) found in general that persons using planful problem solving and positive reappraisal (e.g., seeing adverse circumstances as helping one grow as a person) more often had successful outcomes. Holahan and Moos (1985) divided subjects who had high exposure to stressors into those who responded with high distress and those who did not. The "stress-resistant" individuals used avoidance-oriented coping less. Suls and Fletcher (1985a) did meta-analyses of coping outcome studies. They indicated that avoidance is usually more effective in the short run than attention to threat but that, in the long-term, the attention strategy is superior to avoidance. Bukstel and Kilman (1980) have suggested that persons with poor coping skills may adjust relatively well to prison because that environment provides physical necessities and social structure.

Kobasa and colleagues (e.g., Kobasa, 1982) have described *hardiness* as a personality characteristic associated with resistance to stress. Hardiness consists of commitment, a sense of control, and a sense of challenge. It has been associated with reduced psychologic symptoms and pathology under stress. The Type A behavior pattern is also related to control and challenge, but it seems to imply compulsion and driven-ness, not the resilience of Kobasa's hardiness.

Type A's are highly susceptible to many stress responses (e.g., Glass, 1977), including hostility and aggression (Holmes & Will, 1985). It has been suggested by Eliasz and Wrzesniewski (1988) that the consequences of the Type A behavior pattern depend upon other aspects of personality or temperament. They hypothesized that the Type A behavior pattern will be associated with dysphoric emotion and disease susceptibility in individuals who are high in "reactivity" (roughly, high in biological predisposition to introversion). The social environments of these persons will have imposed the Type A behavior pattern on them despite its incompatibility with their underlying temperament.

Peterson and Seligman (1984) refer to "explanatory style" and provide some evidence for individual consistencies in attributions for bad events. Greenberg and Pyszczynski (1986) found an association between depression and the degree to which subjects focused on themselves after failure. Increased self-focus following failure might make internal attributions more likely.

Oatley and Bolton (1985) emphasized the importance of threatened roles to a person's self-concept. They argued that losing a self-defining role, without having other roles to which self-definition can be transferred, will lead to depression. Retirement may produce depression in someone for whom career is the central aspect of life, but not in someone whose self-definition rests elsewhere, for example in family roles or avocations. By Oatley and Bolton's thesis, individuals whose self-concepts rest upon multiple roles should be relatively resistant to depression.

In a study of control and adjustment to disease by Timko and Janoff-Bulman (1985), mastectomy patients' beliefs that their breast cancers were avoidable predicted their anticipation of future freedom from cancer. Attributions of the original tumor to their own personalities or to other people was negatively related to belief in the success of their surgery. Belief in success of surgery and in future freedom from cancer in turn predicted depression.

There are also studies relating individual differences to physiologic aspects of affective stress response. Cook (1985) studied skin conductance in subjects asked to give a talk about themselves to a video camera. Those with an approach coping style had stronger reactions after getting irrelevant information (a preliminary tape on pigs) than relevant information (a tape of someone else's talk). "Approachers" appeared to use relevant information to reduce stress responses. In a rather novel approach to individual differences, it was found that subjects who were facially expressive when viewing an industrial accident film showed, nine weeks later, less heart rate and respiration change to the threat of shock (Notarius & Levenson, 1979). Increasing arachnophobics' perceived self-efficacy in dealing with spiders reduced their EP and NE responses to items from a hierarchy of spider-approach tasks (Bandura et al., 1985). Wilson (1985) found that the combination of greater ability to engage in problem-focused coping (high danger control) and low ability to control emotions (low fear control) was associated with surgery patients' general level of arousal, as indicated by the need for greater amounts of sodium pentothal in preparation for general anesthesia.

Stress and Performance

Stressors undoubtedly influence performance on tasks requiring skill or concentration. Performance can be affected because the task itself is stressful or because the person must perform it under the influence of an extraneous stressor. Performance can be impaired or improved under stress. One venerable generalization is that performance is impaired at both very low and very high levels of general emotional arousal (see, e.g., Cohen, 1980; Humphreys & Revelle, 1984). However, performance deterioration at high arousal has received the lion's share of attention.

Stress can affect both the ability and the motivation to perform, although in a given situation it may be difficult to decide which is involved. Keinan (1987) studied performance on analogies using a multiple choice format in which subjects could display one possible answer at a time and could switch back and forth among answers freely. Subjects under the threat of (noncontingent) electric shock used less of the available information and scanned the information they did use less systematically. They often chose an answer without even displaying the correct one. Keinan noted that these findings could mean either that shock threat occupied enough of the subjects' attention to prevent full consideration of the task or that subjects simply wanted to get out of the situation quickly.

Cohen (1980) discussed several mechanisms by which stress may impair cognitive function. One is cognitive fatigue or a general depletion of "psychic energy" by the work of coping. Another notion is that task requirements or extraneous stressors are distractors—can overload attentional processors, preventing some necessary internal or external information from being utilized. We mentioned distraction as a type of emotion-focused coping. In that context something else distracts attention from a stressor, but in stress-induced performance impairment it is the stressor or stress response which distracts the individual.

Stress can also focus attention. As Cohen (1980) noted, this may underlie the fact that the optimal level of arousal is higher for simpler tasks. If a task requires the use of only a few cues, narrower attention might reduce the likelihood that distraction will harm performance. However, if there are many task-relevant stimuli, attentional focusing may mean that some necessary cues cannot be processed.

Memory processes change under stress. Eysenck (1976) drew two general conclusions from research on arousal and memory. High arousal focuses attention on the physical attributes of stimuli at the expense of their information content, consequently reducing the storage of the information content in memory. High arousal promotes the retrieval from memory of more accessible material over less accessible material, something which may reflect narrow attention to internal information. The effect of arousal on retrieval suggests that judgmental biases which depend upon the dominance of easily available information (Tversky & Kahneman, 1983) might be worsened under stress; decision makers can become more susceptible to bias just when it is most dangerous, namely in an emergency (Spettell & Liebert, 1986).

There are numerous possible ways for motivational aspects of stress to affect performance. We have already alluded to the idea that if stress or arousal is quite low (in Lazarus and Folkman's [1984] terms, if the individual perceives little threat or challenge), there may be no reason to attempt a task or do it well. Cohen (1980) mentions two other possibilities. One component of learned helplessness (see below) is a motivational deficit. If the organism comes to expect on the basis of past stressful encounters that no actions will be effective in producing desired outcomes, there is little reason to perform.

A somewhat more subtle possibility involves cognitive consistency. Suppose, for example, that a person becomes involved in stressful circumstances without a strong reason to do so and also believes that he/she does not lightly choose to be discomforted. Consistency theory would predict that the individual will interpret the situation as relatively benign and not be too highly disturbed by it (e.g., Zimbardo, 1969). ("I didn't have to learn alligator wrestling, and I'm not dumb enough to risk my appendages for nothing. So this can't be too dangerous.") By responding to the consistency motive in this fashion, the person reduces emotionality (i.e., engages in emotion-focused coping) and therefore eliminates some of the demand on attention. Performance should then not be drastically impaired.

Deliberate failure is still another way for motivation to affect performance. It is possible to fear the consequences of letting others believe that one is competent. One may see one's abilities as inadequate and not want to risk embarrassment when others learn the truth or not want the responsibility that might follow when others realize one's competence. In either case, one might perform a task poorly in order to lower others' expectancies. Such exceptions to the usual desire to look good have been documented (Baumgardner & Brownlee, 1987).

Stress effects on performance may vary with time. If cognitive fatigue produces performance decrements, the decrements should not be apparent at once. Stress may even improve performance initially (Broadbent, 1978). Further, stressor-induced impairment might not show up until after the stress episode (Cohen, 1980). Delayed effects of stress on performance can be mediated by some of the same factors that affect performance during stressor exposure. One process which has more relevance to aftereffects is *transfer* (the effect that dealing with one situation has on learning and performance in another). Someone may adopt particular strategies (e.g., social withdrawal or haste) to counter the effects of a stressor (Cohen, 1980; Poulton, 1978). If such strategies persist, out of habit or due to anticipation that they will be needed in a new situation, later performance could suffer (negative transfer) or benefit (positive transfer), depending upon the particular strategies learned and the similarities of the tasks.

Effects on performance should vary with the type of stressor. Noise can mask auditory stimuli and perhaps the language of inner thought as well (Poulton, 1978; cf. Broadbent, 1978). Similarly, stressors involving visual stimuli may obscure visual cues. Hancock (1986) reviewed studies of heat and vigilance (tasks requiring sustained attention in order to detect occasional stimulus variations). *Changes* in body temperature reduce performance because they make demands on attention, but sustained hyperthermia typically improves performance.

If emotions, motives, and cognitive processes mediate stress effects on performance, then individual differences in any of those classes of variables may alter the stress effects. The anxiety-prone perform less well on complex tasks, and this tendency increases under pressure. Moreover, they may make more internal and stable attributions of failure (Arkin et al., 1983). Performing poorly in order to lower others' expectations is also characteristic of anxious individuals (Baumgardner & Brownlee, 1987). Field-dependent persons may repress threatening information and therefore learn stressful material less well than field-independent individuals (Goodenough, 1976). There is evidence that persons with relatively high epinephrine responses to task demands tend to perform better (Frankenhaeuser, 1975). Perhaps the higher hormonal response means that they are nearer the peak of the arousal-performance curve.

Humphreys and Revelle (1984) have a complex theory relating personality to performance. Their article illustrates well the intricacy of stress effects. They propose that effort and arousal are major determinants of performance and that anxiety, achievement motivation, and impulsivity (a component of extraversion) affect performance via their influences on effort and arousal. Stress-relevant factors come into the Humphreys and Revelle model at two points: First, high trait anxiety and low impulsivity increase arousal, thereby impairing short-term memory function and increasing the efficiency of internal information transfer. Second, success or failure interacts with trait anxiety to affect state anxiety, and can influence momentary achievement motivation.

Social Behavior

All of the results of stress which we have mentioned have social implications. People's emotional reactions and task performance impact others, at least indirectly. In this section, we give some examples of stress responses which have direct effects on others.

Affiliation, seeking to be with others, has long been known to be affected by threatening circumstances. In a classic finding (Schachter, 1959), subjects anticipating electric shock were more likely than others to choose to await their fate in the company of their fellows. When others are the source of discomfort, however, social withdrawal is more likely. Baum et al. (1978) found that students living in functionally crowded dormatories came to perceive less control over their situations and also used a withdrawal strategy in playing a competitive game. A review by Cohen (1980) concluded that loss of sensitivity to others is a frequent aftereffect of stress.

Previous experience and individual characteristics may interact in determining how much social contact individuals seek. Hansson et al. (1982) studied opinion-sharing among residents of a flood plain. Among those who had not been flooded, talking with neighbors about possible future floods increased with belief in being able to cope with a flood. For those who had been flooded, opinion-sharing was higher as their sense of helplessness (and anger) was greater. Perhaps having had the experience and coped poorly with it increased the desire to exchange information.

Rofé (1984) attempted a utility theory of stress and affiliation. In this theory, several factors contribute to cost-benefit judgments and hence to whether one will affiliate under stress. If the negative outcome is avoidable external danger, if one feels helpless, and/or if the potential affiliates are judged able to help, the tendency to affiliate will be greater. Since one's judgments about types of stress, helplessness, and others are themselves subject to many influences, predicting when stressors will actually produce affiliation should be difficult.

Reactance may be an interpersonally relevant consequence of stress. It is based on a motive to protect one's freedom to behave and believe as one chooses. Because many stressors demand particular responses, they can threaten freedom of choice and consequently arouse reactance. The reactance in turn might be expressed in an unwillingness to cooperate with others. Subjects who believed that they had done badly on a task gave less control to a superior partner when the pair were to work together on the same task (Strube & Werner, 1984). Strube and Werner interpreted this in terms of reactance. ("They think that my bad results will make me turn it over to him, but I'm going to do as I please.") Type A personalities, known to be competitive and to desire control (e.g., Glass, 1977), can be less likely than Type B's to give control to someone else with greater competence (Miller et al., 1985; Strube et al., 1985).

PSYCHOSOCIAL CONTRIBUTORS TO THE STRESSFULNESS OF SITUATIONS

We turn now to some examples of psychologic and social variables that help determine how stressful situations will be. As noted previously, psychologic aspects of stressors are often difficult to separate from psychologic responses to stress; therefore some variables mentioned in the preceding section will come up in this one.

Psychologic Stressors

Psychologic stressors are stressors because of their meanings, not their direct effects on tissues. Even stimuli which inflict direct damage can be stressful partly because of the psychologically relevant stimuli they generate (e.g., Mason, 1971). The stressfulness of disease (e.g., Moos, 1982), for example, can stem from the meanings given to symptoms as well as the damage done by the pathology.

THE VARIETY OF STRESSORS

Consider the hunted Elias Openshaw's terrified reaction to dried seeds in Arthur Conan Doyle's "The Five Orange Pips." Part of the difficulty with stress is the huge variety of cues that can act as stressors. The cognitive complexity and extensive learning experiences of humans all but guarantee that weak and subtle cues can be stressors. Some undramatic or unobvious potential stressors are cognitive inconsistency (Higgins, 1987; Kiesler & Pallack, 1976), decreases in the frequency of reward (Goldman et al., 1973), attentional self-focus (Carver et al., 1979), pressure to improve health behaviors (Becker, 1986), relaxation training(!) (Heide & Borkovek, 1983), homeliness (Hansell et al., 1982), and the mere fact of having been bothered by an earlier stressor (Ellis, 1978). Answering a questionnaire dealing with weight significantly lowered adjustment scores in women with overweight body images, but significantly raised the scores of those whose body weight images were normal (DelRosario et al., 1984). This study illustrates the methodologic problems of administering multiple measures as well as the influence of seemingly innocuous stimuli.

Classical conditioning demonstrates that obscure cues can elicit stress responses. A neutral stimulus, if paired with one already capable of eliciting a response, will often come to elicit a conditioned response much like that evoked by the originally potent cue. Both emotions and stress-relevant endocrine responses can be so conditioned (e.g., Brady, 1975; Brush, 1971; Stanton & Levine, 1988; Woods & Burchfield, 1980). Reported pain can be increased by pairing a placebo "analgesic" with a painful stimulus (Voudouris et al., 1985). Classical conditioning has its limits and complexities, of course, but the conditioning of stress responses illustrates the impracticability of trying to produce authoritative classifications of stressors.

Naturally, that impracticability does not keep writers in the field from their classifying. Cohen et al. (1982) differentiated acute time-limited stressors; sequences of stressors stemming from some initial event; chronic intermittent stressors which recur at intervals; and chronic continuous stressors. The Lazarus group (e.g., Lazarus & Folkman, 1984) makes a distinction between between major life events and "daily hassles." Major life stressors such as deaths, marriage, divorce, and imprisonment, are rather infrequent and often dramatic. Hassles are more ordinary aggravations such as family arguments and traffic jams. In the end, however, a stressor's meaning and the responses to it are the important things. If the acute, time-limited event of surgery triggers years of worry about health, the brevity of the original situation may not be crucial. There are probably some for whom the hassles of daily marital disputes have greater effects than would the spouse's death.

Stressor effects are not independent of each other. The life events methodology, in which persons indicate which events have occurred to them, assumes that the more numerous the events the greater the impact and also assumes that some events have much more impact than others (e.g., Dohrenwend et al., 1982). Generally, stress response should increase with the accumulation of greater numbers of more drastic events, but it need not increase in a straightforward manner (Perkins, 1982). There may be thresholds (probably different for different responses) below which there is no impact, and upper bounds, beyond which stress responses cannot increase further. Between these upper and lower limits, stressful events may interact (Perkins, 1982). If death of a child has 90 units of impact and loss of employment has 30, the combination may produce 2700 units rather than 120—or, more likely, something less than 2700 but considerably more than 120.

One stressor can increase or decrease the probability of another's occurrence. Entering the Army almost always means taking a trip and making new friends (Dohrenwend et al., 1982). Unemployment all too often results in a reduced quality of family life (though, given certain resources or personalities, it might actually bring family members together).

Related to the assessment of and impact of stressors is their desirability. The original life stress approach assumed that the change in behavior required by an event indexes its stressfulness, regardless of how pleasant the event may be. Intuitively, however, pleasant events should be less stressful than unpleasant ones which entail the same amount of change, and that seems to be the case (see, e.g., Perkins, 1982).

ROLES AND ROLE CONFLICTS

Connectedness is vulnerability. Family life and roles offer numerous possibilities for stress, even beyond such obvious ones as bereavement or threatened bereavement (e.g., McCubbin et al., 1980). Both unanticipated crises and normal family development can present great demands. Divorce and separation have frequently been associated with adverse outcomes. Bloom et al. (1978) noted three potential reasons for those statistical relationships, namely that those at risk for other problems are unable to maintain satisfactory marriages, that marriage provides protection against other problems, and that marital disruption is a stressor. Each of those possibilities probably represents part of the truth.

If family and home are one domain in which stress can arise, work is another. Indeed, for many, work and family together take up most waking hours. In a succinct and useful summary of research on work-related stress, Holt (1982) has made it clear that many aspects of work can be stressful. Direct physical dangers and discomforts are typically limited to particular jobs, but other stressors, such as quantitative or qualitative overload, monotony, job insecurity, and distressing interpersonal relationships at work, can arise in most occupations. Holt also noted the large number of outcome variables, disease among them, which have been associated with occupational stress.

Role conflict can occur at home, at work, and between home and work roles. If an individual is subjected to incompatible demands, the incompatibility will be an additional demand. To us, role conflicts can take two forms. In one, behaviors in different roles or sub-roles are—or seem—inherently inconsistent. A manager may be expected to assert her opinions openly but also to avoid antagonizing her superiors. Teachers are expected to make courses fun (to garner good student evaluations) and also demanding (to maximize education's contributions to students and society).

The supposed tranquility of women's traditional family/home roles may be a myth. Baruch et al. (1987) have argued that these obligations are associated with conflict and indices of stress, noting among other things that non-employed married women report more demands than do those who are employed. The uncertainty, the need to satisfy several other people, and the lack of a structure which limits others' expectations are similar to what can exist in conflictful professions. By providing satisfactions and buffers against home-role stress, work outside the home might actually lower stress for women.

Other role conflicts (role overloads) center on time. In these cases tasks are incompatible because they cannot all be performed (adequately) in the time available. Such conflicts can occur in many situations. Conflicts between work and family roles are obvious examples. In two-job families, there will usually be more total work to be done than in one-job families. One or both partners will face greater overall demand than would occur if only one had an outside job. With higher job time requirements and lower incomes, the problem becomes more severe. If husbands do not share enough in the home and family work, the benefits to wives of working outside may be lost (Baruch et al., 1987). Part of the work-plus-family problem can be a sense of failure, since if combined demands are great, performance of home tasks, career tasks or both will suffer. The plight of working single householders with children is similar to that of two-job families and may be worse. Role conflicts from excessive time demand might be considered daily hassles (e.g., Holahan et al., 1984), but "hassles" seems too anemic a term for the amount of strain they can engender.

Stressor Controllability

As we noted in Chapter 1 and have had to mention occasionally since, a stressor's controllability—or judged controllability—is one of its important qualities. If stress is considered in terms of demands and resources, seeing a stressor as uncontrollable means judging that one's resources are insufficient to prevent a bad outcome. In theory, then, perceived lack of control over adverse events should aggravate stress responses.

The exercise of control is a means of coping, and some authors (not the present ones) use control as almost synonomous with coping in general (see Thompson, 1981). However, the desire for control is probably also a motive in itself (Schorr & Rodin, 1984), and uncontrollable stressors frustrate that motive in addition to the motive to avoid whatever other undesirable outcomes they portend.

Like all appraisals, control judgments must derive from the combination of the actual characteristics of the situation and the characteristics of the individual. All other things being equal, stressors which are in fact uncontrollable should be judged so, but other factors also contribute. Given human self-enhancement tendencies and the potential aversiveness of lack of control, an "illusion of control" (Langer, 1975) is not surprising. Skinner (1985) has suggested that behavior importantly affects control beliefs. In her theory, behavior generates information about the controllability of a situation, and, less obviously, the information is utilized in a biased way. People tend to give excess weight to instances in which they attempt control and too little to instances in which they do not act. Thus, control beliefs and actions are reciprocally related: our behavior (along with its consequences and our interpretations of it) affects our sense of control, and, of course, our sense of control influences our behavior.

Many stress responses have been shown to depend upon control or perceived control. In lower animals, inability to control aversive stimulation has increased weight loss, plasma glucocorticoids, behavioral indications of fear, and stomach lesions (e.g., Seligman et al., 1971; Weiss et al., 1976). In a study which links human stress responses to this large animal literature, Bandura et al. (1988) found an opioid-mediated analgesia in subjects who attempted a computational task too fast-paced for them but not in subjects who could control the pace of the task. Bandura et al. interpreted these data in terms of lowered self-efficacy in the fast-paced group.

One dramatic human demonstration of the possible benefits of control involved assigning nursing home residents to a treatment in which they received plants to tend and a talk from the institution's administrator on taking responsibility for themselves. Both in the short term and at a follow-up, those encouraged to exercise control did better than a comparison group. The differences were seen on several measures, including nurses' ratings of activity, physicians' ratings of health, questions asked after a lecture on aging, and, most provocative, mortality (Rodin & Langer, 1977; see also Rodin, 1986).

Rodin et al. (1978) found that having control in an elevator or a group discussion reduced perceived crowding. (Crowding and sense of control may be reciprocally related; crowding can reduce perceived control [Baum et al., 1978].)

In a study particularly relevant to stress and disease, Felton and Revenson (1984) compared the psychologic well-being of patients with four diseases, two of which, cancer and rheumatoid arthritis, were seen by patients as relatively uncontrollable and two of which, diabetes mellitus and hypertension, were seen as relatively controllable. In multiple regressions, disease controllability significantly predicted emotional adjustment. Coping style was also predictive, with "wish-fulfilling fantasy" related to more negative affect and "information seeking" related to more positive affect.

Many other human studies of stressor control have been done. Perceived and/or exercised control has produced increases in task performance and persistence, reductions in anticipatory arousal (but not necessarily arousal upon actual receipt of an aversive stimulus), decreases in aggression, and increased helping behavior (see e.g., Cohen, 1980; Rodin, 1986; Thompson, 1981).

A most influential formulation of the consequences of uncontrollable aversive events is *learned helplessness theory* (e.g., Maier & Seligman, 1976; Peterson & Seligman, 1984). The original version of this theory was based on infrahuman research using yoked experimental designs (in which one subject could terminate a noxious stimulus for itself and a powerless partner). The theory purported to explain emotional and performance changes resulting from uncontrollable stress. Powerless subjects' experience of noncontingency—of coping attempts being unrelated to the termination of aversive stimuli—was held to teach that future coping responses would be similarly fruitless. Learning that they were helpless induced subjects not to attempt coping in later, controllable, situations. Motivational and emotional deficits, especially apathy, were also seen as part of the learned helplessness syndrome. One interesting aspect of the theory was that prior experience with control would prevent later noncontingency from inducing helplessness (Maier & Seligman, 1976).

Criticisms of the original helplessness theory were based largely on evidence that noncontingency did not always produce the expected results (see e.g., Miller & Norman, 1979) or might not exert its effects through learning (Weiss et al., 1976). Logical criticisms are also possible. The transfer of expectancies from one situation to a new one involves stimulus generalization and would be expected to occur not broadly, but only when the new situation is reasonably similar to the old (Roselinni & Seligman, 1978). Further, if experience with controllable events inoculates against learned helplessness, then helplessness should be rare; few animals or humans manage never to control anything. As we discussed in considering depression as a stress response, some revisions of the theory invoke causal attributions to explain why helplessness and depression do not occur more frequently (e.g., Miller & Norman, 1979; Peterson & Seligman, 1984).

A recent suggestion by Sedek and Kofta (1990) concerns the conditions which actually produce helplessness. These authors propose that it is the inability to generate cognitive schemata or plans for behavior which induces learned helplessness, rather than the lack of relationship between overt responses and reinforcements. In this view, inconsistent information during attempts to perform tasks will result in ineffectual cognitive efforts, thus producing cognitive exhaustion and a reduced ability to function effectively on later tasks.

Given that judged lack of control, or at least judgment of doubtful control, is nearly essential to the idea of psychologic stress, it is not surprising that several influential formulations incorporate it at least implicitly. Bandura's (e.g., 1982) self-efficacy, for instance, is the expectancy that one can successfully control some outcome. Another example is the notion of *inhibited* (or stressed) *power motivation* emphasized by McClelland (e.g., 1989).

Stressor controllability is seldom omitted from discussions of stress and disease. After all, if stress affects illness and uncontrollability aggravates stress, then uncontrollable stressors should have greater effects upon health. Some questions remain, however. Even when attributional factors are taken into account, uncontrollability does not always intensify stress responses (see, e.g., Brewin, 1985). Maier et al. (1986) recently found that control did not affect the glucocorticoid response to electric shock. Telner et al. (1982) reported that controllable shock produced greater prolactin responses than did uncontrollable shock.

The type of stressor, its intensity, and the processes of adaptation might affect how controllability operates. If the stressor is actual damage rather than a warning of damage, then ability to cope may not affect the initial stress responses, only the rate at which they return to baseline. A person unexpectedly struck by an assailant might show strong initial glucocorticoid and catecholamine responses regardless of his/her ability to master the assailant and prevent other blows, but the ability to control the ultimate outcome might greatly influence how long the hormonal responses persist.

Another thing to be remembered is that exercising control has a cost. Controlling events uses time, effort, and often other resources. When exercising control is arduous, it could actually increase stress. Murison et al., (1981) found that prolonged shock avoidance, in which rats could actually prevent the aversive stimuli, increased stomach lesions in comparison to an uncontrollable shock condition.

Controllability and predictability are often related (Dess et al., 1983 cited discussions of this point). If a stimulus is predictable, either because it occurs at regular intervals or because it is preceded by a warning signal, there can be time to prepare for coping. Predictability provides safe periods during which the organism can relax, and some of the benefits of predictability result from safety signals (Hymowitz, 1979). The offset of a controllable aversive stimulus is almost necessarily more predictable than that of an uncontrollable stimulus.

There is a great deal of evidence that unpredictability increases the stressfulness of aversive stimuli (Abbott & Badia, 1986; Abbott et al., 1984; Hymowitz, 1979; Seligman et al., 1971; but see Arthur, 1986). Effects which seem due to uncontrollability may actually be due to unpredictability (Burger & Arkin, 1980). Unpredictability and uncontrollability are not identical in their effects, however. For one thing, the effects of uncontrollability can be immediate under conditions in which the effects of unpredictability are delayed (Dess et al., 1983).

Much remains to be learned about control over stressors. It is unclear exactly what control means and just when its absence will be detrimental. Antonovsky (1979) has argued that controllability per se is not as important as a broader "sense of coherence." The sense of coherence is the belief that the world, however complex and frustrating, is by and large predictable and comprehensible, and that control over one's life outcomes is where it *ought* to be, partly in oneself and partly elsewhere.

Social Support

As lack of control is widely thought to intensify stress responses, so "social support" is widely thought to mitigate them. The term refers to the effects of a person's social network on stress-related events, though we know of no agreed upon definition. It is, of course, inconceivable that family, friends, and acquaintances would be irrelevant to one's level of stress. It is almost inconceivable that their influences would be simple.

Cohen and Wills (1985) provided an excellent review. They advocated a distinction between the *extent* of someone's interpersonal network and the degree to which the network actually performs social support *functions*. An individual could have a large but useless social network, or a very small network which nonetheless provides a great deal of support.

Cohen and Wills also noted that social support may act through either a "buffering" or a "main effect" process. According to the buffering hypothesis, social support enhances well-being by preventing negative effects of stress. Thus stress and social support should interact, with support having an effect only to the degree that persons are under stress. According to the main effect notion social support is beneficial regardless of stress level. There is evidence for both types of effects. The dependent variables employed in the research have usually been measures of psychologic well-being such as affect.

One illustrative report is by Berkowitz and Perkins (1985). They studied reported stress symptoms (e.g., insomnia, shortness of breath) in a sample of farm wives, finding that support from husbands was associated with lower symptom scores, whereas task loads and farm complexity were unrelated to stress symptoms. A partly experimental study (Sarason & Sarason, 1986) demonstrated a social support effect on task performance. Subjects with smaller social networks did less well on anagrams unless they were given support by the experimenter. Subjects with neither large networks nor experimenter support reported more irrelevant thinking during the task, suggesting that social support can reduce distraction.

There are obviously many specific ways in which social support can operate. Other people are capable of affecting both an individual's appraisals and her/his coping processes. They can inform the person that anticipated outcomes are not as adverse as feared (to a child who argued with a playmate, "In a few days, you'll be friends again."). They can intervene to moderate internal, stable, or global attributions of failure (to a disabled friend, "Okay, there are a few things you can't do. But there aren't many."). Others can provide material resources and information on how to perform tasks, can encourage or reward coping (e.g., Doherty et al., 1983), can even take over the job of coping. They can prevent some stressors from occurring, and are, of course, the only realistic cure for loneliness and social isolation.

With regard to the last point, we may wish to consider the possibility that humans are inherently social creatures and that the absence of social connections is thus inherently distressing or damaging. There is certainly evidence to suggest that lack of social contact has deleterious effects on other animals (e.g., Fajzi et al., 1989).

Not unexpectedly, social support interacts with individual difference variables. Locus of control is one of these. Lefcourt et al. (1984) found that support seemed more beneficial for persons who were less affiliative, more autonomous, and more internal in locus of control. They speculated that these independent persons make better use of information from their networks and that, since they are likely to take blame for bad outcomes, they need others to provide hopeful attributions. Complex relations among stress, gender, locus of control, and social support were found by Caldwell et al. (1987). For example, support was less beneficial for men with an external locus of control than for internals or women in that study.

Revicki and May (1985) obtained statistical evidence for a causal model in which depression is predicted by occupational stress, external locus of control, and low family social support. In this model, family support *results from* internal locus of control in combination with low stress. These findings suggest that locus of control may influence the amount of social support offered as well as need for or ability to benefit from support.

Indeed, personal characteristics could hardly fail to affect others' willingness to provide social support (e.g., Dunkel-Schetter et al., 1987). (This is a potential confounding in nonexperimental studies of social support effects.) Individuals who are lonely (Jones et al., 1982; Wittenberg & Reis, 1986) and individuals with small social support networks (B. Sarason et al., 1985) tend to have less social skill and to be judged unfavorably by others. If stress reduces sensitivity to others (Cohen, 1980), then it should affect the amount of social support a person elicits from others. Another potential problem is that there may be individual differences in *perceived* social support. People can believe that they have more or less support than they actually have.

As a final example of a study relating personality to the effect of social support, we cite Kelly and Houston (1985). Among employed women, Type A's experienced more stress and tension, but did not differ from B's in reported social support. Most interestingly, Type A's with higher social support reported being under greater stress. Kelly and Houston noted that stress may lead Type A's to seek more support and that social support may increase the pressure on Type A's to excel.

Kelly and Houston's data bring up the possibility that social support can be deleterious. Social networks have as much potential to aggravate as to assist. Even attempts to be helpful can be counterproductive. Accurate information can hurt as well as comfort. Emotional warmth may be interpreted as smothering. Attempts to help someone cope may be seen by him/her as patronizing, and even if they are appreciated at the time they may, by making learning unnecessary, set the individual up for later failure.

HOLISM REVISITED

In this chapter and the preceding one we have tried to illustrate the variety of phenomena which need to be taken into account in considering stress. It is almost an understatement to point out that the relationships involved are multivariate, interactive, and reciprocal. The stressfulness of a situation for an individual depends partly upon the environment—the demands, the material resources, and the others who impinge upon the person. It depends partly on the individual—her/his personality, skills, behavior, and physical attributes. The members of the person's social environment are themselves persons, subject to all of the influences that affect the individual under consideration, including influence from that individual.

The hyper-numerous elements of this psychosocial matrix influence each other in almost every conceivable way, producing moment by moment changes in the person and simultaneously in his/her environment. Many, perhaps all, of the elements are involved in direct or indirect reciprocal relationships with many, perhaps all, of the others. An individual's behavior, for example, influences her/his physical environment, resources, social environment, and interpretations of all of those. In response to the person's behavior and other characteristics, others alter their interpretations of the person, the demands they make, the comforts they provide, and the physical environment. These alterations in others' qualities and actions impinge upon the person, often within a moment, and another set of effects ripples through the matrix.

Internally, the biologic organisms to which all of this happens are, for practical purposes, at least as intricate as the psychosocial matrix. A host of substances, from simple ions to large proteins, carries information from almost every cellular compartment to almost every other in a network of interactive, reciprocal influences so complex as to beggar the imagination. And the "stressfulness" of relationships in the psychosocial-behavioral realm impinges, sometimes gently, sometimes dramatically, on those internal communications.

It is important to note that many independent variables can have opposite effects on many dependent variables depending upon the context and the levels of the independent variables. Thus glucocorticoids can enhance or depress immune function; stress can impair or improve performance; social support can be helpful or harmful; what is challenging for one person can be threatening to another.

The physiologic world and the psychosocial world together form the context of and the stimuli for pathology. We turn next to incorporating pathology into this holistic context.

A General Schematic for
Stress-Disease Relationships

Our discussions of stress and stress responses have set much of the context for stress-disease questions. We now make a transition between that broad context and stress-disease research per se. In general terms, how *might* stress and disease be connected? Figure 6 is a framework for answers to this question—answers consistent with the complexity of organisms' relations with their environments, and with the fact that both stress and disease involve most of those relations. We shall spend some time with Figure 6; we wish to use it to introduce examples of relevant variables that do not fit well elsewhere as well as to describe paths that can link stress and disease.

The model in Figure 6 (a model in only the loosest sense) depicts relationships among seven very general classes of variables put under the even broader headings of environment, organism, and response. Using a larger number of more specific variable classes could easily be justified but would make the figure impossibly complex. The seven classes of factors are social environment, physical environment, psychologically relevant stimulation, genome, phenotypic organism, pathologic processes, and overt behavior. Because these classes of variables are so general, the distinctions among them are rather artificial at times; there are specific variables whose classification into a particular one of these seven categories is questionable.

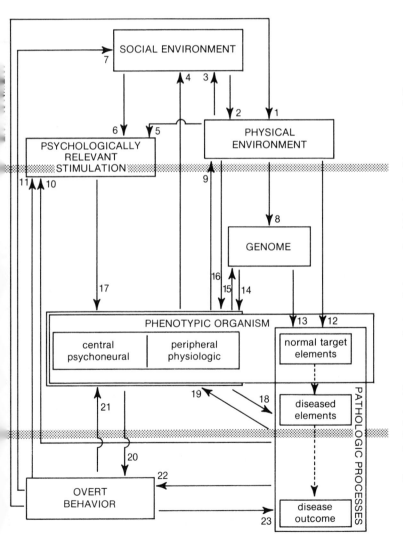

Figure 6. Relationships among the broad classes of variables involved in stress and disease.

The *social environment* in Figure 6 refers to persons, groups, and institutions which might directly or indirectly influence the person whose stressor exposure and health are under consideration.

Physical environment refers to all relevant non-social aspects of the environment. Of particular interest in stress and disease are elements of the physical environment which affect the organism directly, independently of their sensory-psychological impacts. We use the term *exogenous agents* for such directly disease- or stress-relevant factors as dietary elements, infectious organisms, drugs, pollutants, and radiation. A complete list of exogenous agents would be very long. Ames (1983), for instance, has noted the large number of bioactive compounds found in common dietary plants.

As the term suggests, *psychologically relevant stimulation* acts via psychologic processes, usually meaning that the influence begins with sensory receptors. As we discussed in the last chapter, how a person will respond to a particular stimulus depends upon attentional, perceptual, and other cognitive processes as well as upon its sensory impact.

Psychologically relevant stimulation is not always meaningfully distinguishable from the social and physical environments. It is sometimes not important to decide whether a person or object *is* or merely produces psychologically relevant stimulation. In other cases the distinction is important. Many exogenous agents act without producing detectable sensory impacts, and the environment may act upon the individual by altering these nonsensory influences (and by other indirect means as well).

For the most part, the organism can be considered in terms of two general variable classes, the *genome*, and the *phenotypic organism*. *Normal target elements* and *diseased elements* must also be considered part of the organism, even though they also belong with pathologic processes. These distinctions are clearly artificial; they are helpful in illustrating stress-disease relationships, but would not necessarily serve well in other contexts. In addition, it is possible to think of psychologically relevant stimulation as arising from within the organism as well as from the environment.

The term genome refers to DNA structure. It does not include changes in gene expression. Genes are constantly being turned on or off by regulatory processes, but we consider those changes as phenotypic organism functions.

The phenotypic organism includes all "normal" (non-diseased) structures and processes except the genome. It provides the cells, tissues and functions that become deranged in disease, and also provides the milieux in which pathologies must exist. In Figure 6, we break the phenotypic organism down into three subcomponents—the *central psychoneural*, the *peripheral physiologic*, and the *normal target elements* components. The distinction between central psychoneural and peripheral physiologic processes is useful because, as Chapters 2 and 3 have emphasized, central processes mediate a multitude of possible transactions between stressors and pathology.

Normal target elements designate the focal tissues, cells, or substances of the disorder being considered. In many disorders, of course, either many components are involved almost from the beginning, or the focal elements are unknown. However in other cases, there are elements upon which proximal etiologic factors converge in pathogenesis (e.g., pancreatic ß-cells in insulin-dependent diabetes, the vascular endothelium in atherosclerosis). Normal target elements are also considered with the class of variables termed *pathologic processes*, since they are one starting point for pathology. *Diseased elements* merely represent the results of initial and/or progressive pathologic changes. As we indicated in Chapter 1, it can sometimes be difficult to distinguish normal from diseased.

The final subclass of variables under pathology is *disease outcome*. Disease outcome is also included as a form of response. This term represents the disease dependent variables, or the "responses" of the pathophysiologic processes to factors which affect them. It is helpful to be reminded that different indices of pathology may respond differently to such influences as stress. Dechambre (1981) provided an example of divergent responses in which social isolation increased Krebs-2 ascites weight (cancer mass) in mice but paradoxically lengthened survival time (Dechambre, 1981).

Overt behavior, the last class of variable given in Figure 6, refers to the sorts of easily detectable responses which constitute the standard dependent variables of the behavioral sciences. Covert behaviors, such as internal smooth muscle responses and neural responses are considered as phenotypic organism activities for the purposes of this model.

RELATIONSHIPS AMONG GENERAL VARIABLE CLASSES

Figure 6 depicts 23 types of causal influences among pairs of the seven major variable classes. These represent in global terms the influences that must be taken into account in studying, interpreting, or intervening in relations between stress and disease. Since each variable class represents many specific systems, structures, substances, and functions, each type of causal influence in the model stands for large numbers of specific effects. To make reference to Figure 6 a bit easier, the number of a type of effect will be indicated in brackets { } when we discuss it. Two or more numbers in series will indicate a sequence of influences. For example, {17,20} would signify an effect of psychologically relevant stimulation on the phenotypic organism, followed by an effect of the phenotypic organism on overt behavior.

In the schematic, every general variable class has both independent variable and dependent variable roles. We shall order our consideration of the pairwise relationships by taking under the heading of each variable class those relationships in which it serves as dependent variable, but logically we could just as well have organized our treatment by independent variables. We can give only a few examples to illustrate the range of effects represented by each relationship. We need not devote equal space to each relationship. Some have already been discussed extensively; others are obscure or are likely to be important under only a few conditions.

Factors Affecting the Social Environment

In our schematic, the social environment is affected by the physical environment {3}, the characteristics of the phenotypic organism {4}, and the overt behavior of the individual {7}. Physical environment influences on members of an individual's social environment {3} must, of course, be much the same as those on the individual him/herself ({8} or {16}), and those effects will be considered below.

It goes without saying that one's overt behavior influences one's social environment {7}. Much of our behavior is intended to affect those persons and organizations that in turn affect us {7,6,17}. When we model or reinforce behavior, dress in a particular way, or express our frustrations, we affect our social environments whether the consequences are desirable or not. Illness behavior, for example, can elicit either sympathy or irritation on the part of others. In terms of stress, we behave in order to avoid, escape, or reduce the aversive stressors produced by others, or to gain support from others.

Characteristics of the phenotypic organism other than overt behavior have impacts upon others {4}. Others form different impressions and react differently depending upon a person's age, physical attractiveness, sex, size, and skin color. Persons who are discriminated against because of skin color, gender, or disfigurement deal with different stressors than those not so stigmatized (e.g., Herman et al., 1986). Large and ferocious-looking people may have still other problems.

Factors Affecting
the Physical Environment

The physical environment is influenced by the social environment {2}, phenotypic organism characteristics {9}, and overt behavior {1}.

It is obvious that much of our physical environment is built or modified by others. Everything from the asthetics of cities (or the lack thereof) to the thickness of apartment walls and the chemical composition of food is influenced by the actions of large institutions. Members of the individual's personal social network also modify the physical environment. One need think only of such commonplaces as passive smoking (e.g., White & Froeb, 1980), a neighbor having his/her trees sprayed (with the consequent drift into one's kitchen), or a nurse administering an injection.

We think of phenotypic characteristics of the organism as influencing the physical environment {9} at least in terms of a person's ultimate exposure to exogenous agents. Skin pigmentation influences effective exposure to solar radiation. "Natural resistance" to microorganisms includes the physical barrier of the skin, the antimicrobial activities of sebaceous gland secretions and tears, and the actions of the hairs, cilia and mucous of the respiratory tract (Barrett, 1983).

The effects of overt behavior on the physical environment {1} are crucial to stress and disease. They can be thought of in several ways. For one thing, behavior alters the environment in the service of goals, whether those goals involve physiologic needs, asthetic preferences or social values.

Behavior also affects exposure to exogenous agents. This is a major part of what is meant by disease and health as "lifestyle" phenomena. Often, of course, the relevant behavior is undertaking or avoiding self-administration (e.g., drinking alcohol). In other cases, it is a matter of going to the right (or wrong) place at the right time (e.g., moving to a high-pollution area or leaving the scene of a tank car derailment). The AIDS epidemic is making many people more aware that behavior can expose one to significant exogenous agents. To the extent that exogenous agents influence health and stress influences behavior, behavior can mediate the effects of stress on disease and influence the stressfulness of disease ("External Loop Effects," below).

Factors Affecting
Psychologically Relevant Stimulation

Psychologically relevant stimulation is affected by (or produced by) the social environment {6}, the physical environment {5}, overt behavior {11}, and pathologic processes {10}. The first two of these relationships hardly need extensive discussion here. Much of behavioral and social science deals with environmental stimulation and its effects. Only the effects of overt behavior and pathology require comment from us.

Behavior produces stimulation directly by activating distance receptors (we hear what we say and see what we do), and internal sense receptors such as those for pain, pressure and kinesthesia. An illustrative effect is for response-produced stimuli to take up cognitive channel capacity and thus reduce access to other information (Quattrone, 1985).

We noted previously that behavior is subject to interpretation. A classic example of the importance of that fact is an experiment by Zimbardo et al. (1969). They studied subjects who participated in a task involving electric shocks and volunteered for a second session immediately following the first. The experimenter gave half of the subjects only a weak justification for participating in the second experiment; the others were given a more persuasive justification. Shock-induced disruption of learning in the second experiment was less among the weak-justification subjects than among those given the strong justification. The weak-justification subjects also had lower galvanic skin responses (GSR) in the second experiment than the first, whereas the opposite was true for the strong-justification subjects. In other words, those who had less reason to expose themselves to the shock seemed behaviorally and physiologically less disturbed by it.

This is a cognitive consistency phenomenon (see Chapter 3). The experience of the second shock was brought into line with the implications of participating. Subjects given the weak justification for the second shock session might have reasoned (consciously or not) that, "I don't put myself into painful situations without a good reason. Since I chose to take part in this second session without much reason to, these shocks can't be very bad."

Our interpretations of our actions and choices can change us. If we are provoked to aggression, we may conclude that we are more hostile than we had thought. If we surmount a difficulty, our belief in our own abilities might increase. Later behavior, including responses to stressors, will reflect such changes.

In the Zimbardo et al. study, choice behavior affected the functioning of the organism. However, other types of behavior can also influence internal functions. One possible example is from Notarius and Levenson (1979). Subjects who were more facially expressive when viewing an accident film exhibited less heart rate and respiration change when threatened with shock nine weeks later. In an experimental study of posture effects (Petty et al., 1983), subjects who received persuasive messages while reclining were more persuaded by cogent arguments and less persuaded by weak arguments than were standing subjects. Petty et al. suggested that reclining improved processing of the arguments, possibly because it produced fewer distracting stimuli. Related effects may occur with exercise, but because exercise has many direct effects on the organism {21} we shall consider it in a subsequent section.

If internal sense receptors produce and/or receive psychologically relevant stimulation, then we must consider pathology capable of producing psychologically relevant stimulation {10}. Pain, pressure, and nausea, for example, can reflect the influence of pathology. Those stimuli, like all others that are attended to, can be interpreted and acted upon. They can be stressful and can also alert an individual to changes that require attention.

Factors Affecting the Genome

Figure 6 depicts the genome as susceptible to influence by the physical environment {8} and the phenotypic organism {15}. We reiterate that in our division of variable classes, alterations in gene expression are considered to be phenotypic organism processes. The most important physical environment effects on DNA are those of exogenous agents. Such agents are often pathogens. Viruses add DNA or RNA to the cells which they infect, and viral DNA can sometimes be incorporated into host cell chromosomes (see Chapter 5). Chemicals, radiation, and viruses can mutate existing genes.

It seems possible that effects beyond the most obvious ones might occur through exogenous agents' modifications of the genome. If a wide variety of agents are at least mildly mutagenic (Ames, 1983), then subtle variations in disease susceptibility, and conceivably even in psychological characteristics, may result from differences in exogenous agent exposure. If such things do happen, they would be most likely to occur early in development.

Exogenous agent effects on the genome can be beneficial. Some cancer chemotherapy agents kill neoplastic cells via DNA alterations such as chain breakage and crosslinking of DNA strands (Calabresi & Parks, 1975). These agents are toxic to normal cells as well as cancerous ones, particularly to dividing cells.

The effects of the organism on DNA {15} can be seen in DNA repair. Enzymatic mechanisms recognize and restore damaged DNA in various ways, as by excising defective bases from one strand and using the information on the other strand to insert the proper bases (Freifelder, 1983). There is evidence that stress can interfere with DNA repair mechanisms (see Kiecolt-Glaser & Glaser, 1987). Therefore psychologic conditions may be able to produce (or allow) permanent genetic changes {17,15} at least in occasional cells.

Factors Affecting the Phenotypic Organism and Pathologic Processes

In this section we treat some influences on the normal organism and on pathology together because they can be difficult to distinguish. (Should the effects of dietary fats on blood cholesterol be considered to be on pathology or on normal function? It is difficult to say). In some cases, moreover, we may know that a particular genetic or environmental factor produces disease but not know whether the effect is a direct production of pathology or a modification of host resistance. As long as we keep in mind that pathogenic factors can affect disease outcome by acting upon normal function (e.g., {16,18}) and also by producing pathology directly (e.g., {12}), we need not assign every effect to one of those categories.

We shall concentrate in this section on influences that are not treated extensively elsewhere in the book. Thus we shall not dwell on stressors' effects or upon the etiologies of the diseases that we discuss later.

GENOMIC EFFECTS ON NORMAL FUNCTION AND PATHOLOGY

Genomic influences on the organism {14} are ubiquitous by definition. Of course what are often meant by genetic influences are genetic individual differences, not genetic characteristics which are shared by all members of a species. Evidence on genetic individual differences is difficult to obtain in humans because heredity and environment are very often confounded. In lower animals, of course, much clearer conclusions can be drawn. New methods are making information available at the level of chromosomes and actual DNA sequences, and difficult human genetic questions will get definitive answers.

Hundreds of disorders are directly traceable to genetic defects or show familial patterns suggesting genetic influence {13} (Robbins et al., 1984). Genetic factors can affect structural proteins, enzymes, or regulatory molecules, and depending on the precise defect, the results can be mild or devastating.

In familial hypercholesterolemia, cells cannot take up low-density lipoprotein (LDL) because of a mutation in a gene which codes for cell membrane LDL receptors. Profound susceptibility to atherosclerosis can result (Robbins et al., 1984). As another example, Robbins et al. list eight enzyme deficiencies that disrupt glycogen metabolism with widely divergent results. In McCardle's syndrome the deficiency is confined to muscle and, despite pain, longevity can be normal; in generalized glycogenosis, death can result in two years from cardiac and respiratory failure.

In the diseases just mentioned, and in many others, the link with genetics is strong; pathology is nearly inevitable. In other disorders, both genetic and environmental factors are greatly involved. There seems to be a genetic component in alcoholism (Schuckit, 1985). Obesity is known to be familial, and adoptees' obesity is more closely related to their biological parents' overweight than to their adoptive parents' (Weight Disturbances, 1986). Individual differences in DNA repair capacity are related to cancer (Setlow, 1983). One of the best known of these syndromes occurs in xeroderma pigmentosum, the victims of which develop skin cancer from solar radiation.

The evidence for genetically determined differences in stress response is less than for disease susceptibility, but it does exist (see, e.g., Ciaranello et al., 1982; Hamburg et al., 1975). Spontaneously hypertensive rats respond differently to stress than do normotensive controls (LeDoux et al., 1983). Monozygotic twins are more alike than dizygotics in cardiovascular responses to some stressors (Carmelli et al., 1985). Relevant personality factors such as altruism and aggressiveness may also have genetic components (Rushton et al., 1986).

Genomic influences need not be obvious. A mutation can produce a protein which, while not normal, is still partly functional. A normal protein can be in short supply in heterozygotes who have one normal and one defective copy of a gene. With a defect in an enzyme that catalyzes one step in a biosynthetic pathway, precursors can build up because they are not used. Stress will sometimes alter the levels of those precursors. A partial defect in adrenocortical 11 ß-hydroxylase, for instance, can produce excessive androgens under stress, because ACTH enhances production of compounds that are precursors to both glucocorticoids and adrenal androgens (Hamburg et al., 1975).

PHYSICAL ENVIRONMENT EFFECTS
ON NORMAL FUNCTION AND PATHOLOGY

Exogenous agents provide most of the direct influences of the physical environment on the phenotypic organism {16} and pathologic processes {12}. Like genes, exogenous agents affect everything. We shall not discuss infectious agents or those that produce trauma; their influence is too obvious. We shall mention drugs, diet, and environmental toxins. Some agents might fall under more than one of these headings.

Drugs

We need not discuss the fact that therapeutic agents are very often beneficial. However, most medicines have undesirable, if unavoidable, side effects (see Gilman et al., 1980; Gilman et al., 1985; Robbins et al., 1984, from which our examples are taken unless otherwise indicated).

Antibiotics can reduce normal gut flora and any resistance to pathogens those flora ordinarily provide. At least in rats, antibiotics can protect against stress-induced gastric ulcers (Rosoff & Goldman, 1968). The reduction in gut flora seemingly reduces stomach secretions. Specific antibiotics can be toxic to specific organs. Antibiotic-induced anaphylaxis can be fatal.

Exogenous hormones are used for a variety of purposes, and can have many undesirable effects. They can speed the growth of some established cancers and can act like chemical tumor promoters (Furth, 1975). Cancer has been an issue with birth control pills, especially the older forms. Oral contraceptives are also associated with cardiovascular disorders, but there is some evidence that postmenopausal estrogen reduces all-cause and myocardial infarction mortality (Henderson et al., 1986). Corticosteroids are used as antiinflammatory agents, as immunosuppressives, and in some cancer chemotherapies. They can increase risk of infection and suppress symptoms of infection.

Some persons with eating disorders use cathartics or emetics to excess. Excessive cathartic use can damage the bowel and produce severe constipation. Emetine (in syrup of ipecac) is toxic to the gastrointestinal system and the heart; its overuse use can be fatal.

Neuroactive drugs alter behavior, psychologic processes and peripheral physiology. ß-adrenergic blockers, used in treating hypertension and cardiac ischemia (reduced blood supply to the heart), may induce depression and lethargy and impair task performance (Durel et al., 1985). Antipsychotics are well known to induce the secretion of prolactin. Antianxiety agents can blunt the adrenal cortical stress response (Lahti & Barsuhn, 1974).

Even over-the-counter analgesics are not without problems. It is well known that aspirin participates in the etiology of Reye's syndrome. (Reye's typically appears in children following viral infection; its major manifestations are liver dysfunction and potentially fatal neurologic involvement.) Aspirin seemingly protects against heart attacks and occlusive stroke but might promote hemorrhagic stroke (Steering Committee, 1988). Long-term overuse of some combination analgesic products can produce chronic nephritis. (Robbins et al., 1984).

The undesirable effects of many "recreational" drugs are well known. Some, like opiates and such sympathomimetics as amphetamines and cocaine, are similar or identical to drugs with medical uses. Illicit use often carries extra hazards from drug combinations and dangerous forms of self-administration. Some "recreational" drugs have been tolerated if not actually encouraged by society despite their adverse effects. Prominent among these are ethyl alcohol and tobacco. Caffeine may be considered a drug, although its effects are relatively minor.

Ritchie (1985) provides a concise description of ethanol's effects. It alters energy metabolism and cell membrane function. At a more molar level, ethanol can depress neural function by reducing postsynaptic potentials; lead to the accumulation of fat and protein in the liver; and increase plasma catecholamines, at least partly by reducing neuronal reuptake of norepinephrine. It lowers internal body temperature by increasing blood flow to the body surface. Alcohol can produce a rather direct blood pressure increase in normotensives (Puddey et al., 1985). Its actions on the hypothalamic-pituitary axis reduce the outputs of several hormones. Alcohol can depress bone marrow and immune function, which may explain the susceptibility of alcoholics and fetal alcohol syndrome victims to infection. Ethanol disrupts the transport and metabolism of the vitamin folic acid. It tends to inhibit lead excretion. In a meta-analytic review of ethanol's behavioral effects, Hull and Bond (1986) confirmed the usual conclusions of impaired cognitive and motor performance, improved mood, and increased aggression. Alcohol expectancies—beliefs about alcohol's effects and that one has taken it—increase sexual arousal and actual alcohol consumption.

Not surprisingly, ethanol is a risk factor for a number of disorders, among them cardiac myopathy, hypertension, stroke, cancers (mouth, esophagus, pharynx, larynx, liver, and lung), and of course cirrhosis of the liver. The use of alcohol by nursing mothers appears capable of adversely affecting infant neural or neuromotor function (Little et al., 1989). There is also evidence for a negative effect on osteoblast (bone-forming cell) activity and bone density (Diamond et al., 1989). Moderate use may reduce ischemic heart disease risk, perhaps by lowering the ratio of low density to high density lipoproteins (Ritchie, 1985). The range of its effects suggests that ethanol can contribute to stress and disease in a variety of ways.

Tobacco is a major scourge. We take our brief discussion largely from Jaffe (1985) and Taylor (1985a). Tobacco smoke is not one drug. It contains hundreds of delectables, including heavy metals, ammonia, hydrogen cyanide, and formaldehyde (Jaffe, 1985). Nicotine is presumably the addictive substance. Nicotine, carbon monoxide (CO), and the components of "tar" are the important pathogenic elements.

Nicotine stimulates one type of acetylcholine receptor (the nicotinic receptor, of course) (Taylor, 1985a). The initial effects include stimulation of adrenomedullary output, muscles, CNS and heart, and an increase in blood pressure. However, initial stimulatory effects are often followed by depressive effects, seemingly because target cells remain depolarized. The depressive impact on muscle occurs very rapidly. Beneficial or reinforcing effects include mental alertness, reduced irritability, and in smokers an increase in euphoria (Jaffe, 1985). Tranquilizing effects of nicotine may derive from muscle relaxation or from inhibition of pain perception (Fertig et al., 1986; Gilbert, 1979).

Some of the other effects of tobacco smoking include increases in cholesterol and low density lipoproteins (Perkins, 1985), and interference with ciliary and immune function in the respiratory system. Smoking is associated with atherosclerosis, myocardial infarction (MI), peptic ulcer, emphysema, bronchitis, perinatal mortality and several cancers (lung, larynx, mouth, esophagus, pancreas, kidney, and bladder). Smokers who suffer acute MI are otherwise less ill than nonsmoking MI patients (Kelly et al., 1985), presumably reflecting the fact that smoking induces heart attacks in persons who otherwise would not have them.

Caffeine has not been strongly associated with pathology, although there is evidence that it affects experimental tumor systems, sometimes enhancing and sometimes inhibiting neoplastic processes (Pozniak, 1985). Caffeine is a methylxanthene, as is the asthma drug, theophylline. Xanthenes appear to have several mechanisms of action, including mobilizing calcium ion from intracellular stores (recall that Ca^{2+} has a major role in intracellular regulation); inhibition of cyclic nucleotide phosphodiesterase and therefore augmentation of cAMP and cGMP actions; and blockade of adenosine receptors (Rall, 1985). Caffeine can alter the cell division process, producing early condensation of chromosomes (Schlegel & Pardee, 1986).

Caffeine and theophylline are strong CNS stimulators. They interfere with fine motor control and in high doses can produce insomnia, tremors and convulsions. Their complex cardiovascular actions can result in tachycardia (increased heart rate), arrhythmias, increased peripheral blood flow, and increased blood pressure. Other xanthene actions include adrenomedullary activation, increases in plasma renin, relaxation of smooth muscle (hence theophylline for asthma), diuresis, increased gastric secretion, augmentation of the insulin response to gastric hormones, inhibition of mast cell anti-inflammatory activity (Rall, 1985), and augmentation of the adrenocortical and catecholamine responses to stress (Henry & Stephens, 1980).

Diet

Much has been claimed for proper diet, but much of what has been claimed is not well supported by data. Diets grossly inadequate in overall calories or in specific nutrients produce pathology rather directly. Moderate deficiencies may have more subtle effects, but less is known about them.

Obesity results, of course, from an excess of calories over need, but the derangements which contribute to it are quite complex. It is interesting that rats are easily made obese by free access to the highly palatable foods that constitute too much of the American diet (Sclafani & Springer, 1976). Even more striking is the finding that dietary restriction lengthens the life of laboratory rodents considerably, slows the decline of immune function with age, and retards the aging of structural proteins (e.g., Harrison, 1982).

Diet affects many stress- and disease-relevant systems. Low cholesterol diets seem to reduce blood cholesterol (Hegsted, 1986). The unsaturated fatty acids in fish oils (eicosopentanoic and docosahexanoic acids) have been said to protect against coronary thrombosis by inhibiting platelet aggregation and increasing the ratio of high density to low density lipoproteins, but the evidence is inconclusive (Fish Oil for the Heart, 1987). Protein-calorie malnutrition and specific vitamin deficiencies impair some aspects of immune function; vitamin A deficiency can reduce the protective function of the skin; excess iron intake can promote, and iron deficiency retard, the growth of some bacteria (Barrett, 1983). Plasma cortisol is increased in malnutrition because its clearance is reduced, and in obese persons cortisol production is directly correlated with amount of dietary protein (Bondy, 1985). Protein-calorie malnutrition is associated with high levels of growth hormone (GH) but low levels of somatomedins. Fasting reduces the somatomedin response to GH (Underwood & Van Wyk, 1985). Fasting or carbohydrate deprivation diminishes the synthesis of triiodothyronine from thyroxin (Ingbar, 1985). Low dietary tryptophan (the amino acid precursor to serotonin) increases depression and lowers task performance (Young et al., 1985). Adequate prenatal and early postnatal nutrition may increase later social involvement, curiosity and initiative in children (Barrett & Radke-Yarrow, 1985).

Dietary factors have, of course, been associated with specific pathologies. It could be said that excess food intake contributes to those disorders for which obesity is a risk factor: gallstones, hypertension, hyperlipidemia, diabetes mellitus (e.g., Van Itallie, 1979). Persons taking tryptophan as a dietary supplement or over-the-counter medication may develop an eosinophilia-myalgia syndrome (Hand, 1990) which can include muscle pain, severe neuritis, and dermatosclerosis (hardening and thickening of the skin). Several patients have apparently died from this disorder, but the problem may have been with impurities in the commercial preparations rather than with tryptophan itself.

Some dietary elements are related to cancer. Among the carcinogens are aflatoxin from a mold that commonly grows on grain, nitrosamines that can be synthesized internally from nitrites, and polycyclic hydrocarbons from broiled food. Possibly protective are low dietary fat, high dietary fiber, vitamin A and related compounds, selenium, vitamin C, and various antioxidants produced by edible plants (e.g., Ames, 1983; Committee on Diet, Nutrition, and Cancer, 1982).

Sodium has been considered a causal factor in hypertension. Salt intake is cross-culturally associated with blood pressure, and salt reduction can reduce high blood pressure at least in the short term (Schlundt & Langford, 1985). However, salt may be more a problem in people *with* hypertension than an etiologic factor (Shapiro & Goldstein, 1982). There is evidence that magnesium deficiency contributes to vascular reactivity (Altura et al., 1983), and that potassium may protect against hypertension (Treasure & Ploth, 1983). In one large study high blood pressures were associated with low intake of sodium, calcium, potassium, vitamin C, and vitamin A. (McCarron et al., 1984).

Environmental Toxins

Industrial pollutants and household chemicals affect psychoneural and peripheral biologic processes (e.g., Weiss, 1983). Alterations of normal function can occur at exposures that do not produce large increases in pathology. Insecticides are of interest because exposure is so common; small amounts are present in foods and many persons are exposed through home and garden uses. Organophosphate insecticides are similar to "nerve gasses"; they interfere with the degradation of acetylcholine at cholinergic junctions. Thus they increase acetylcholine activity and alter CNS, autonomic nervous system and muscle activity (Klaassen, 1985; Taylor, 1985b).

There are many other substances to which people may be exposed without thinking about the consequences. Among them are gasoline vapors, nitrites, lead, halogenated hydrocarbons which can be produced by the chlorination of drinking water, and the particularly vicious polychlorinated biphenyls (better known as PCB's).

Everyone is aware that exposure to high levels of pollutants as a function of occupation or accidents can produce illness, but seemingly innocuous background levels can also be important. Levels of lead which had been thought safe may not be (Robbins et al., 1984). Since lead accumulation may be slow and derive from unobvious sources, occult lead poisoning could contribute directly or indirectly to many disorders. Another subtle environmental effect is suggested by the finding that cancer mortality in Louisiana is higher in areas using Mississippi river water for drinking (Page et al., 1976). There is evidence that moderate radiation doses can have significant effects on normal functions, as by speeding up aging (Bertell, 1977).

Combinations and Interactions

Our concern is not solely with the pathology which exogenous agents can induce directly; it is also with the possibility that exposures insufficient to produce detectable pathology may alter host resistance or psychoneural functions and therefore alter susceptibility to diseases with other primary etiologic agents or to stress.

Exogenous agents might serve as stressors by producing direct biologic demands and discomforts, alterations in appearance (e.g., hair loss and skin lesions with cancer chemotherapy), and decrements in cognitive or motor skills. The mere anticipation of aversive drug effects can induce patients to forgo treatment (Burish & Carey, 1984).

Exogenous agents can reduce stress when they relieve pathology or restore coping skill.

Given that exogenous agents can, albeit often mildly, affect normal functions and can serve as stressors, a holistic emphasis suggests that unobvious exogenous agent effects may well be interactive or, at least, may occur with combinations of agents. Of course the number of interactions and combinations is huge. We have not systematically searched for them, but we can give a few examples. Caffeine augments the antiinflammatory effects of compounds such as aspirin and indomethacin (Rall, 1985). Ethanol increases the gastric irritation produced by aspirin and has additive effects when combined with many neuroactive drugs (Ritchie, 1985). DDT and phenobarbitol enhance carbon tetrachloride (CCl_4) toxicity by inducing enzymes that convert CCl_4 to its active metabolite. Ethanol augments CCl_4 effects because both compounds disrupt cell membranes. CCl_4 increases cardiac susceptibility to arrhythmias induced by catecholamines (Klassen, 1985). CO may increase blood cholesterol only in conjunction with a high cholesterol diet (see Perkins, 1985). Citrate increases the absorption of aluminum from the intestine and can be toxic in combination with antacids which contain aluminum (Kirschbaum & Schoolwerth, 1989).

We cannot say how much subtle effects like these contribute to disease susceptibility or stress. But one can ask what might be the results of such a common combination as aspirin, antihistamine and sympathomimetic taken for a cold if that combination is added to a touch of garden insecticide, a good dollop of alcohol, some nicotine, and a few slugs of caffeine. Common exogenous agents affect most normal functions short of outright disease. What do they do in concert at low to moderate exposures?

EFFECTS OF OVERT BEHAVIOR ON NORMAL FUNCTION AND PATHOLOGY

It is difficult to distinguish between the direct influences of behavior on the organism ({21}, {23}) and those influences mediated by response-produced stimulation ({11,17}). Self-inflicted damage would fall into the former category. We shall consider the effects of exercise at this point, although some of them are surely mediated through sense receptors.

Exercise is stressful; it is a demand, sometimes an extreme demand, upon the organism's resources. Its usual physiologic effects include increases in adrenocortical activity, in sympathomedullary activity, and in free fatty acids (see Landsberg & Young, 1985; Rose, 1980).

Dimsdale et al. (1984) reported that plasma norepinephrine continues to rise after exercise. In their data, it reached approximately 10 times baseline. The post-exercise epinephrine (EP) increase was not significant, but EP levels did triple during exercise. Although the corticosteroid and catecholamine responses to exercise may adapt, other responses may not. A case in point is amenorrhea in athletes. This effect on the pituitary-gonadal system may occur because intense, prolonged exercise reduces body fat (Reichlin, 1985).

The fact that exercise produces classic stress responses is an interesting contrast to its seeming benefits. It has been associated with better blood lipid profiles, greater cardiopulmonary efficiency (Martin & Dubbert, 1982), and increased vigor in older persons (Kasch et al., 1985). Obesity is associated with inactivity, at least in adults, and exercise is frequently used in treating it (Brownell, 1982). The fat loss may be produced by catecholamines (see Thompson et al., 1982), something worth keeping in mind because catecholamines are often cast as villians in disease promotion by stress. There is some evidence that an increased metabolic rate persists for a considerable time after a bout of exercise (Bielinski et al., 1985). Exercise can increase interleukin-1, thus inducing fever (Cannon & Kluger, 1983), enhance natural killer cell activity (Targan et al., 1981) and increase plasma interferon (Viti et al., 1985). The idea that stress can be biologically beneficial seems well exemplified by exercise.

In terms of pathology, exercise is thought to be helpful in preventing or treating a number of disorders (Martin & Dubbert, 1982). Cardiovascular disease has received the most attention, but there is also reason to believe that exercise may be beneficial in diabetes, chronic lung disease, asthma, and osteoporosis.

Psychologic benefits may be among the several virtues of exercise. Tomporowski and Ellis (1986) reviewed the effects of exercise on cognition. They suggested that light exercise may increase general arousal and thus improve cognitive performance. They also noted that one's level of fitness is likely to influence the direction of the exercise effect on performance and that exercise may be psychologically stressful for non-exercisers. Older data suggested that exercise improves self concept and mood, but many studies were methodologically inadequate (Folkins & Sime, 1981). However, a study by McCann and Holmes (1984) provides rather clear evidence that exercise reduces depression.

The psychologic effects of exercise could be produced in many ways. Folkins and Sime suggest the release of endogenous opioids, distraction from dysphoric emotions, compensatory reductions in muscle tension, and a sense of mastery. Improved physical appearance could also play a role. With the current evidence, we cannot tell which effects are directly due to muscular exertion and which are produced indirectly by altered capabilities, changes in body image, altered reactions to the exerciser by the social environment, or the mere expectancy that exercise will be salutary.

Not all of the effects of overt behavior on pathology are exercise effects. Some disorders involve skeletal muscle activity in a primary way (e.g., muscle tears, some types of spasm-induced pain). Scratching directly exacerbates skin lesions. Palpation or gross muscle activity may assist in tumor metastasis by physically straining the tumor (Bammer, 1981).

EFFECTS OF THE PHENOTYPIC ORGANISM ON PATHOLOGIC PROCESSES

This general relationship {18} is central to the whole idea that stress and disease are linked. Many, perhaps by definition all, systems of the phenotypic organism have defense against pathology as major functions. So intimate is the relation between normal function and pathology that, as we have noted, it is often difficult to distinguish between them. Clearly, then, variations in normal function, including variations produced by stressors, should be associated with variations in pathology.

In Chapter 2, we emphasized the neuroendocrine and immune systems because they are the phenotypic organism systems most often mentioned as mediating stress effects on disease. The possibilities are obvious for traditional immunologic functions but, except for their immunoregulatory roles, may be less so for neuroendocrine functions.

Sympathoadrenomedullary (SAM) activation produces vasoconstriction both directly and by increasing renin output from the juxtaglomerular cells of the kidney. It stimulates renal sodium retention by several mechanisms. It increases heart rate and contractility, thereby increasing cardiac output and the oxygen needs of the heart muscle. The effects on sodium, cardiac output and blood vessels could contribute to hypertension. The effect on myocardial oxygen demand certainly contributes to cardiac ischemia. Other SAM effects, such as increases in serum cholesterol and in platelet aggregation, could enhance atherosclerosis (e.g., Herd, 1981). The tendency for catecholamines to enhance platelet aggregation and clotting factor VIII (antihemophilic globulin) may contribute to the formation of thrombi (abnormal clots in blood vessels) and emboli (free thrombi), thus reducing blood flow to the heart or to other tissues. However, catecholamines can also increase the levels of plasminogen activator, a factor which participates in the dissolution of blood clots by producing the proteolytic enzyme plasmin (fibrinolysin).

Reduction of intestinal motility by SAM activation could contribute to some gastrointnestinal disorders and, if it slows the transit of material through the intestine, could lengthen the contact of nutrients, bacteria, drugs, and carcinogens with the bowel. The mobilization of glucose and inhibiton of insulin secretion by SAM activation might be of significance in diabetes mellitus.

Glucocorticoids potentiate the catecholamine mobilization of lipids; they block prostaglandin synthesis, thereby tending to produce vasodilation and hypotension; they can either enhance or depress immune function (Bondy, 1985); they inhibit certain types of chemical carcinogenesis (Slaga, 1980); they alter the effects of some viruses and the permeability of blood vessels (see Newberry et al., 1984). Estrogens increase levels of very low density lipoproteins and of hormone-binding proteins in the blood; they can inhibit the secretion of bile in susceptible individuals (Ross, 1985). Estrogens and androgens inhibit the development of some cancers and enhance that of others. There are hundreds of other endocrine examples. In addition to contributing to the environment in which pathology might develop, the endocrine system is subject to pathology involving the hypersecretion or hyposecretion of nearly every hormone (Wilson & Foster, 1985).

EFFECTS OF PATHOLOGIC PROCESSES ON THE PHENOTYPIC ORGANISM

If pathology did not influence normal functions {19}, it would hardly be pathology. Like the effects of everything else on everything else, those of pathology on the phenotypic organism can be dramatic or subtle, direct or indirect. But because it is tautological to say that such effects occur, a catalog of them would be an encyclopedia of disease. Our interest is limited to making the point that disease effects on the organism are relevant to stress and the development of yet more pathology.

Many kidney disorders (e.g., Robbins et al., 1984) affect blood pressure because the kidneys regulate both fluid volume and, through their hormones, arteriolar constriction. The kidneys' role in ion regulation means that changes in bone and calcium-regulating hormones can occur. Reductions in renal erythropoetin output and increases in blood urea can affect bone marrow function. Uremia is also associated with neuromuscular dysfunctions.

In infections, bacterial toxins and endotoxins (the latter being components of bacterial cell walls rather than secreted products) are responsible for many symptoms (Von Lichtenberg, 1984), and attenuated effects can presumably occur in subclinical infections. Diptheria toxin, for example, prevents protein assembly by cells. Tetanus toxin blocks inhibitory neurotransmission in the spinal cord. Endotoxins produce many of the nonspecific effects of bacterial infections.

Many pathologies influence the CNS. These effects may be due to specific substances (e.g., toxins, hormones) released in the pathologic process, to fever, or to hypoxia, as well as to direct involvement of the CNS in the disorder (Drudge et al. 1986; Tarter et al., 1986). Hypertension lowers mental performance (Shapiro et al., 1987). It is now clear that CNS involvement in AIDS is common (Holland & Tross, 1985; Price et al., 1988).

Peripheral biologic demands, the organism's uncertainty as to whether it can manage those demands, dysphoria produced directly by CNS dysfunction, behavioral disabilities produced by pathology, stimulation of sense receptors (and the interpretations of all of these) can make pathology stressful. In addition, disease victims are often put under stress by receiving a diagnosis, by therapy, or by others' reactions to their disorders. It is hardly a surprise that people who are physically ill can have psychologic problems (Dobkins & Morrow, 1985/86; Stewart et al., 1989).

EFFECTS OF PSYCHOLOGICALLY RELEVANT STIMULATION ON THE PHENOTYPIC ORGANISM

We shall not repeat Chapters 2 and 3, but, because psychologically relevant stimulation constitutes a major class of stressors, these influences {17} are central to our topic. In the schematic of Figure 6, psychosocial stimulation affects pathology through its effects upon normal function {17,18} rather than directly.

We have said that there can be few stimulus distinctions which are guaranteed not to involve differences in stressfulness. However, some stimulus effects are more difficult than others to attribute to stress in any conventional or clear way. Some of these are subtle or unexpected. We would put the very existence of placebo effects (e.g., Ross & Olson, 1982) into this category, as we would the classical conditioning of drug effects on the immune system (Ader & Cohen, 1984). The ability of enriched environments to increase brain complexity (Uphouse, 1980), the effect of the mere exposure to stimuli on preference for them (Zajonc, 1980), and the effect of a communicator's posture on persuasion (McGinley et al., 1975) also illustrate the power of psychologically relevant stimulation to produce less-than-obvious effects. Nonobvious influences are relevant to pathology; constant light prolongs life in hamsters with heart disease (Tapp & Natelson, 1986).

Factors Affecting Overt Behavior

Overt behavior in Figure 6 is affected by the phenotypic organism {20} and pathology {22}. The first of these effects is too obvious for anything but a discussion more detailed than we can pursue; organisms generate behavior, and differences among organisms—whether produced by genetics, exogenous agents, psychologically relevant stimulation, or pathology—produce differences in behavior, including differences in responses to stress. Most paths from pathology to overt behavior would probably be indirect (e.g., {19,20} or {19,4,6,17,20}). Including a direct effect of pathology on overt behavior {22} merely accounts for the possibility that something like a tumor mass could prevent a motor response from occurring even though the nerves and muscles were intact.

One would expect pathology and individual difference variables to interact in their effects on behavior, including health and illness behaviors. That this is so is suggested by Miller et al. (1988). They investigated the dimension they call "monitoring," which is the tendency to seek and attend to information about potentially threatening situations. In their study, high monitors tended to seek medical care for milder problems than did low monitors. In addition, the high monitors wanted more medical tests to be run and wanted more detailed information about their conditions. Miller et al. noted that monitors may be either more sensitive to bodily symptoms or more sensitive to the possibility that mild symptoms could signal significant disease.

COMBINATIONS AND INTERACTIONS IN RELATIONSHIPS INVOLVING STRESS AND DISEASE

In discussing the relationships presented in Figure 6, we have taken them one at a time, alluding only occasionally to more extended sequences of effects. This section and the next return to holism and deal more explicitly with the implications of a network of relationships that are extended, multivariate, reciprocal and interactive.

Every variable class in Figure 6 is acted upon by more than one other class; the status of any structure or process is determined by multiple factors. This idea is hardly profound, but it is useful to keep in mind. If, for example, hypertension develops partly from intense, sustained adrenergic constriction of arterioles, then accounting for hypertension means considering *all* the factors that influence arteriolar adrenoreceptors.

Regarding reciprocal influences, in Figure 6 every variable class can influence itself via its effects on other classes of variables. Some reciprocal effects are direct, as in the relations between pathology and the phenotypic organism {18,19,18...}. The indirect possibilities are vastly more numerous.

Numerous feedbacks involve psychologic stressors and behavior, for example. Worry can contribute to insomnia, and insomnia becomes another worry (Borkovec, 1982). Type A behaviors are presumably partly responses to stress (Glass, 1977) and may also get persons into stressful situations (Byrne & Rosenman, 1986). Alcohol contributes to aggression and its stressful outcomes (Taylor & Leonard, 1983), and stress seems to stimulate drinking (Sher, 1984). Stress-induced decrements in task performance are stressful. Lonely persons tend to be deficient in social skills (Jones et al., 1982), and that deficit might both contribute to and be exacerbated by lack of social contact. When stress stimulates coping attempts, those attempts can improve coping skills and self-efficacy, which improvements allow further improvements to occur.

In the examples just given, the feedback is positive; an existing situation becomes more extreme. Some effects of stress involve negative feedback. If stress induces someone to seek social support, the support may reduce stress (and possibly then reduce the tendency to seek support). If stress improves task performance, that improvement may reduce stress (and possibly then reduce motivation to perform).

The types of behavioral reciprocities we have just illustrated are in addition to reciprocal relations involving other variable classes (e.g., between the social and physical environments) and those within a variable class (e.g., within the set of normal neuroendocrine and immune functions). Thus the psychobiology of health and disease involves a very large number of reciprocal influences, influences which are almost necessarily more difficult to analyze and understand empirically than are unidirectional influences.

Interaction effects also complicate matters. We have mentioned situation-personality interaction effects on behavior. We have noted interactions among hormones in the so-called permissive effects of one hormone for the actions of another. We shall mention a few more examples here. Some are obvious; the effect of antibiotics on body temperature will depend upon whether the individual has an infection. Others are not so obvious. A deficiency in glucose-6-phosphate dehydrogenase need not produce pathology, but anemia can result if persons with this deficiency take the anti-malarial drug primaquine (Robbins et al., 1984). Smoking and stress may interact in affecting diastolic blood pressure (Dembroski et al., 1985). Smoking increases myocardial infarction (MI) risk more for persons with a family history of MI than for those without (Khaw & Barrett-Connor, 1986). Dietary restraint—the cognitive tendency to resist eating—interacts with situational factors in determining food intake; restrainers tend to increase eating under stress (Ruderman, 1986). If stress alters variables relevant to disorders with genetic predispositions, then genetics and stress will interact in determining the outcome.

It is as important to keep in mind that the status of any variable involves extended sequences as to note that it involves multifactorial, reciprocal, interactive causation. Everything about an individual grows out of the whole history of the person and the culture. On a much smaller time scale, momentary changes reflect causal chains with large numbers of links. How many biochemical steps would need to be described in accounting *fully* for the adrenocortical stress response?

Obesity illustrates the idea that the determination of one characteristic of persons can be quite complex. Both genetic and environmental factors seemingly contribute to overweight (Price, 1987). The importance of balance between food intake and utilization is supported by the finding that obesity is becoming more prevalent in children and that, though obese children may not consume more or exercise less than their lean peers, they do watch more television (Weight Disturbances, 1986). There is good reason to believe that diet palatability contributes to overeating (Brownell, 1982), and this may relate to the changes seen when people migrate to regions in which obesity is common (see Jeffrey, 1987).

Underlying the dietary and cultural influences, and reflecting the genomic ones, is a maze of physiologic factors. At least some of the variables involved in hunger and satiety have been identified. Stricker and Verbalis (1987) argue that hunger depends upon the absence of peripheral satiety cues—cues which arise from stomach distention, from the liver, and from certain hormones (probably including cholecysto-kinin, oxytocin, and insulin) which are secreted during the digestion and storage of food.

Additional factors must be invoked to explain obesity, of course. Much thinking centers on the idea of a biologic set point for weight and the relation of the set point to fat cell size and/or number (see Brownell, 1982; Kolata, 1986). Organisms seem to "defend" their set points; energy expenditure tends to increase with high food intake and decrease with low intake. Increased efficiency of food utilization at low intake is one thing that makes weight loss difficult. Fat cells can apparently signal their condition to the CNS (Flier et al., 1987), and this helps to indicate whether the individual is at, above, or below the set point. Those who successfully maintain large weight losses may for ever after receive peripheral hunger signals and show some metabolic characteristics of the undernourished; the set point may not change.

It is apparently not yet clear how organisms come to develop overweight set points. Possibly, genetic predisposition and overeating due to the availability of too-palatable foods increase adipocyte size/number or alter the signalling process. The factors that produce obesity need not always be the same as those that maintain it. When obesity results from disturbances in lipid metabolism, hyperphagia is a secondary phenomenon (Stricker & Verbalis, 1987).

Rodin (1985) described the interplay of some behavioral and physiologic events which lead to obesity. In this analysis, a number of factors contribute to a spiral which increases the amount of stored fat. Included among those factors are individual differences in the efficiency of food utilization; individual differences in the tendency to experience hunger in response to the sight of food; insulin secretion in response to the mere sight of food and to eating; insulin-induced hunger; and increasing resistance of cells to insulin. Particularly interesting is the idea of a bidirectional positive feedback between eating and insulin such that eating increases insulin levels and insulin stimulates hunger. Rodin's is an excellent example of how the interplay of diverse variables might push organisms toward disease—in the case of Rodin's analysis, toward non-insulin-dependent diabetes among other things.

We have now looked at the context of possible stress effects on disease. We have tried to emphasize the fact that stress and pathology exist in, and are of, a system of systems that includes the environment, the organism, pathologic processes, and behavior. At every level, these systems appear to respond to each other in a multifactorial, reciprocal, interactive fashion that we believe deserves the label holistic. It may be somewhat overstated, but is not terribly far off the mark, to say that everything affects everything else and does so through multiple sets of causal links.

WAYS IN WHICH STRESS
MAY AFFECT DISEASE

We can now describe some of the plausible types of links between stress and disease, making more specific what Figure 6 presents in very general terms and drawing upon the implications of what we have discussed.

In terms of the model, stress can arise from the physical environment {16} in terms of exogenous agents or contact with physical objects; from psychologically relevant stimulation that signals threat, frustration, pain and the like {17}; from behavior that makes demands directly {21} or produces stressful stimulation {11,17}; from pathology that produces demand directly {19} or produces stimuli that signal demand psychologically {10,17}. The effects of all of these potential stressors depend upon the biologic, psychologic, and social state of the organism.

In Figure 6, pathologic processes are influenced by the physical environment (principally exogenous agents) {12}, the genome {13}, the phenotypic organism {18}, and behavior {23}. Thus any effect of stress on pathology must be via one of those variable classes, and any stressor which alters one of those four types of factors might affect disease. (Note that behavior and the physical environment are sources of stress as well as influences on pathology, and that the characteristics of the phenotypic organism are major modulators of stress.)

Figure 6 allows for multitudes of paths from stress to disease. We count 101 single-pass paths leading to pathologic processes in that diagram, a single-pass path being one which is as long as possible without any variable class appearing more than once before the path ends at pathologic processes. Embedded in these paths are 187 shorter paths. Of the 101 single-pass paths, 70 begin with a variable class that is rather clearly capable of serving as a stressor. When extended, reciprocal paths are considered, the number becomes very large.

Complex paths including stress and disease do not occur just in diagrams. Take a study of adherence to prednisone treatment in leukemic children by Lansky et al. (1983). Among boys, parental anxiety was associated with medication compliance; among girls parental anxiety was not predictive, but their own anxiety was. One can attempt to reconstruct what might have led to these findings. The children's genomes largely determined their gender assignments. Those assignments, together with cultural values, the parents' personalities, and probably the children's behaviors, helped to determine the degree to which the parents gave the children responsibility for their own medication. On average, the parents seem to have given more responsibility to the girls, and the girls' anxiety, affected presumably by genome, culture, and stressors, thus predicted their compliance and possibly the outcomes of their disorders. We hold no strong brief for this particular interpretation, but it illustrates the number of factors that might combine in stress-disease relations.

Internal Loop Effects

It is probably not useful to attempt an exhaustive classification of paths from stress to pathology. However, we would like to mention one useful distinction which we have taken from Weiner (1977), namely a distinction between *internal loop* and *external loop*.

Most discussions of stress effects on disease emphasize internal loop paths. In these cases the organism's internal responses to the stressors change the milieux of pathologic processes (e.g., {17,18}). Thus an internal loop effect is, roughly, a psychosomatic effect. A case in which the stress response affects pathology via effects on the genome (e.g., DNA repair) is a variant of the internal loop. There are many possible internal loop effects. Failure at an important task could increase plasma catecholamines thereby enhancing platelet aggregation at a point of damage to vascular endothelium and potentiating atherosclerosis. Bereavement-induced glucocorticoid increases could prevent the transformation of a normal cell to a cancer cell by a carcinogen. Immunodepression from new job responsibilities could allow an infection or neoplasm to get out of control.

External Loop Effects

In the external loop case, the central feature is an effect of the organism on the environment, with the result that exogenous agent exposure is altered. The change in exogenous agent exposure then affects pathology directly or via alterations of normal function. In the simplest external loop effect, stress changes the self-administration of exogenous agents (e.g., {17,20,1}). In smokers, smoking is used to reduce negative emotions, and beginning to smoke probably reflects social pressure and anxiety (Leventhal & Cleary, 1980). Stress might also increase smoking by promoting the excretion of nicotine (Schachter et al., 1977). Stress can lead to drinking alcohol, but the strength of the effect depends upon other factors (Sher, 1984). Meaninglessness, perceived lack of control (Newcomb & Harlow, 1986) and emotional distress (Swaim et al., 1989) predict adolescent drug use to some degree. Stress may affect food intake, and the effect of distress on eating varies with obesity (e.g., Ruderman, 1983). Fear of violating weight norms can induce dieting even in children (Weight Disturbances, 1986). In anorexics and bulimics, the patterns of food intake and the use of cathartics and emetics are partly responses to a fear of not meeting society's standards of thinness (Schlesier-Stropp, 1984).

Stress should be able to affect exposure to almost any exogenous agent. It might affect the decision to work in the garden and use pesticides, to remove old lead-based paint from the walls, to take a job in a less polluted city. Stress might affect adherence to medical regimens, for example by distracting people from completing courses of antibiotics, leading them to care less about taking medications, or even strengthening their resolve to take their medications. It is worth remembering in the context of health behavior that freedom from illness need not always be a dominant value (Lau et al., 1986) and that people may knowingly respond to demands with self-harmful acts.

Other Types of Effects

Many possible influences of stress on disease cannot be classified as simple, unambiguous internal or external loops. As one example, the effects of exercise (e.g., {21,18}) involve behavior but need not involve exogenous agents. Also, stress-induced behavior can affect the social environment with consequences for both exogenous agent exposure and psychoneurally mediated change. Thus social support for a stressed intimate might include the offer of a double martini, a glass of carrot juice, or a leftover benzodiazepine tablet. Similarly, one's behavior can lead one's social environment to increase or reduce the level of psychologic stress it imposes: a stressed employee's altered performance or expressions of affect might lead a boss to fire the employee—or perhaps to give her/him a day off.

Behavioral responses to stress can affect the individual's contacts with the health care system just as with any other part of the social environment (e.g., Berkanovic et al., 1988). If stress delays treatment-seeking, it affects possible exposure to therapeutic agents, to reassurance, or to the stressor of receiving a diagnosis. It also gives the pathology time to progress. Stress could result in earlier diagnosis or treatment as well as delay, either because the person is bothered by the physiologic symptoms of the stress response or because stress heightens concern with the symptoms of disease. One example of the possible outcomes of stress-related encounters with the health care system is an increase in injuries from anxiolytic drugs (Ray et al., 1987).

In short, it is not difficult to think of ways for stress to affect disease. If there is a problem, it is a surfeit of plausible connections.

Stress, Disease, and Holism

All of the putative effects implied by Figure 6 involve or are conditioned by the complex of psychoneural and peripheral physiologic changes brought about by a particular stressor, by the individual's characteristics and environment, by the nature of the particular pathologic processes involved, and by the interactions among these. Moreover, with every factor, it is reasonable to fear that the details may be important. A stressor that provokes growth hormone secretion may have a different effect from one that does not. Cancer clones that differ slightly in hormone responsiveness or immunogenicity may well respond differently to the same stressor. The individual's precise previous history with a particular type of stressor may determine the influence a stress episode has on a disease outcome.

It should be clear, then, why holism is a desirable starting point in considering stress-disease relationships. The relevant factors are very numerous and disease outcomes presumably result from the *pattern* of their influences. It should also be apparent why we argue for a dynamic and analytic holism. A "feeling for the whole person" is no substitute for the psychobiology of kidney function or for discovering whether psychologic factors influence DNA repair.

However, a holistic viewpoint as we have outlined it is not completely optimistic. It provides no guarantee that the study of any small set of psychobiologic variables will greatly improve our ability to predict and control disease. The variety of individual differences, environmental circumstances and pathologies may well produce too many causal patterns to be apprehended quickly or easily. This does not mean that research should not try to isolate those variables that have the greatest influence. It means only that we should cast our nets widely and not be too surprised if the relationships we identify are somewhat weak.

Nothing about a holistic or biopsychosocial approach dictates the *direction* of stress effects upon disease; stress should be able to protect against disease as well as exacerbate it. Given the number of physiologic changes which stress can produce and the diversity of diseases, one would expect to find even straightforward internal loop effects that inhibit pathology. When external loop and more complex paths are considered, there is even less reason to expect only disease exacerbation. Adverse situations can improve health behavior as well as worsen it, can produce better self-images as well as worse ones, can strengthen coping skills and perhaps directly induce biologic toughening. In other words, stress can have growth-enhancing potentials (Cohen et al., 1982). What is more, the data on stress and disease indicate that protective effects can occur. Some of those data will be discussed subsequently. The literature deemphasizes the logical possibility for beneficial effects of stress and the data suggesting such effects. It is misleading in that regard.

A holistic viewpoint and the possibility of bidirectional stress effects suggest that current research may underestimate the contribution of stress to disease. If research does not take into account the diversity of links between stress and pathology, then different influences may tend to cancel each other out in any set of data. This idea has been mentioned by Fox (1982) with regard to cancer, and it applies in principle to other disorders as well.

Good estimates of the strength of stress effects, and even the clear demonstration that there are stress effects, require demonstrating causality. As we noted in Chapter 1, that is most difficult to do in human studies, and its difficulty often seems to go unrecognized. One virtue of models like that of Figure 6 is that they draw attention to what is necessary for causal conclusions to be drawn. The idea that stress affects disease can be accepted only to the extent that disease effects on stress and effects of third variables on both stress and disease are controlled for. The more specific the hypotheses, the greater the number of alternatives that need to be ruled out.

A final thing to keep in mind regarding the connections between stress and pathology is that public awareness of stress-disease relationships may change the relationships. We have emphasized the importance of beliefs, expectancies and attributions as influences on human stress responses. People who believe stress is a threat to health may well respond differently than people who do not believe that. Thinking that stress exacerbates disease can create more stress and/or trigger coping processes which improve health.

Findings of Relations between Stress and Disease

We can now concentrate upon research relating stress-relevant variables and disease. We shall sample mostly relatively recent findings, but even so, we shall be able to mention only a fraction of the literature. Many general treatments are available to lead the reader further (e.g., Bunney et al., 1982; Cohen, 1981; Friedman & Booth-Kewley, 1987; J.P. Henry, 1982; Natelson, 1983; Rowland, 1977; Syme, 1984; Wallston et al., 1983; H. Weiner, 1977, 1985; Zegans, 1982).

We must consider studies of individual differences and disease as well as studies of stressors and disease. Nearly all psychologic individual differences are relevant to stress, if only because stress is relevant to nearly all psychologic processes. Thus a finding that hardiness, Type A behavior, or depression predicts disease might well mean that persons who differ in personality respond differently to everyday levels of stress, choose differentially stressful situations, or have had differentially stressful situations imposed upon them.

After noting some limitations on the types and strength of stress effects as suggested by the literature, we shall discuss stress-disease research in terms of outcome variables. The first group of studies to be considered involves illness or symptoms in general rather than particular diseases. Subsequently we shall look at cardiovascular disease, infectious diseases, diabetes mellitus, and cancer, beginning each of the

162

discussions with a short presentation of the pathophysiology. Finally, we make briefer mention of several disorders for which there is less in the way of recent information. We shall consider mostly the human research, but some animal findings will be cited. Our discussions of specific studies will often mention their limitations as well as their virtues. Unless indicated otherwise, the relationships we describe when discussing specific studies reached the conventional .05 level of statistical significance by one or another test.

SHOULD STRESS ALWAYS AFFECT DISEASE?

One goal of the preceding chapters has been to suggest that stress effects on pathology should not be simple either biologically or psychologically, and there seems to be some agreement that this is the case (e.g., Cronkite & Moos, 1984; Suls & Fletcher, 1985a). If stress effects are complex, then stressors should sometimes fail to affect pathology significantly.

Unfortunately, the existing data do not indicate too clearly when stress will and will not be associated with disease outcomes. The characteristics of stressors, individuals, background conditions, and diseases should all contribute. Too few studies have looked at broad enough ranges of stressors, mediating factors, and diseases for clear patterns to emerge. There have been too few replication attempts, and it is not clear how many findings will hold up. There are, however, some general considerations which might serve to guide both the design of future research and the interpretation of the research which has been done.

Stressor severity could hardly fail to be important, as we have noted previously. The psychologic and biologic changes provoked by mild demands will often differ from those provoked by more severe demands. Related to the severity of stressors is the likelihood of adaptation. If the organism does not adapt to protracted stressor exposure, the consequences for health could be more extreme simply because stress responses will be more prolonged (cf. Baum et al., 1981; Folkman, et al., 1986b). However, there seems to be little information on when adaptation will fail to occur.

We have already noted that a wide variety of individual difference factors can affect the characteristics of stress responses. Friedman and Booth-Kewley (1987) have done meta-analyses which suggest that roughly similar personality patterns are associated with a variety of diseases. Individual differences in biologic disease susceptibility may also be important. Natelson (1983) has suggested that stress is likely to worsen disease outcomes only when there is preexisting disease or predisposition to disease.

Even if stressors always produced the same pattern of endogenously and exogenously induced biologic changes, it is unlikely that all pathologies would respond similarly to those changes. As pointed out in Chapter 1, general characteristics of disease dynamics such as the rate of disease development and the reversibility of pathology should affect whether, and when, stress effects are observed. The specifics of etiology and pathologic processes should also be important. For example, pathology resulting from over-vigorous or misdirected immune system activity might be ameliorated by stress-induced immunosuppression and stimulated by stress-induced immunoenhancement. The consequences of stress effects on pathology from gram-positive and gram-negative bacteria might well be different because of the mechanisms by which gram-negative endotoxins act. Cancers with differing hormonal responsivities might well respond differently to stressors. A careful consideration of pathophysiology would probably reveal many differences among disorders in their expected responses to the physiologic changes commonly accompanying stress.

The timing of stressor exposure relative to the stage of disease development should be critical under some circumstances. There is evidence from animal model research that stress before the induction of pathology can have an effect opposite to that produced by stress after the induction of pathology (e.g., Plaut & Friedman, 1981; Riley, 1981). In the cases of cancers and infections, it is possible to think of a point at which host defenses and pathogenic processes are in balance. At such a point, stress might have greater effects on disease outcome than it would have either earlier or later. There may be similar points in other types of diseases, as for example diseases involving cell loss from systems which normally have excess functional capacity.

Relationships between stress-relevant variables and disease are often rather anemic even when they are statistically significant. It is not uncommon to find stress or stress-related personality variables accounting for less than 10% of the variance in disease dependent variables. The weakness of these associations has been noted repeatedly (e.g., Friedman & Booth-Kewley, 1987; Rabkin & Struening, 1976), and the need to improve the prediction of disease variables by psychosocial factors has been a major reason for the development of more complex models (e.g., Cronkite & Moos, 1984).

There are probably many reasons for the observed associations between stress and disease being unimpressive. For one thing, the number of factors contributing to illness may be so great and their influences so interactive that, even though few of them are totally irrelevant to stress, their effects will not be picked up by the usual predictor measures. If pesticides make a small contribution to disease, and if stress causes some people to garden as a way of relaxing, that particular contribution of stress is going to be difficult to detect with the types of global measures often used. More generally, whenever multiple influences contribute to some phenomenon, the relationships between single independent variables and the dependent variable are not likely to be strong (Ahadi & Diener, 1989).

A second reason for the flabbiness of the reported relationships between stress and disease may be that with some combinations of stressors, individual characteristics and pathologies, stress protects against disease. As we have noted, the complexity of stressors' relationships to biologic and psychologic variables suggests that stress should be able to impede pathology as well as promote it. If a piece of research includes cases of stress-induced illness enhancement and stress-induced protection, the overall observed association could well be weakened.

We should also mention measurement problems as possible reasons for weak correlations between stress and illness (e.g., Rabkin & Struening, 1976). Low reliability (in measures of stressor occurrence, personality, or pathology) attenuates observed associations. Reliability and other factors contribute to the validity of a measure—the degree to which it measures what it is supposed to measure. The question of validity is complicated by the fact that some important variables, particularly stress and personality variables, are abstractions whose "true" nature is unknown and partly arbitrary. In any case, it is obvious that the use of measures with low validity could weaken observed associations between disease and stress or personality.

Low validity might also be able to produce *over*estimates of the strength of stress-disease relationships. This may occur when measures of stress reflect disease. Even items on life stress questionnaires such as, "had problems in school or training program," (Dohrenwend, et al.,

1982) might be endorsed because the person has been ill. Kobasa et al., (1981) reported that life stress was significantly associated with illness only when prior illness was not controlled for.

On the other side of the equation is the possibility that measures of health status are contaminated by psychologic distress or other psychologic sequelae of stress. We noted earlier that measures of pathology such as reported symptoms and utilization of health care services can reflect persons' psychologic states as well as actual pathology (cf. Costa & McRae, 1985; Kellner, 1985; Mechanic, 1972; Wagner & Curran, 1984). Persons who are under stress may conclude that they are ill because of their psychobiologic stress responses or their search for attributions for their psychologic discomfort. Moreover, some illness report instruments include psychologic disorders and psychophysiologic stress responses as illnesses (e.g., Wyler et al., 1968). To the extent that measures of stress reflect disease (even past disease) and/or measures of disease reflect the psychologic aspects of stress, we can hardly fail to detect supposed stress-disease associations, but those associations can be partly or wholly artifactual (e.g., Brett et al., 1990; Schroeder & Costa, 1984; Watson & Pennebaker, 1989).

Some danger accompanies attempting to purify the assessment of stress and disease. The psychobiologic responses to stressors may reflect the beginnings of disease, and removing their influences from disease dependent variables may remove part of an actual effect of stress upon disease. The attempt to remove disease effects from stress measures is even more problematic. Disease is stressful, and stress assessments which fail to include disease-induced stress cannot be wholly adequate. The best course is to treat different types of stressors and different types of "illness" separately and make the problem one of interpreting complex relationships rather than one of instruments with obscure meanings.

The problem of cross-contamination in measures of stress and disease is one more consequence of having to use correlational methods in dealing with multifactorial, interactive, reciprocal causation. This difficulty only adds to the more basic problem that a stress-disease association may reflect, not a stress effect upon disease, but the stressfulness of disease or the effects of other variables on both stress and disease (cf. Krantz & Glass, 1984).

STUDIES OF NONSPECIFIC ILLNESS

A large amount of stress-relevant research has involved several diseases simultaneously or used nonspecific outcome variables such as utilization of health care services, total reported illnesses, or general symptomatology. By and large, these studies have found positive correlations between stress and illness.

Some nonspecific illness studies have focused almost exclusively on stressors, instead of emphasizing moderating factors such as personality. Godkin and Rice (1981) analyzed data from over 20,000 patients seeing primary care physicians. They used anxiety, depression, marital conflict, and child abuse to classify patients as "cases" of stress. Standardized morbidity ratios were higher among stress cases than among the rest of the sample for a variety of disorders. There were differences among stressors, however. For example, acute bronchitis was significantly associated with abuse or neglect in children, with marital conflict, and with anxiety, but not with depression. Low back pain was associated with depression but not anxiety. Obesity was associated with abuse/neglect, marital conflict and depression, but not with anxiety.

Hoiberg (1982) reported rated job stressfulness and hospitalization rates across U.S. Navy job classifications. Although Hoiberg did not estimate the strength of association between job stressfulness and hospitalization rates, an association of at least moderate strength is apparent in her data. It is also apparent that the pattern of specific disease susceptibility varies considerably from one occupational group to another. In the second enlistment of Hoiberg's 1966 cohort, for instance, mess management specialists, whose job was rated as among the most stressful, were the most likely to be hospitalized for hypertension, but among the least likely to be hospitalized for diabetes. Of course, job classifications may well have been related to preexisting individual differences in disease susceptibility.

Other studies have attempted to look at more theoretically important characteristics of stressors. Stern et al. (1982) found that life event controllability contributed significantly to the ability of multiple regression to account for reported illness. DeLongis et al. (1982) found that daily hassles were more strongly associated with illness than were "major" life events and added significantly to prediction of health status even when the effects of the major events had already been accounted for (see also Zarski, 1984).

Much recent research on the relation of stress to general health has incorporated more than one type of predictor in order to refine the ability to account for disease with psychosocial variables. As we have emphasized, the greater the number of variables taken into account simultaneously, the fewer are the possible confounds in reported stress-disease associations.

It would not be surprising to find gender differences in stress-disease relationships. Differences between males and females in endocrine and immune systems, in longevity, and in society's impositions of roles and opportunities all provide opportunities for stress-relevant differences in health. It has been suggested that women generally experience more illnesses and symptoms than do men (see citations in Bishop, 1984).

Georgas and Giakoumaki (1984) reported on stress and illness in a sample of particularly successful Greek teachers. They found overall that reported life stress was positively related to reported symptomatology in women but not in men. A study of British executives (Cooper & Melhuish, 1984) presented multiple regressions of bad health risk (medical laboratory values) on a number of stress-relevant predictors. More factors were predictive for women than for men, and stressors of a psychosocial nature seemed to play a greater role for women. Bishop (1984) studied a small sample of men and women serving in Army administrative and combat support units. The men and women were matched on several demographic variables. Women reported more health problems retrospectively than did men, but there were no overall gender differences in symptom reporting in a subsequent diary. Type of unit and sex did interact in predicting symptom types, however. There was, for example, little difference between administrative and combat support units in females' reports of respiratory symptoms, but a considerable difference was found for males.

Stroebe and Stroebe (1983) have reviewed the evidence for sex differences in illness and mortality following the deaths of spouses. They noted that women seem more prone to illness than men, but less prone to serious illness. Following bereavement, there appears to be excess illness and mortality in men, and the excess seems to be greater among younger widowers. In accounting for the greater disease risk among men, Stroebe and Stroebe emphasized sex differences in constitutional susceptibility to illness and males' probably greater loss of social support after bereavement.

One personality variable to have received a fair amount of attention as a possible moderator of stress-disease relationships is *hardiness*. In an initial study, Kobasa (1979) found personality differences between high life-stress executives who did and did not become ill. The low-illness subjects tended to be more hardy—to have a greater sense of control, less self-alienation (greater "commitment"), and a greater tendency to react to life events as challenges. A subsequent investigation confirmed this finding with a prospective design (Kobasa et al., 1982). In an analysis of covariance in which earlier illness was controlled for, hardiness and life stress interacted rather dramatically in predicting reported illness, illness scores being considerably higher among subjects classified as simultaneously high on life stress and low in hardiness. Among the other findings with this variable are that exercise and social support add to the prediction of illness when hardiness is accounted for (Kobasa et al., 1985), and that the Type A behavior pattern and hardiness may interact in their association with reported illness (Kobasa, Maddi, & Zola, 1983).

Hardiness and its measurement have come in for some criticism. Hull et al. (1987) suggested on the basis of their psychometric data that Kobasa's challenge and control measures are not particularly useful. In addition, they pointed out that lack of commitment and control may be thought of as stressful in themselves rather than as personality variables which act to modulate the effects of other stressors. Funk and Houston (1987) also emphasized the lack of evidence that hardiness is a single construct. In addition, they found that the relationship of hardiness to reported illness disappeared when corrected for general maladjustment.

A number of other stress-relevant individual differences have been related to health. Scheier and Carver (1985) found that higher *optimism*, as measured by a brief questionnaire, was prospectively associated with lower reported symptoms in college students, even when original symptom levels were controlled for. They see optimistic persons, who by definition expect favorable outcomes, as more likely to continue coping efforts when they meet difficulties in attaining their goals, and therefore as likely to experience less severe psychobiologic responses to stressors. Interestingly, Scheier and Carver found that symptoms did not predict later optimism. This may reflect the fact that the study involved only minor illnesses.

Peterson et al. (1988) reported that *explanatory style* can predict illness over the long term. Academically successful, physically sound, mentally healthy Harvard students were assessed psychologically while in school and then followed for 35 years. Peterson et al. studied 99 of these 268 fortunate individuals. Interviews from the beginning of the study were coded for pessimism of explanatory style (stable, global, and internal explanations given for bad events). The composite pessimism of subjects' styles was correlated with later physician health ratings. (The description of the procedure did not indicate the degree to which the health ratings could reflect mental health.) Beginning approximately 20 years after the interviews, but not earlier, pessimism was negatively correlated with rated health. This finding calls into question results in which individual differences predict health in the short term.

Linville (1987) investigated *self-complexity*, assessed in terms of the number and independence of subjects' self-aspects as derived from sortings of trait descriptors. Over a 2-week prospective period, stressful events and the stress by self-complexity interaction predicted symptom reports. The interaction reflected a tendency for symptoms to be lower in high complexity subjects than low complexity subjects under high stress but to be higher in the high complexity subjects under low stress. In Linville's theory, threats involving one or a few areas of an individual's life should affect a smaller proportion of the self in high-complexity persons and therefore should be less deleterious. Regarding the positive association between self-complexity and symptoms under low stress conditions, Linville suggested that maintaining a complex self-representation might itself be somewhat stressful, and that positive affect, like negative, might be less extreme or pervasive in those of high self-complexity.

Private self-consciousness (PSC; that is, attention to self) was hypothesized by Suls and Fletcher (1985) to weaken stress effects on disease. In these authors' view, persons high in PSC should attend more readily to internal stress responses and should therefore cope earlier and more adequately with stressors. (We add that these persons might also recognize disease symptoms earlier.) Suls and Fletcher found that stressful events predicted subsequent illness among low PSC subjects but not among high PSC subjects. Scheier and Carver (1985) found that the negative association between optimism and later symptom reports was slightly stronger for subjects high in PSC than for those low in PSC.

Watson (1988) has suggested links among negative affect, stress, and symptom reports. He studied between-subjects and within-subjects correlates of everyday somatic complaints. Subjects completed daily reports on physical problems, stress, and mood. They also responded to several global measures. In several analyses, the expected sorts of positive associations were found involving somatic complaints, negative mood, and the trait of negative affectivity. However, physical symptoms were not related to average perceived stress. General somatic complaints (but not frequency of discrete illnesses such as colds or flu) were related to negative affect. In discussing his findings Watson emphasized the possibility that negative affect, subjective stress, and physical symptom reporting all reflect the same trait tendency to look for and communicate the unpleasant.

As we noted in Chapter 3, social support may buffer the effects of stressors. It may also improve well-being more directly (Cohen & Wills, 1985), perhaps in part because it means that one's social network is not a source of threat. The effects commonly attributed to social support certainly suggest its relevance to pathology. Wallston et al. (1983) reviewed studies on social support and physical illness. They noted more than a few problems with the conceptualization and assessment of social support and with the research. However, they concluded tentatively that social support tends to be associated with beneficial outcomes, and that the association has been more clearly shown for recovery and coping with illness than for the development of illness.

As an example of recent work on social support, we can take a study of submarine school students by I.G. Sarason et al. (1985). In one group, reported negative life events over the previous year correlated significantly with self-reported illness in that year, though not with illnesses indicated in medical records. A second group was asked to distinguish between the first and last 6 months of the preceding year. In this group, negative life events from the earlier period were associated with both self reported and medically recorded illnesses in the later 6-month period. Sarason et al. studied social support in their combined groups. For isolated (but not for chronic/repeated) illness, the relation between life events and illness was significantly stronger among subjects who were less satisfied with their social support.

Some research has employed variables which, though they might not be considered explicitly as reflecting social support, nevertheless seem connected to it (e.g., B.R. Sarason et al., 1985). Friedman and

Booth-Kewley (1987) included sociability (i.e., extraversion) in their meta-analytic review of personality-disease studies. This class of variable was positively related to ischemic heart disease, was negatively related to ulcers and arthritis, and was not significantly related to asthma or headache.

Reis et al. (1985) related students' four year health center records to variables taken from two-week social interaction diaries and to a variety of measures of social skills, social strategy and social distress. Multiple regression analyses clearly indicated that health center use was related to the psychosocial variables. However, the relationships were complex; they depended upon the subjects' sex and the type of disorder. Thus, infections were related to psychosocial variables for women, but not for men; blood and circulatory disorders were significantly negatively related to quality and quantity of social interaction for women but were significantly positively associated with such variables among men.

Stuart and Brown (1981) reported a study of life stress, social coping ability, and reported illness in college students. Life stress was positively associated with illness scores, but neither social coping nor the stress by coping interaction added to the amount of illness variance accounted for. These results seem at least superficially contradictory to the general findings of Reis et al. (1985).

Anger, hostility, and persons' reactions to those represent another relevant class of person variables. We noted in Chapter 4 that anger and hostility are possible consequences of stressful encounters, and we shall mention them again when we consider specific diseases. For the moment, we draw attention to two articles. The Friedman and Booth-Kewley (1987) meta-analyses indicated positive associations between anger/hostility and heart disease, asthma, and arthritis. Julius et al. (1986) found that subjects with a tendency to suppress anger suffered excess all-cause mortality. The relationship held across age, sex, and educational level, and also when a number of medical risk factors were controlled. Further, anger suppression interacted with blood pressure. Among subjects with systolic pressure at or above 140 mm Hg, there was a dramatic increase in mortality with increasing anger suppression, but that association was not found among those with lower blood pressure.

Exercise has been associated with better health. Paffenbarger et al. (1986) reported data on over 16,000 Harvard alumni. There were clear trends for lower all-cause mortality as exercise level increased. Taking the relative risk of death as 1.00 in those whose exercise was estimated to consume less than 500 kilocalories of energy per week, that relative risk lessened monotonically to .46 in persons with activity indices of 3000-3499 kcal. Activity of 3500 kcal or greater was associated with a somewhat higher risk (.62). Paffenbarger et al. found that activity level predicted mortality over several years of follow-up, noting that that increased the likelihood that their data reflected an actual protective effect of exercise.

We have mentioned the Kobasa et al. (1985) study of hardiness and exercise. Roth et al. (1989) did a self-report study of illness as predicted by life events, hardiness, and fitness. By multiple regression, life stress, fitness, and gender were related to illness reports in the expected ways, but neither hardiness nor any interactions added to the prediction of illness scores. Structural equation analyses suggested that hardiness might contribute to illness by influencing the occurrence of or responses to stressful events.

In a nine-week prospective study using undergraduates (Roth & Holmes, 1985), subjects reported recent negative life events, were tested for fitness, and kept a log of health problems. Total reported illness severity on the health log was predicted by stress and fitness. Illness was also predicted by the stress/fitness interaction when that was entered last in a multiple regression. Increasing life stress was associated with greater reported health problems among the less fit but not among the more fit. Interestingly, fitness was not related to illness as reported on a health questionnaire covering retrospectively the same time period as the log. This dependence of results on the assessment method bears keeping in mind.

One issue with respect to moderating variables in stress-disease associations is the degree to which different investigators are giving different names to the same or similar factors. It is not uncommon for researchers to report the correlations of their favorite variables with others, and the usual result is a sizeable proportion of significant correlations. We are not aware of much detailed work on the possibility that measures of hardiness, social support, anxiety, optimism, locus of control and so forth are all to an extent tapping the same underlying "moderator." We need better information on how many *independent* psychosocial moderators of stress-disease relationships have actually been discovered and on the nature of whatever is left over when anxiety, general negative affectivity or maladjustment has been removed statistically.

The investigations we have cited certainly indicate that a variety of factors enter into the network of associations involving stress and disease. A study by Cronkite and Moos (1984) illustrates the type of research that is likely to be needed in sorting these relationships out. They used a large number of variables to predict physical symptoms in 267 married couples. The research was based on a complex model of stress which included "predisposing" factors (social status and prior functioning) and "moderating" factors (family support, self-esteem, and coping responses) in addition to stressors (negative life events and spouse's functioning).

Cronkite and Moos found physical symptoms to be predicted somewhat better for wives than for husbands in main effect multiple regressions. Moreover, different variables made significant contributions for the two sexes. For the wives, low education, prior physical symptoms, negative life events, and low family support were all significant. Husbands' physical symptoms were related only to their earlier physical symptoms. When interactions between stressors and avoidant coping styles were assessed, none were significant for husbands. Wives' symptoms were predicted by the life stress x avoidant coping interaction and the interaction between husband's alcohol consumption and avoidant coping. In yet another set of analyses, husbands' physical symptoms were associated with the interaction between their levels of approach coping and their wives' levels of self esteem, and by that between their levels of approach coping and their wives' levels of avoidant coping. None of the interactions in this set of analyses was significant for the wives' symptom levels. Data such as these make it clear just how much we still need to learn.

Each of the studies we have cited thus far in this section has provided reason to suspect associations between illness and stress or stress-related individual differences, and there are many other such studies. However, some published findings give the opposite impression. Bieliauskas (1980) found that neither life stress nor defensiveness was associated with illness (physician visits or hospitalization) among firefighters. Aagaard (1982) studied the relationships of numerous family variables and clearly stressful life events to rehospitalization in a sample of 307 previously hospitalized children. In a series of 46 bivariate tests only three (being an only child, arguments with peers, and death of a close relative) were significant. Such things as low socio-economic status, hospitalization of family members, parental unemployment, and increased family arguments were not associated with rehospitalization. A similar shortage of significant associations was found with a health questionnaire filled out by parents for the children. Funk and Houston (1987) could obtain significant relationships of life stress and hardiness to health only when retrospective data were used and subjects' psychologic maladjustment was not controlled for.

The lack of illness findings when maladjustment is controlled (Funk & Houston, 1987) is consistent with the possibility that psychologic status may affect illness reporting in addition to (or instead of) actual illness. A related issue may be seen in studies finding relationships between stress-relevant predictors and indices of psychologic discomfort but no comparable associations with illness measures. Funk and Houston (1987) found that depression related to hardiness when illness did not. Folkman et al. (1986b) found that married couples' appraisal and coping strategies in response to stressful events were not significantly related to physical health by multiple regression analysis, but were related to psychologic symptoms. Bereaved parents were found to differ from controls in behavioral and psychologic symptoms but not physical health (Miles, 1985). Greene et al. (1985) administered a life stress measure to adolescents attending a clinic. The only diagnostic groups with life events scores higher than a routine examination control group's were those referred for behavior problems or for pain with no apparent organic etiology.

To summarize, studies of nonspecific and multiple illness measures clearly tend to report positive associations between stress and illness. Moreover, there is sufficient evidence to warrant the working hypothesis that individual differences moderate those relationships, though the exact nature of these moderating influences still seems quite unclear. The literature on nonspecific/multiple illness is far from uniform, however. Stress-illness associations have failed to occur often enough to suggest caution about drawing blanket conclusions. Occasional findings suggest that stress is associated with better health. Even within a study, there are often seemingly inconsistent results. There may also be some biologic naivete in many of these reports. It is not clear to us what biologic properties widely disparate disorders could share which might make them all responsive to stressful conditions in the same manner (cf. Depue & Monroe, 1986).

CARDIOVASCULAR DISORDERS

Cardiovascular diseases have been the focus of more research and discussion in relation to stress variables than has any other group of disorders. This effort has concentrated on hypertension and ischemic heart disease. The seeming relation of the Type A behavior pattern to coronary atherosclerosis and heart attack has probably been the single most visible topic in behavioral medicine. A supplement to the journal *Circulation* (July, 1987) contains good summaries of the literature on stress and cardiovascular disease.

Pathophysiology of Cardiovascular Disorders

HYPERTENSION

Hypertension (HT) is quite a common disorder—so common that Eliot (1979) wryly wondered whether something was being put into water supplies. About 10% of cases are secondary to other disorders such as endocrine or kidney diseases (Robbins et al., 1984). The rest fall under the heading of *essential* or *primary hypertension*, meaning that the etiology is unknown. It is essential HT which researchers have attempted to relate to stress and which we shall discuss as HT.

Arterial blood pressure (BP) is a function of cardiac output and vascular resistance to blood flow (total peripheral resistance). Anything that increases either of these will elevate BP unless there is a compensatory reduction in the other factor. The control of BP is vested in several interrelated systems (e.g., Guyton, 1986). Guyton emphasizes the distinction between short-term and long-term BP regulation, with disturbance of the latter leading to HT.

Some of the shorter term mechanisms are reflexes that produce vasodilation and reduce cardiac output when stretch receptors (baroreceptors and low pressure receptors) in artery walls and the atria are activated by increased pressure. Chemoreceptor reflexes increase BP when arterial chemoreceptors sense reduced O_2 levels. Other mechanisms include reflexive contraction of abdominal muscles to increase venous return to the heart; release of catecholamines and vasopressin; and activation of the renin-angiotensin system. Shifts of fluid from capillaries to the extracellular fluid or in the reverse direction can lower or raise BP, respectively.

Guyton sees long-term BP control as primarily a product of body fluid volume and kidney function. In this view, the kidneys' role in maintaining optimal sodium concentrations and body fluid volume is central. With increased BP, the renal excretion of water and sodium will increase until reduced fluid volume reduces cardiac output and therefore BP. With low BP, the kidneys' excretion of water and sodium decreases, allowing fluid to accumulate and raising BP. The renin-angiotensin system has a long-term role in BP regulation via angiotensin's direct effects on the kidneys and its stimulation of aldosterone secretion. Both of these angiotensin effects increase salt and water retention and therefore blood volume and cardiac output. Increased blood flow in a tissue produces a constriction of the arterioles in that tissue, preventing hyperperfusion but also increasing resistance.

Guyton (e.g., 1986) sees HT as resulting primarily from abnormalities in renal function. The kidneys' capacity to excrete sodium and water is impaired, so that high arterial pressures are required to produce normal fluid volume and composition. In this view, only altered kidney function can produce true long-term HT; vasoconstriction or increased resistance are seen as primary etiologic factors only when they reduce renal blood flow and thereby produce kidney dysfunction.

There are other perspectives, however. In one (e.g., Folkow, 1987), the primary etiologic process is structural change in arterioles. Hypertrophy of these vessels increases total peripheral resistance and this produces sustained HT. Folkow emphasizes repeated vasoconstriction via SAM activation, in conjunction with salt intake, as producing the vascular hypertrophy. HT almost certainly involves genetic predispositions, and Folkow sees central and peripheral SAM hyperreactivity as a critical genetic factor. The Folkow hypothesis would seem to allow a greater scope for associations between stress-relevant variables and HT than would the Guyton hypothesis.

ATHEROSCLEROSIS AND ISCHEMIC HEART DISEASE

Ischemia is a reduction in blood flow to a tissue, implying insufficient oxygen to meet the tissue's needs. Thus ischemic heart disease (IHD) involves inadequate blood flow to the heart muscle. Nearly all IHD occurs in persons with severe coronary *atherosclerosis* (AS), and the term coronary heart disease (CHD) is often used as equivalent to IHD.

IHD can manifest itself in several ways (Robbins et al., 1984). *Myocardial infarction* (MI) refers to the death of heart cells due to severe, sudden ischemia. Although the precipitation of acute MI is not fully understood and is likely to vary from case to case, it may involve thrombi (blood clots), vasospasm, and/or platelet aggregation in coronary arteries already severely narrowed by atherosclerosis. *Angina pectoris* refers to episodes of pain which result from ischemia just short of the severity needed to produce infarction. The term *sudden cardiac death* usually implies arrhythmia that leads to death within minutes or hours of initial symptoms. It can arise in any type of IHD, but the precipitating event is often unclear.

Because coronary AS underlies most IHD, a great deal of effort has been directed at understanding its development. AS is the most important type of arteriosclerosis (Robbins et al., 1984). It involves the development of atheromata—plaques of fatty material with fibrous caps—in the intimal layers of larger arteries. (The tunica intima is, with the exception of the monolayer of endothelial cells, the innermost layer of the arterial wall.) With the progression of AS, the arterial lumina can become greatly obstructed. Further complications can include calcification, rupture of the plaques and release of microemboli, thrombosis on the plaques, and weakening of the underlying layers of the vessel.

There have been several theories of AS etiology. The predominant one postulates injury to the arterial endothelium as the initial event. This endothelial injury allows pathogenic substances or cells to contact the intima. Several subsequent processes contribute to the development of atheromata. Included among them are alterations in intimal cell membrane function; intimal cell death and/or proliferation; infiltration of the vessel wall by blood monocytes and their differentiation to macrophages; the appearance of lipid-filled foam cells derived from macrophages and smooth muscle cells; further endothelial injury; platelet adhesion and aggregation; and the release of growth factors that promote cell proliferation at the site of the lesion (Clarkson et al., 1987).

Risk factors for AS, and therefore for IHD, include smoking, obesity, high blood cholesterol, hypertension, diabetes mellitus, and family history. At least the first three of these present obvious possibilities for psychological/behavioral influences on AS.

Stress, Behavior and Hypertension

It is clear that stress can evoke short-term increases in BP, but whether stress and related psychogenic factors can produce human essential HT has not yet been settled (Dustan, 1987). A number of rather plausible mechanisms have been suggested (e.g, Folkow, 1987; Light, 1987). Stress can decrease renal excretion of salt (and therefore of water). This would increase fluid volume and thus tend to increase cardiac output. SNS stimulation of the kidneys, with activation of the renin-angiotensin-aldosterone axis and constriction of renal arterioles, is presumably involved in this effect. Pituitary vasopressin (antidiuretic hormone) may also contribute. Folkow cited evidence that, in lower animals at least, stress increases salt intake and Na in turn intensifies SNS stimulation of the cardiovascular system.

A second possibility is that stress contributes rather directly to increased vascular resistance (Folkow, 1987). Acute increases in BP might induce vascular hypertrophy if they are intense and repeated. Catecholamines can accentuate this effect by increasing the excitability of and stimulating the proliferation of vascular smooth muscle cells.

McCubbin et al. (1985) implicated endogenous opioids in protection against HT. The opioid antagonist naloxone increased the BP response to mental arithmetic in subjects with low BP, but not in those with high BP. McCubbin et al. suggested that endogenous opioids normally protect against excessive BP responses to stress and that the weakening of this protective mechanism may contribute to the development of HT. (The protective effect of endogenous opioids proposed for HT contrasts with the deleterious effects proposed by Shavit and Martin [1987] for immune function and neoplasia.) McCubbin et al. also found that subjects with higher resting BP did more poorly on the mental arithmetic task (cf. Shapiro et al., 1987).

There are probably still other stress-relevant mechanisms for HT. Insulin has been mentioned. In obese women, fasting insulin level correlated with both diastolic and systolic BP, even when age, serum glucose and weight were controlled (Lucas et al., 1985). Recall, however, that stress is usually assumed to decrease insulin output.

As is true of other diseases, it is reasonable to think that stress might affect HT through external loops as well as the internal loops we have been discussing. Sodium intake, but also potassium, calcium, alcohol, and caloric intake have been implicated in HT (e.g., citations in Chesney et al., 1987).

The fact that HT is often asymptomatic allows some speculations about how stressors might affect diagnosis and subsequent adherence to treatment. Hypertensives may subscribe to naive models of illness in which treatment is undertaken in response to symptoms and is finished when the disorder is "cured" (Meyer et al., 1985). Hypertensives who reported that medication affected their "symptoms" were more likely to take it, and new patients who reported symptoms when they were diagnosed were more likely to stop treatment. If psychophysiologic stress responses can lead persons to see physicians, then those hypertensives who present with such symptoms may not comply with recommended treatment. On the other hand, low stress, and hence few psychophysiologic stress symptoms, might be associated with delay in diagnosis, since such persons would have fewer reasons to seek medical attention. Therefore, at least among individuals with existing HT, the disorder's relationship to stress may be complex.

There is no shortage of findings consistent with the hypothesis that stress participates in the development of HT. One type of evidence concerns animals predisposed to HT. Stress has been implicated in the HT of spontaneously hypertensive rats (SHR's) (e.g., Folkow, 1987). At least some SHR strains are highly reactive when exposed to stressors, showing greater heart rate, cardiac output, and renal nerve responses than do control strains. This reactivity is apparent even before the animals develop HT. Further, stressors speed the development of HT in SHR's and in SHR x control hybrids. Cox et al. (1985) demonstrated that shock-induced HT development in such hybrids is reduced by exercise.

The evidence on humans is also relatively consistent in showing positive associations between stress-relevant variables and HT. The earlier literature has been presented by Weiner (1977). Reasonably prolonged, though not permanent, elevations in BP have been associated with such obviously stressful circumstances as natural disasters and war. Weiner carefully noted that essential HT may have a variety of origins; that studies of persons who already have HT may detect the behavioral consequences of the disorder, not etiologic factors; and that the research he reviewed was not entirely consistent. Nevertheless, he favored a role for psychosocial factors, noting that anger and stressful conditions such as social disorder and separation may at the least act to exacerbate incipient HT.

There is evidence for a positive association between psychophysiologic responsiveness and cardiovascular disorder in humans (Krantz & Manuck, 1984). Like young SHR's, young humans with family histories of HT tend to react strongly to stressors (e.g., Folkow, 1987; Light, 1987). Light et al. (1983) reported that subjects who were predisposed to HT and were simultaneously high in heart rate response showed reduced sodium excretion in response to competitive tasks. (Although the complete statistical analyses were not presented, it seems that high heart rate reactors who were low in HT predisposition actually increased their sodium excretion under stress. This raises the possibility that stress might have a protective influence in some people.)

Another line of evidence comes from studies of culture change (James, 1987). As usual, the findings are not wholly consistent, but a number of investigators have reported increased BP among members of traditional cultures undergoing contact with modern societies. This finding may represent changes in diet or in other pathology, but it may also represent the demands of novel social conditions or frustrated desires for higher standards of living.

Presumably stressful work situations have also been associated with elevated BP. In a classic study, Cobb and Rose (1973) found that HT was more common among journeyman air traffic controllers than among airmen, and was particularly common among controllers at high-traffic centers. Cooper and Melhuish (1984) reported that frequent job changes and high employment-related stress predicted BP among women executives, but not men. Job loss has also been related to elevated BP (and to other disorders; Weiner, 1977).

Relationships between stress-relevant individual differences and human HT have also received much attention. We have already alluded to individual differences in cardiovascular and CNS reactivity as possible predictors of HT. This reactivity is probably related in some fashion to personality. We have also noted that the Type A behavior pattern has been associated with greater reactivity to some stressors.

Coping style may well be related to HT. Linden and Feuerstein (1983) found that hypertensives tended to interpret situations as less stressful than did normotensives. They suggested that this might reflect a repressive form of cognitive coping, though it might also reflect a belief in one's own efficacy. James (1987) interpreted some of the literature as reflecting an association between HT and circumstances which demand a great deal of active coping. In line with this, he has found evidence that the trait of *John Henryism*—a tendency to tackle demanding circumstances actively—interacted with level of education in predicting BP among black men. The lowest BP's were in subjects high in both education and John Henryism; the highest were in subjects low in education but high on John Henryism. Perhaps the determination to cope is beneficial if resources are adequate but harmful if they are too limited. (We mentioned earlier that coping may not be an unmitigated good.)

There has long been speculation that anger, hostility, and/or conflicts involving these are associated with cardiovascular disorders. The possible role of this individual difference constellation in HT has been reviewed by Diamond (1982) and mentioned by most writers who have discussed psychologic factors in human HT. A variety of studies support this idea, and one thread running through them is the possible importance of ambivalence about anger. Some studies have suggested overt complaisance and low overt anger as characteristics of hypertensives. Such findings might indicate that hostility-centered conflict—the combination of high anger and inability to express that anger—might be critical.

We can use a study by Cottington et al. (1986) to illustrate the type of relationships that have been found. These authors investigated HT (diastolic BP of 90 or more) in men working at two manufacturing plants. Data from men on hypertension medication were excluded from the analyses. HT was most prevalent in those who reported both high job stress (particularly ambiguity about future job status) and a strong tendency not to express felt anger ("anger-in"). This general pattern was supported by logistic regression analysis with several relevant factors (e.g., age, smoking, family history) controlled. Cottington et al. did not report how much anger their subjects actually experienced though they seem to have collected that information.

We should mention the relevance of psychologic intervention data to the stress-HT question. The available evidence suggests that relaxation and biofeedback are in fact capable of reducing BP, at least in mild hypertensives (for reviews, e.g., Chesney et al., 1987; Shapiro & Goldstein, 1982). There is some reason to believe that this lowering of

BP can be sustained. The effectiveness of such interventions is quite consistent with the hypothesis that stress participates in the development of HT, although it is not definitive evidence.

Stress, Behavior, IHD, and Sudden Death

POSSIBLE MECHANISMS

Pituitary-adrenocortical and sympathoadrenomedullary stress responses are thought capable of promoting IHD in several ways (e.g., Herd, 1981; McKinney et al., 1984; Williams, 1984): Damage to the arterial endothelium might result from shear pressure with increased BP or HR. Catecholamines may damage the endothelium and myocardial cells directly. Increases in blood lipids and cholesterol occur under the influence of catecholamines and glucocorticoids. Platelet aggregation can be increased, thereby promoting atherosclerosis or thrombosis. Vasospasm from catecholamines or other vasoconstrictors may produce ischemic attacks. Increased cardiac work will increase myocardial O_2 requirements and potentiate ischemia. Abnormalities in cardiac rhythm may precipitate sudden death.

Speculation can extend beyond the rather frequently mentioned mechanisms which we have just listed. Williams (1985) found that testosterone levels were higher in Type A than Type B student subjects and noted that exogenous testosterone has been found to stimulate the development of atheromatus plaques.

One can also speculate about a role for stress-induced immunomodulation in IHD. The most obvious possibility is perhaps that the failure of the immune system to contain infections would subject the organism to the general stress of the infections. More specific to IHD is the role of monocytes/macrophages as components of atheromata. Any situation which alters the functions of those cells might affect the progress of atherosclerosis.

Another possible immune system connection is via the toxicity of certain cytokines. Tumor necrosis factor (TNF; a.k.a. cachectin) is secreted by macrophages in various diseases and is particularly strongly stimulated by the endotoxins of gram-negative bacteria. TNF seems to have several effects which might promote IHD, including damage to vascular endothelium, stimulation of platelet aggregation, enhancement of coagulation, and increases in blood lipids (see Beutler & Cerami, 1988; Morrison & Ryan, 1987). If stress-induced immunosuppression allowed a serious gram-negative infection to develop, the resulting high TNF levels might significantly enhance atherogenesis. On the other hand, stress might suppress TNF secretion as it can suppress other aspects of lymphoreticular function, in which case the result could well be protective. If and when stress enhances immune function, the opposite possibilities arise.

The mechanisms we have just discussed are all internal loops, but there are external loop possibilities. As we noted in Chapter 4, both beginning to smoke and continuing to do so are partly responses to stressful situations. Smoking is well known as a risk factor for IHD, and there are several possible mechanisms for its actions (e.g., Perkins, 1985). Carbon monoxide (CO) can seemingly raise serum low density lipoproteins, lower high density lipoproteins, and damage vascular epithelium. It can reduce the O_2 available to the heart. Nicotine can also have adverse effects on serum cholesterol. Further, it increases catecholamine levels, with all that that implies for IHD. Perkins also suggests that smoking interacts with diet and cholesterol in determining risk. Dembroski (1984) and colleagues have found that smoking and the arousal that stems from playing a video game have at least additive, and possibly synergistic, effects on HR and BP.

One notable thing about IHD and HT is that most of the internal loop mediators which have been suggested point to exacerbation of disease with the classic sympathoadrenomedullary and adrenocortical stress responses. To be sure, possible external loops might have beneficial effects; some persons might improve their diets in response to stressors, for example. However, the IHD/HT situation seems rather different from something like cancer, where there seem to be numerous internal loop possibilities for protective effects of stress.

STRESSORS AND IHD

The study of personality (see below) has overshadowed the study of stressful circumstances where IHD is concerned, but there is a literature on stressors and IHD. Lown (1987) and Tyroler et al. (1987) have cited much of the relevant evidence. Low socioeconomic status and education, work-related stress, lack of social support, bereavement, and life change have been associated with MI or sudden cardiac death. We shall give some examples of recent studies not cited by Lown or Tyroler et al.

Hendrix (1985) studied traditional risk factors and stress variables as predictors of the ratio of total cholesterol to HDL cholesterol in a sample of 225 working adults. A high ratio should indicate IHD risk. Although gender, overweight, smoking, and dietary fruit had the expected associations with cholesterol ratio, stress-related factors (role conflict, workload, job boredom, job stress, and life stress) did not. With another sample and somewhat different predictors, Hendrix found that "microsupervision" by a supervisor predicted higher ratios, but a number of other variables (e.g., organizational climate, job satisfaction, intergroup conflict, job autonomy) apparently did not.

Magnus et al. (1983) used more definitive outcome measures and obtained results more in line with expectations. They studied all MI's and fatal coronary events in four Dutch communities, excluding persons over 70 and those who had previous MI's. The cases were compared to a stratified random sample. Self-employed men were over twice as likely to suffer acute coronary events as employed men; self-employed women were nearly six times as likely as housewives to suffer such events. In addition, men who considered themselves as self-driven were much more likely to have MI's. Neither excessive working hours nor time pressure were associated with coronary events.

Byrne and Whyte (1980) were interested in the possibility that the interpretation of life events is more closely related to MI than is their mere occurrence. They compared 120 patients discharged after MI with 40 admitted for possible MI but not so diagnosed. Neither number of life events nor population-based measures of their impacts discriminated the groups, but some responses to events did discriminate. MI patients described their responses to events as more strongly characterized by upset, depression, and hopelessness.

A study by Rozanski et al. (1988) illustrated that ischemia can occur in response to stress. Coronary artery disease patients and controls were given three laboratory stressors (mental arithmetic, the Stroop color-word task, and speaking about their personal flaws). They also exercised heavily on a bicycle ergometer. The psychologic stressors produced abnormalities in patients' ventricular wall motions that indicated reduced blood flow to areas served by narrowed arteries. The ischemic effects of giving the self-critical speech were nearly as severe as those of the exercise.

The question of psychologic factors and IHD has not received as much attention in women as in men, but there are studies. Haynes

(1984) noted that clerical work is positively related to IHD in women, something that may reflect a lack of autonomy and recognition among those workers. Cottington et al. (1980) investigated bereavement and women's sudden death from coronary disease. All cases occurring over eight months in a single county were investigated. Information on cases was gained from the next of kin. Neighborhood controls provided information on themselves. Cases were more likely than controls to have suffered the death of a significant other during the six previous months. They had also experienced less positive life change and less chronic illness, but did not differ from controls in negative life change.

We mentioned that sudden death can result from abnormalities of cardiac rhythm, particularly in persons with IHD. A large literature suggests that stress can trigger arrhythmias in both infrahumans and humans (Kamarck & Jennings, 1991; Lown, 1987; Verrier, 1987; Verrier & Lown, 1984). Blood supply to the heart and the balance between sympathetic and parasympathetic actions on cardiac cells appear to influence the heart's resistance to electrical instability. One good example of the relationship between stressors and electrical abnormalities is a study by Haughey et al. (1984). Patients with known or suspected arrhythmic tendencies provided 24-hour ambulatory EKG data and diaries which included notations of emotional episodes. Several types of electrocardial aberrations were more likely during emotional episodes. Reported one-year life stress was not associated with EKG abnormalities.

Consistent with its anomalous status as a stressor, exercise cuts both ways in IHD. There is evidence that exercise is associated with lower IHD morbidity (Eichner, 1983; Martin & Dubbert, 1982; Oberman, 1985) and can reduce the reinfarction rate in persons who have suffered one MI (Naughton, 1985). These putative benefits may derive from improvements in blood pressure and lipid profiles. At the same time, however, exercise can precipitate acute events such as anginal pain, ischemia, and death in those suffering from IHD (e.g., Eichner, 1983; Rozanski et al., 1988).

PERSONALITY AND IHD

The story of personality and IHD is largely the story of the Type A behavior pattern (TABP). The TABP is characterized by ambition, aggressiveness, competitiveness, concern with deadlines, a feeling that there is not enough time for everything, and the endeavor to overcome obstacles in order to achieve (Chesney et al., 1981; Matthews, 1982). The TABP is as frequent in women as in men of similar social status, even though IHD is more frequent among men (Baker et al., 1984).

The best assessment of the TABP is by a structured interview (SI) derived from the original work of Friedman and Rosenman (1959). The SI is intended to elicit Type A expressive behavior in addition to tapping Type A content in subjects' responses. Many aspects of its scoring refer to such things as interrupting the interviewer, sighing, and speech style (Chesney et al., 1981). There are several questionnaire measures of TABP. The Jenkins Activity Survey (JAS), which was developed from the SI, is the most prominent of these. The questionnaire measures are less closely associated with heart disease than is the SI (Booth-Kewley & Friedman, 1987; Chesney et al., 1981; Dembroski & Costa, 1988).

Matthews (1982) has discussed psychologic theories about the TABP. One view depicts A's as excessively concerned with controlling events, struggling to control them (thus appearing competitive, etc.), and becoming helpless if convinced that control is beyond them (see Glass, 1977). A second view emphasizes self-involvement as an underlying psychologic characteristic of A's which enhances the salience of discrepancies between goals and attainments. Matthews' own approach is more developmental and considers individuals' criteria for evaluating productivity. A's are seen as having a high need for productivity but not having clear standards for assessing whether they measure up. The result is said to be incessant striving and a sense of there being too little time to do what needs to be done.

Mechanisms for TABP Effects

There may be several ways in which the TABP could contribute to IHD (and to other disorders as well [Suls & Marco, 1990]). The predominant idea is that A's respond more strongly than B's to stressors (Contrada & Krantz, 1988; DeQuattro et al., 1985; Glass, 1977; McKinney et al., 1984). Contrada and Krantz (1988) concluded that stress reactivity differences between A's and B's are clearest for systolic BP and epinephrine. They also cited evidence for greater cortisol responses in A's. Contrada and Krantz emphasized that A's and B's might not respond differently to all stressors; A's may be most likely to overrespond in situations which elicit anger or engage their tendencies to exert control.

A study by Ward et al. (1986) is illustrative. They assessed the systolic BP, diastolic BP and HR responses of A and B men to six stressors. There were no A/B differences at baseline, but A's had significantly greater change scores on 6 of 18 comparisons. The significant differences were found for the four more "psychologic" stressors (concept formation, reaction time, videogame play, mental arithmetic) but not for the hand grip and cold pressor tasks.

It is also reasonable to think that the overt behavior of A's might contribute to their IHD risk. A's may encounter (i.e., may generate) stressful situations more often than B's. Competitiveness, ambition, hostility, time urgency, and need to control could well lead to frequent frustration and/or interpersonal friction. A's report more stressful life events (and stronger responses to them) than do B's (Byrne, 1981; Byrne & Rosenman, 1986). In direct observations of police dispatchers at work, Kirmeyer et al. (1988) found that subjects higher on the JAS initiated more tasks for themselves and had more tasks imposed upon them by others.

The behavior of A's might also affect exposure to exogenous agents. Lombardo and Carreno (1987) found that Type A smokers had higher alveolar CO levels and longer durations of inhalation than Type B smokers. This suggests greater exposure to toxic smoke components among A's. (It also illustrates that simple measures of exogenous agent exposure need not be accurate indices.) There is evidence as well that Type A individuals consume more alcohol than do Type B's (Folsom et al., 1985).

Finally, we cannot forbear pointing out that the TABP might illustrate extended (long-term) reciprocal relationships involving stress. Matthews and Woodall (1988) have suggested that the TABP might originate partly from stressful conditions. The parents of Type A children have been found to push them to greater levels of performance and to provide less verbal reinforcement. The children make more negative statements about themselves when they are not given clear standards against which to evaluate their performances. It may be, in other words, that certain types of early stressful situations engender personality and behavior patterns which promote high reactivity to stress and the creation of stressful situations in later life. Stress begets stress.

Type A/IHD Findings

The story of the initial success of the TABP as a predictor of IHD has been told and retold. We need not detail it here. The reviews and discussions we shall cite provide ample references (see Haynes & Matthews, 1988, for a good, brief treatment). The key findings were of a significant prospective relationship between TABP and IHD in large studies, a relationship that was maintained when other risk factors were controlled (or seemingly controlled; cf. Lombardo & Carreno, 1987). In various studies, the TABP has been positively associated with initial MI, reinfarction, and CAD as assessed by angiography. It has appeared as a risk factor in women as well as men (Haynes, 1984).

As additional data became available, however, the TABP/IHD relationship seemed more confusing (see Booth-Kewley & Friedman, 1987; Haynes & Matthews, 1988). Some seemingly well-conducted studies have failed to show the expected relationship. Shekelle, Hulley, et al. (1985) reported prospective structured interview (SI) findings on over 3,000 men in the Multiple Risk Factor Intervention Trial (MRFIT) from 1973 to 1976. There was no support for TABP as a risk factor in first coronary events (cardiac death or nonfatal MI). Data from over 12,000 MRFIT subjects indicated no relationship between JAS TABP and coronary events. In another study Shekelle, Gale, and Norusis (1985) found that the JAS did not predict major coronary events among 2,300 participants in the Aspirin Myocardial Infarction Study. Even more interesting are data such as those of Ragland and Brand (1988). They studied cardiac mortality in a 22-year follow-up of subjects from the original Western Collaborative Group Study who has shown IHD in that study. TABP had been assessed by SI. Among the 231 original subjects who had survived their initial event for more than 24 hours, those assessed as Type A had significantly *lower* mortality from subsequent coronary events. TABP was not related to mortality during the 24 hours after the initial event.

A broader perspective on the TABP issue can be gained from the meta-analyses of Booth-Kewley and Friedman (1987). Among many other things, they showed that beginning around 1975 the variability in TABP/IHD findings increased dramatically and the size of the average effect declined. The overall relationship between TABP and all IHD measures is +.112 (expressed as a correlation coefficient). That for prospective studies is +.045. The SI appears to be considerably more strongly related to IHD outcomes than the JAS (+ .062 vs. + .009 in prospective studies).

The existence of significant discrepancies in the TABP findings has provoked significant discussion. Dimsdale (1988) called the history of the TABP a "topsy-turvy career for a risk factor" and argued against a simple TABP-IHD connection. Haynes and Matthews (1988) looked for ways to explain the discrepant findings and noted several factors which might contribute: the use of questionnaire TABP measures, small samples, the lack of appropriate control groups, societal changes in health behaviors, and the possibility that the TABP is not predictive for persons who are at high IHD risk for other reasons. We presume that these considerations would call into question some positive studies as well as some negative or null result studies.

From a holistic perspective, the idea that the TABP has a complex relationship to coronary disease is not surprising. The relationship might be expected to shift with changes in such things as sample characteristics, the medical treatment given to coronary patients, and the public's awareness of psychologic risk factors.

Other Personality Variables and IHD

Questions about the TABP have led to consideration of other variables in its stead, particularly variables which appear related to the TABP. Hostility has come in for much recent attention (e.g., Williams, 1984). It is possible that hostility of some sort is the core of coronary-prone behavior and that the TABP is associated with IHD because hostility is one of its components. The possible association between hostility and HT is consistent with a hostility-IHD relationship.

Williams et al. (1980) gave 424 angiography patients the TABP SI, the MMPI, and six other measures the day following their arteriograms. A's were more likely than non-A's to have at least one coronary artery occluded by 75% or more. In addition, patients at the low end of an MMPI hostility (Ho) scale (Cook & Medley, 1954) were less likely to meet the 75% occlusion criterion. Williams et al. concluded that this hostility measure is related to coronary atherosclerosis more strongly than, and independently of, the TABP. They did not report the associations between angiogram results and their other psychosocial measures.

MacDougall et al. (1985) found that "potential for hostility" and "anger-in," as assessed by supplemental scoring of the SI, predicted the number of coronary vessels occluded in angiography patients. Time pressure was negatively related to the dependent variable, but no other predictors, including overall TABP, were related.

Booth-Kewley and Friedman (1987) located 13 studies which examined the relationship between MI and anger, hostility, or aggression. Their meta-analysis indicated that these variables are significantly related to MI.

However, not all studies have found hostility-IHD associations. In a 25-year follow-up of 478 physicians who had taken the MMPI during their medical school interviews, McCranie et al. (1986) found no relationship between Ho and IHD as indicated by angina, MI, or IHD death. McCranie et al. noted that applicants' desires to look good may have lowered their Ho scores; when they attempted to correct for this using MMPI K (defensiveness) scores, IHD remained unrelated to Ho. Leon et al. (1988) could not find an association between Ho and cardiovascular outcomes in a 30-year follow-up of 280 businessmen.

The association between Ho and other health related psychosocial variables was investigated by Smith and Frohm (1985). Using undergraduate subjects, they found Ho to be positively related to anxiety, neuroticism, depression, locus of control, questionnaire TABP, negative life events, and daily hassles. Ho was negatively associated with social desirability, interpersonal trust, hardiness, and social support measures. From these data, the cynicism and suspiciousness evident in the Ho items (Cook & Medley, 1954) fit into an overall pattern of negative affectivity and self-reported unfortunate circumstances. If there is a general relationship between stress-related psychosocial variables and cardiovascular disorders, Ho might be a reasonable summary index.

That there may be such a general relationship is suggested by meta-analyses (Booth-Kewley & Friedman, 1987). When all coronary outcome measures were considered, depression, anxiety, and extraversion, as well as hostility and TABP, were associated with disease. Depression appears, in fact, to be at least as strongly associated with coronary disease as is TABP. Booth-Kewley and Friedman cautioned against overinterpreting meta-analyses. Their work and many others' make it clear that much remains to be learned about relations among stress-relevant individual differences and cardiovascular disorders. Not least, we need more information on the relationships among the individual difference variables themselves.

Interventions

As with hypertension, there is some evidence for the effectiveness of psychologic interventions in IHD (Barr & Benson, 1984; Blumenthal & Levenson, 1987; Johnson, 1982; Levenkron & Moore, 1988). It appears that the TABP, blood lipids, and arrhythmias can all be reduced. For our purposes, however, the critical endpoints are hard indices of IHD, and there the data are relatively few, if encouraging.

Friedman et al. (1984) reported on a large, complex behavioral intervention designed to reduce Type A behavior and clinical coronary events in patients who had had an infarction. The intervention reduced the nonfatal cardiac recurrence rate significantly in comparison to controls. However, it did not significantly affect mortality.

A smaller, simpler intervention study was reported by Frasure-Smith and Prince (1985). They studied 453 MI patients randomized into control and stress-intervention groups. Intervention subjects were contacted by telephone each month and given a brief stress questionnaire. If the stress score exceeded a specified criterion or the patient was readmitted, he was visited by a project nurse, and intervention and support were provided. At the end of one year, controls were significantly ($p = .051$) more likely to have suffered cardiac death. The authors noted, however, that despite randomization their intervention group differed from the controls on several relevant variables.

In sum, the evidence for stress-induced exacerbation of human cardiovascular disease is considerable. The preponderance of human data are consistent with that hypothesis. Animal model work shows clearly that such effects can occur. What is known about plausible mediating mechanisms also suggests that internal loop stress effects should potentiate hypertension and ischemic heart disease, if anything. Much remains to be learned about every aspect of this topic, but we expect research to continue supporting the general idea that stress-related factors are positively associated with cardiovascular disease outcomes.

We turn now to areas where less is known.

INFECTIOUS DISEASES

Infectious Agents

A multitude of organisms and almost-organisms are capable of living (or almost-living) in higher vertebrates and causing disease. We cannot describe even a tiny proportion of them or the pathologies they induce. It may be helpful, however, for readers to get a sense of the range of pathogenic agents which occur. We shall mention viruses and bacteria because they are given the most attention, but fungi, protozoa, and helminths are also important. This brief discussion is taken from Krieg (1984), Luria et al. (1978), and Robbins et al. (1984) except as otherwise indicated.

VIRUSES

There are about twenty families of viruses which can cause disease in humans (e.g., picornaviruses in polio and the common cold; orthomyxoviruses and influenza; poxviruses and smallpox). Many of these families contain numerous species with diverse pathogenic potentials. It has been rather common over the years for viruses to be suggested as causal agents in disorders whose etiologies are unknown.

Intact virus particles (*virions*) are basically genomes (DNA or RNA) surrounded by protein *capsids*. In addition, they often have outer *envelopes* composed of lipid membranes and membrane-bound proteins. The envelope membranes are derived from the membranes of previous host cells; the envelope proteins are often coded for by viral genes. More complex virus particles will have larger genomes and/or will carry important enzymes in addition to their genomes.

Viruses are not alive, strictly speaking. They are not cells and cannot carry out metabolic or reproductive processes except within host cells. They must have host cell energy substrates, enzymes, chromosomes and/or other constituents in order to function. Exactly what host cell components a virus uses depends upon the virus, but their needs are always extensive. Virions are basically non-functional, except that they can manage to have their components taken into host cells. Virions disassemble upon infecting a host cell, and only then can they use the host's resources.

In many viral infections there are *latent* periods during which there are few signs of virus presence. Some viruses insert DNA into host genomes, and the viral genes may be unexpressed (or expressed at very low levels) for long periods, conceivably decades. It is also possible for viruses to remain dormant without their DNA being integrated into host chromosomes. Whatever the form of latent viruses, they can become activated and then produce overt disease. Recurrent genital and oral herpes eruptions are perhaps the best known examples of this.

Herpesvirus disorders have been studied rather extensively in relation to stress. Herpesviruses are enveloped and have a double stranded DNA genome. They multiply in cell nuclei. This virus family contains several members known to cause human disease. Herpes simplex 1 and 2 (HSV-1, HSV-2) are responsible for "fever blisters" and genital herpes, respectively. Varicella-zoster virus (herpes zoster, HZV) is the agent of chickenpox. Its reactivation in adults produces shingles. The Epstein-Barr virus (EBV) is responsible for infectious mononucleosis and has been associated with Burkitt's lymphoma (a type of malignant tumor originating in lymphoid cells and particularly common in parts of Africa). The EBV genome can become integrated into B-lymphocyte chromosomes and apparently immortalize those cells. Cytomegalovirus (CMV) infections are usually referred to as cytomegalic inclusion disease. (The term "inclusion" refers to microscopically visible evidence of the virus in cell nuclei.)

The *human immunodeficiency viruses* (HIV) (Fauci, 1988) are far different from the herpesviruses. HIV-1 and the more recently discovered HIV-2 are *retroviruses*. The virions are enveloped and carry two copies of a single stranded RNA genome. They are the agents of AIDS. The older HIV-1 has received most of the study, and what we say may apply only to it. HIV-1 had other names early in its career (e.g., HTLV-III for human T-lymphotropic virus or human T-cell leukemia virus; LAV for lymphadenopathy virus). As with all retroviruses, HIV's RNA genome must undergo *reverse transcription* (that is, transcription into DNA), and the resulting DNA must be integrated into host cell chromosomes for the viral "life" cycle to be carried through. When the retrovirus exists only as a segment of integrated DNA it is called a *provirus*.

HIV-1 is *T-lymphotropic*. It has an affinity for T-cells, particularly T-cells with the CD4 protein on their surfaces. CD4 apparently serves as a receptor for viral proteins, allowing the virus to infect the cell. The $CD4^+$ lymphocytes are helper T-cells, and a serious diminution in their activity would be expected to have serious consequences.

CD4$^+$ lymphocytes are not the only targets for HIV-1. Monocytes, macrophages, brain glial cells, and B-lymphocytes are among the cell types that may be attacked (e.g., Barnes, 1986; Gartner et al., 1986; Koyanagi et al., 1987). This may mean that there are CD4-like molecules on some of these cells or that there are other receptors for the virus. The virus seemingly mutates readily, and different strains are differentially capable of infecting different cell types. Viruses isolated from infected individuals change over time, becoming more virulent (Cheng-Mayer et al., 1988). The genesis of AIDS from HIV infection is still imperfectly understood (Blattner et al., 1988; Fauci, 1988).

The case definition of AIDS has been revised and will probably continue to be (Blattner et al., 1988). Major elements contributing to the diagnosis of full-blown AIDS are the presence of antibodies to HIV (indicating that the person has been infected), low numbers of CD4$^+$ lymphocytes, generalized lymphadenopathy (swelling of lymph nodes), and the presence of opportunistic diseases such as pneumonia caused by the protozoan *Pneumocystis carnii*. (Opportunistic diseases are those against which normal host defenses are almost always adequate and whose appearance therefore indicates that the defenses are weak.) Certain cancers, such as the otherwise rare Kaposi's sarcoma, are also frequent in AIDS.

It has been clear for some time that neuropsychiatric and psychologic symptoms are important in AIDS. Primary causes are the direct manifestations of CNS infection by HIV and opportunistic CNS infections following the immunodeficiency. Progressive dementia is a well documented component of AIDS (Price et al., 1988). There are indirect effects as well, of course. The very existence of the disease has been a profound source of threat in some high-risk groups. A positive antibody test or a diagnosis produces justified fear for one's continued existence and, for many, fear of discrimination as well (e.g., Coates et al., 1987; Holland & Tross, 1985).

BACTERIA

Bacteria represent if anything a larger variety of pathogens than do viruses. They are much more complex than viruses and are definitely living cells. Bacteria are prokaryotes, meaning that they lack the definitive nuclear membrane, the internal membranous structures, and the chromosomal complexity of eukaryotes. Bacteria can be considered more primitive than eukaryotes, as long as primitiveness does not connote lack of adaptive success.

Almost without exception, bacteria possess rigid cell walls outside the cell membrane. Many also have gelatin-like capsules outside the cell walls to help protect them from phagocytes. Some bacteria can form spores. The spores have greatly reduced metabolic activity and can persist for long periods in unfavorable environments. Adaptive genetic change within many bacteria is aided by the transfer of extra-chromosomal DNA (plasmids) during conjugation. The development of antibiotic-resistant strains can presumably be hastened by the spread of plasmids containing resistance genes.

The advent of vaccines and antibiotics has reduced the impact of infectious diseases, but that impact is still considerable. Effective treatments or vaccines are not yet available for many infections, and resistant strains can develop in any case. In addition, it is possible for infections to become so disseminated within the host that treatment does not avail; bacterial *septicemia* (i.e., *sepsis*, in which the microbes or their toxins are distributed through the blood) is often fatal. Those of us in developed countries also need to keep in mind that infectious disorders are a much greater burden in less developed lands, where resources are scarcer and where conditions can favor some particularly obnoxious pathogens.

Stress and Infectious Diseases

The requirements for specific pathogens in infectious diseases makes some possible types of stress effects more salient than in disorders whose basis is more strongly endogenous. One thing is behavior which exposes the person to infectious agents. Stressors should render one more or less likely to contract infectious disorders as they steer one toward or away from situations in which the agents are encountered. For instance, someone who experiences low self-esteem and responds to it by seeking large numbers of sexual partners should be at relatively great risk for sexually transmitted disease. Someone who responds to the same low self-esteem with social withdrawal should be at lower risk. The integrity of the body's physical barriers can also be critical. Stressful conditions which damage the skin or mucous membranes (e.g., accidents, surgery) create risks from agents which have little capacity to breach or evade these defenses on their own.

Naturally, other mediating sequences, both internal loop and external loop, are also relevant. Health behaviors are always important. Medical treatment might promote infectious disease in several ways. Hospitalization can expose people to strains of pathogens which have been selected for survival in hospitals and are difficult to control. Another possibility is that surgically implanted prostheses such as artificial joints and heart valves promote infection (Gristina, 1987). These devices must provide good adherence for patient tissues, and therefore they also provide good sites for bacteria. The resulting infections can be difficult or impossible to control. In these cases, we can say that the original pathology and its treatment, both easily considered stressors, promote infectious disease. Notice the reciprocity; attending to one problem increases the individual's risk for others.

The immune system has been regarded as the primary mediator of internal loop links between stress and infectious disease (Jemmott & Locke, 1984). There may be internal loop possibilities which do not involve the immune system, but we have not encountered discussions of them. Immunomodulation by stressors may either increase or decrease susceptibility to infectious agents, however. We pointed out in Chapter 2 that there is some evidence for immunoenhancement under stress. Something else that is seldom appreciated is that the activity of the immune system can occasionally promote infectious disease. As an example, the presence of antibodies to dengue viruses can enhance the infection of monocytes/macrophages by the viruses and convert a relatively mild disorder into a life-threatening one (Halstead, 1988). There is also evidence that some antibodies to HIV can promote that infection (Barnes, 1988). In such cases, one might speculate that stress-induced immunodepression would be protective.

Immunodepression by stress might slow AIDS development by another mechanism. It has been found that stimulation of the immune system by cytokines, mitogens, and other infections can increase the production of HIV (Barnes, 1987; Folks et al., 1987; Siekevitz et al., 1987; Zack et al., 1988) and might therefore move infected persons toward clinical manifestations. Presumably, this occurs because transcription of proviral DNA is increased along with the transcription of other genes. To the extent that stress reduces immunocytes' ability to respond to stimulation, it might slow the progression of the disease.

On the other side of the HIV coin is the more obvious possibility that stress immunodepression can limit host capacity to deal with the virus. The course of AIDS may be one of initial high virus titers, followed by largely latent infection because immune defenses have dealt with most overt virus, followed in turn by a weakening of immune competence and a resurgence of virion production (e.g., Price et al., 1988). If this is so, then the effect of stress-induced immune depression might vary with the stage of the disease.

HUMAN STUDIES OF STRESS AND INFECTIOUS DISEASE

Although research is being reported, infectious disorders do not appear to be a major focus of stress-health research at the moment. More attention is being given to chronic/degenerative diseases.

Jemmott and Locke (1984) and Cohen and Williamson (1991) have reviewed studies of stress and infectious disease. Life events, mood, and stress-relevant personality variables were among the predictors studied. Among the outcome variables were number of upper respiratory infections, virus shedding, herpes simplex recurrence, incidence of and duration of mononucleosis, and hypersensitivity reactions to vaccines. Despite methodologic weaknesses in some of the studies and occasional null findings, stressor exposure and personality characteristics which indicate stress susceptibility tend to be positively correlated with infectious disease, and particularly with illness behavior.

One topic which has been studied recently by several research groups is the relationship of stress-relevant factors to recurrence in herpesvirus infections. Recall that these viruses are known for their ability to exist in a latent state and then break that latency.

Glaser et al. (1985) studied loneliness and medical school examinations as these related to antibodies (Ig's) to three herpesviruses—HSV-1, EBV, and CMV. Blood samples were taken one month before students' final examinations, at the exam time, and upon return from the ensuing summer vacation. The main analyses were of Ig's to two EBV antigens. With capsid antigen, Ig levels were lowest at the post-vacation sample and appeared about equally high at the pre-exam and exam samples. Overall, loneliness was associated with higher levels of anti-capsid Ig. With EBV "early antigen," the three sampling times did not differ significantly, but high loneliness subjects had significantly higher titers. Ig's to HSV and CMV were analyzed only for the exam and post-vacation samples. Ig levels to both viruses were significantly lower post-vacation. Loneliness was not related to HSV Ig titers and was not assessed with CMV.

Higher antiviral Ig titers in these studies are taken as indices of immunodepression as well as infection status; Ig levels are assumed to increase when cell-mediated immune function is weakened and unable to control virus activity. We note, however, that these increases in Ig's with stress imply that stress does not greatly impair the function of memory B-cells or of any mechanisms required to stimulate those cells.

Glaser et al. (1985) found that self-reported loneliness related to antiviral Ig in a manner similar to presumably stressful situations. Other individual difference variables have also been looked at in the context of response to herpesviruses. To the extent that the Type A behavior pattern (TABP) reflects a hyperresponsiveness to stress or a high frequency of stressful encounters, it should be associated with multiple disorders. Barton and Hicks (1985) reported a retrospective study of Jenkins Activity Survey TABP and self-reported experience of mononucleosis (EBV). Nearly 20% of college student A's reported having had mononucleosis, as compared to about 5% of B's. Depression also seems to fit well into the general scheme of informal stress theory (e.g., maladaptive attributions, high ACTH levels). Thus one might expect depressives to have high herpesvirus Ig titers, but that was not found by Amsterdam et al. (1986).

Relationships between psychologic variables and genital herpes (presumably largely HSV-2) were reviewed by VanderPlate and Aral (1987). (They also cited studies on oral herpes). They emphasized the stressfulness of having genital herpes. They noted that the data on stress and herpes recurrence are inconclusive, but suggestive that stress predicts recurrence.

At least one study not cited by VanderPlate and Aral has suggested a relationship between stress and the recurrence of genital herpes (Schmidt et al., 1985). Subjects with recurring herpes took a number of questionnaire measures on two occasions—one when they had no lesions and again shortly after lesions appeared. Scores on several presumably stable measures (e.g., Jenkins Activity Survey, social support, coping style) were not significantly different on these two occasions. However, differences were found on some state variables (to which subjects responded the second time with reference to the week before recurrence). They reported having been more anxious (on two measures) and having had more hassles and stressful life events during the week before lesions appeared (as indicated by one-tailed t-tests). Several other state variables (e.g., well-being, depression) were not different on the lesion and no-lesion occasions, however. More-over, hassles and one anxiety measure would not have discriminated significantly by two-tailed t-tests with the proper degrees of freedom.

Kemeny et al. (1989) looked at several potential predictors of genital herpes recurrence over a 6-month period. Neither stress (a rather thorough composite measure) nor mood was related to recur-rence overall. However, depressed mood was positively correlated with recurrence among those subjects who reported few other infec-tious diseases. Percentage of suppressor/cytotoxic T-cells was nega-tively related to herpes recurrence, but percentage of helper/inducer cells was not.

In a completely retrospective study, Lacroix and Offutt (1988) found that TABP (Jenkins Activity Survey) was unrelated to reported frequency of genital herpes recurrence, but that A's did report their recurrences as more severe.

Longo et al. (1988) compared a behavioral intervention (which included stress management, imagery, and relaxation) to social support and a wait-list control condition, using self-reports of genital herpes recurrence as dependent variables. The behavioral intervention did reduce follow-up reports of recurrence frequency, severity, and dura-tion, but social support had no effect.

Although studies relating psychologic variables to herpesvirus infections appear to have been the most common recently, other types of infectious diseases have been investigated. Research by Graham et al. (1986) provided some prospective evidence for stress as a predictor of respiratory symptoms. Subjects kept 6-month respiratory symptom diaries and were also asked to contact the investigators when respira-tory illnesses occurred. With bivariate correlations, initial life stress scores predicted the number of reported symptom days but not the number of illness episodes. In a multiple regression analysis, initial frequency of daily hassles was significantly associated with number of subsequent respiratory illnesses when entered after sex and age. It is not clear whether the study controlled for factors such as smoking.

Williams and Deffenbacher (1983) reported a retrospective in-vestigation of life stress and yeast infections in college women. The reported number of yeast infections, concern about them, and number of physician visits for them were positively correlated with life stress. A number of other variables, including overall physician visits and, most interestingly, actual yeast infection as assessed by laboratory test were not related to stress, however. When antibiotic use was separated from life stress in analyses of variance, no measure of yeast infection or of response to it was significantly related to life stress.

ANIMAL STUDIES OF STRESS AND INFECTIOUS DISEASE

There does not seem to be much current research on stress in animal models of infectious disease. However, such research was pursued in rather lively fashion a few years ago. Some relatively recent discussions of that literature are available (Jensen, 1981; Plaut & Friedman, 1981, 1982), and we shall rely upon those.

One major conclusion to be drawn is that the effects of stressors on animal infectious disease are complex. The outcome depends upon the infectious agent, the genetics of the host, the type of stressor, and the background conditions. In reporting investigations from his research group, Jensen (1981) noted that intense sound enhanced the susceptibility of mice to vesicular stomatitis virus if the viral inoculum was given shortly before the stressor, but if the virus was given just after the stressor, the stressor had a protective effect. In another study shock-avoidance increased monkeys' resistance to poliovirus. Plaut and Friedman (1981) cite studies from their group's research to similar effect. Living in larger groups accelerated the death of mice infected with malarial parasites but retarded death from encephalomyocarditis virus. Light-shock pairings reduced resistance to Coxsackie B virus but increased resistance to malaria.

These research programs provided much evidence for promotion of infectious disorders by stressors, but just as important is the evidence that those effects are not straightforward. Plaut and Friedman (1982, p. 281) emphasized "the need to consider a multitude of interacting variables." Jensen (1981) made the same point and went so far as to suggest that researchers limit their attention to one simple model as a way of coping with the complexity of the phenomena.

We see a point here which seems to be ignored by many who write about stress and disease. Well controlled animal studies suggest that stress effects upon disease depend on a "multitude of interacting variables" and can change with a small shift in any of numerous parameters. Since this is so, more poorly controlled correlational studies of humans need to be interpreted with the utmost caution, particularly since, as we have just seen, those human studies contain inconsistencies. Thus in the case of infectious diseases, there is good reason to believe that stress plays a significant role, but some all-important details elude us. Is the relationship as complex as the animal data make it appear, and if so, why?

DIABETES MELLITUS
Pathology

The hallmark of diabetes mellitus is hyperglycemia resulting from abnormalities in the availability and/or function of insulin and, possibly secondarily, from excess glucagon activity. (Here, the term "diabetes" will mean diabetes mellitus; diabetes insipidus is an entirely different disorder based on a deficiency in antidiuretic hormone.) Our treatment of the pathology of diabetes mellitus comes from Robbins et al. (1984) and Unger and Foster (1985) unless indicated otherwise.

There are several types of diabetes. We shall not attempt to follow all of the finer distinctions. However, we have to deal with the difference between *insulin-dependent diabetes mellitus* (IDDM; roughly equivalent to "Type 1" or "juvenile-onset" diabetes) and *non-insulin-dependent diabetes mellitus* (NIDDM; roughly equivalent to "Type 2" or "maturity-onset" diabetes).

INSULIN-DEPENDENT DIABETES

In IDDM there are few if any insulin-producing ß-cells in the pancreatic islets, and little if any insulin is produced. There is more to the consequences of insulin lack than just the failure of glucose to be taken up by cells. Insulin's restraining influence on glucagon secretion is removed and as a result the production of glucose and ketones is enhanced. (Ketones are derived from free fatty acids, and are released in large amounts in the absence of insulin. Ketones can be used as energy substrates.) The major acute results of untreated IDDM are hyperosmolality (excess solutes in body fluids) and ketoacidosis. The exit of water from cells as a result of hyperosmolality and the increased acidity of the blood have fatal results. We shall consider the long-term consequences of diabetes below.

The etiology of IDDM is not well understood. It appears most often in children. There is no pronounced tendency for it to run in families, but it is significantly associated with certain major histocompatibility types and possibly other genetic variants. It thus appears that both genetic predispositions and environmental factors are involved.

Evidence suggests that autoimmunity plays a part in the destruction of ß-cells. Infiltration of lymphocytes into the pancreatic islets sometimes accompanies the onset of IDDM. Antibodies to ß-cell constituents are also found. The fact that IDDM tends to appear following viral infections is consistent with a role for autoimmunity, assuming that virus-infected cells can stimulate the production of anti-self Ig's. It is also possible, of course, that autoimmunity develops as a consequence of ß-cell damage and is not the primary cause of it.

NON-INSULIN-DEPENDENT DIABETES

In NIDDM, ß-cell destruction is not the primary problem. In fact, insulin levels can be above normal in NIDDM. However, insulin levels often do not increase with exogenous glucose administration, suggesting that insulin regulation is abnormal. Glucagon levels may also be high and may not drop in response to glucose as they should. Another characteristic of NIDDM is *insulin resistance*; tissues do not respond to insulin with increased glucose uptake. Insulin resistance may involve reduced numbers of insulin receptors on cells or abnormalities in the intracellular consequences of receptor binding.

Untreated NIDDM does not usually result in ketoacidosis, possibly because there is enough insulin to block glucagon's stimulation of ketone production. Hyperosmolality alone is therefore the major acute threat. Glucose appears (through ingestion and internal production) faster than it can be metabolized and/or excreted. The results are extreme hyperglycemia, dehydration, and severe upset of osmotic balance.

As with IDDM, the origins of NIDDM are obscure. Unger and Foster emphasize the possibility that there are two types of NIDDM— one which resembles IDDM and may progress to it, and the second, more common, form which is the classic type 2 diabetes. NIDDM may have a strong constitutional component; the concordance rates among identical twins are very high. There are also striking (about 40-fold) racial/cultural differences in prevalence, with rates being particularly low in Japan and quite high among some American Indians. Environmental influences are suggested by the fact that improvements in the economic status of disadvantaged populations are associated with increased rates of NIDDM. That increase may reflect the best known risk factor for NIDDM, namely obesity. It is not clear whether the initial defect in NIDDM is insulin resistance accompanying obesity, a pancreatic problem which results in hypersecretion of insulin, or something else. Autoimmunity is apparently not involved in NIDDM to an important degree.

THE CHRONIC COMPLICATIONS OF DIABETES

Advances in the therapy of diabetes have reduced the dangers from acute crises. Therefore the more slowly developing consequences take on great importance. These long-term complications are poorly understood, but they are quite threatening.

Vascular disease (*angiopathy*) in diabetics involves pathology such as thrombosis and aneurysms in small vessels, increased permeability of capillaries, and atherosclerosis. Both damage to vascular endothelium and lipid abnormalities may contribute to the rapid progress of atherosclerosis in diabetics. Diabetic *retinopathy* is closely related to the angiopathy. It takes two forms. Background retinopathy involves retinal aneurysms, hemorrhages, vascular constrictions, and the exudation of lipids and proteins from retinal capillaries. More serious is proliferative retinopathy. This begins with the development of new retinal blood vessels. It can result in hemorrhage into the eye, retinal detachment, and eventual blindness. Renal dysfunction (*nephropathy*) is common in diabetics and is an important cause of death. It most commonly centers on the glomerular apparatus—the functional part of the kidney which initially removes fluid from the blood. *Neuropathy* in diabetes most often affects the extremities. The combination of angiopathy and neuropathy is largely responsible for diabetics' susceptibility to gangrene. It is possible that uncontrolled glycosylation of proteins (the adding of glucose to protein molecules, thereby possibly altering their function) is important in several of the chronic complications of diabetes.

Stress and Diabetes

POSSIBLE MECHANISMS

The etiology that is operating and the stage of the disease should determine which potential mechanisms for stress effects are the most influential. Stressor effects on immune function could be involved in the initial development of IDDM. If the sequence of events is from viral infection to anti-ß-cell autoimmunity, then immunodepression might promote the initial infection and later limit the immune system attack on ß-cells. Remember also that interleukin-1 is directly toxic to pancreatic endocrine cells (Bendtzen et al., 1986). When stressors alter food intake and body fat, they would be expected to affect the development of NIDDM. Surwit (1988) has suggested that sympathetic nervous system hyperreactivity may be associated with NIDDM, even in the absence of severe stress.

Most discussion of stress and diabetes (e.g., Surwit, 1988; Surwit & Feinglos, 1984; Wing et al., 1986) has concerned events after the disease has developed. Several stress hormones produce exaggerated glucose increases in the absence of insulin, reduce the insulin/glucagon ratio, and can materially worsen the status of some patients (Surwit & Feinglos, 1984; Unger & Foster, 1985).

We must also note the strong possibility that stress and related factors might affect the consequences of existing diabetes by affecting adherence to treatment. It is not yet clear how well careful adherence to treatment protocols can protect against the long-term complications of diabetes (Santiago, 1984; Unger & Foster, 1985) but it surely can to some degree. The management of diabetes requires the patient's careful participation. Following special diets, taking medications at the proper times, monitoring blood glucose, and exercising are all components of treatment (e.g., Wing et al., 1986). Stressful events, as well as attitudes, personality, and social support, could hardly fail to affect such a complex of behaviors. A holistic view would suggest, of course, that stress might sometimes be beneficial; bereavement, for example, might jolt a careless diabetic into a greater appreciation of life's precariousness and strengthen his/her resolve to comply with complicated medical recommendations.

FINDINGS

Despite the fact that there are several experimental models of diabetes, few animal stress studies appear to have been reported. The scattered studies cited by Surwit and Feinglos (1984) include cases of disease exacerbation and of disease inhibition, but the methods were too different to allow general conclusions. Surwit (1988) summarized research on animals predisposed to NIDDM. His discussion suggests that stress produces exaggerated glycemic responses in such animals.

Some human research has examined the glucose response to stressors in diabetics. Diabetics can seemingly have either higher or lower glucose stress responses than controls (Surwit & Feinglos, 1984). Naliboff et al. (1985) compared NIDDM patients' and normal controls' responses to standing for 10 minutes, to a handgrip test, and to mental arithmetic. Although they found the expected increases in catecholamines with their tasks, as well as some changes in glucagon, blood glucose levels remained virtually constant in both the controls and the diabetics. On the other hand, Surwit and Feinglos (1984) described research in which relaxation training and biofeedback improved glucose tolerance in NIDDM patients.

There has been some research on stress and the onset of IDDM. Leaverton et al. (1980) collected data on highly salient life events (e.g., parental loss, and severe family turmoil such as intense marital discord) in the families of a representative sample of diabetic children and a group of matched controls. Parental loss before the age of cases' diabetes onset was more frequent for the diabetics.

Post-diagnosis IDDM status seems to have received more attention in relation to psychologic factors than has the origin of the disease. Young patients at a diabetes summer camp were studied by Brand et al. (1986). They responded to life events and locus of control scales on the first day of camp. Criterion measures derived from the repeated monitoring done by camp staff, and included fasting blood glucose, urinary glucose, and urinary ketones. Demographic variables were correlated with the outcome measures, and therefore a series of partial correlations for various subgroups was used to assess relationships with life events. The only significant associations were with ketones; urinary ketones were positively related to life stressors among internals but not externals, males but not females, and 10-12 year olds but not 13-17 year olds. If this pattern of results were to be replicated, it would pose a pretty problem of interpretation.

Another study of young diabetics (Hanson et al., 1987) used percentage of glycosylated hemoglobin (HgA) as a measure of diabetic control. (HgA, reflecting as it does the reaction of excess glucose with protein molecules, is often employed as a measure of blood glucose over the preceding 1.5-2.5 months.) Life stress predicted HgA even when adherence to treatment was controlled. The stress-HgA relationship was buffered by social competence. Both parental support and social competence were positively associated with treatment adherence. The Hansen et al. results on HgA do not agree with the lack of urinary and blood sugar effects reported by Brand et al. (1986). It is possible that stress effects on blood glucose levels are idiosyncratic (Gonder-Frederick et al., 1990; Halford et al., 1990).

Edelstein and Linn (1985) reported relationships between diabetic control and perceived family qualities among older insulin-dependent men. It is not clear what if any prospective interval was used. The outcome measure was a single score combining HgA, fasting blood glucose and blood lipids, making the results difficult to compare with others. Multiple regression indicated that family achievement orientation was associated with better diabetes control, while conflict and family organization were associated with poorer control (total R^2 = .13). Seven other family measures did not relate to the dependent variable.

Jacobson et al. (1985) studied links between stress variables and diabetes complications. They studied HgA in patients with ("cases") proliferative retinopathy (PR) and without it ("controls"). The PR cases evidenced poorer diabetes control on several measures. They also reported significantly more psychiatric symptoms. Interestingly, negative life events scores were correlated with HgA in PR cases but not in the controls, and this association was further limited to cases with recent PR onset. The relation between negative events and HgA in the recent PR group persisted when several medical variables and psychiatric symptoms were controlled. Jacobson et al. suggested that patients with recent PR onset may still be uncertain about how severe the consequences of their retinopathy will be, and that life events may add sufficient stress to this already aversive situation to compromise glucose control.

The development of a general model of diabetes control was attempted by Peyrot and McMurry (1985). They divided relevant variables into two groups. Factors involved in "direct effects" on diabetes control act in what we term an internal loop manner, by altering endocrine and metabolic function. "Indirect effects" in this scheme are those which influence health care behavior (similar to the idea of external loop actions).

To put it simply, Peyrot and McMurry listed, in the context of diabetes, the broad classes of psychosocial variables likely to affect biologic function and behavior. They did not set out a detailed path description for the interrelationships among their variables. However they did assess the associations of some of them with diabetes control (HgA) in adult IDDM subjects. By one-tailed (!) t-tests, several factors differentiated good control from poor control subjects. External health locus of control, extremity of anxiety, lack of knowledge about diabetes, tolerance of symptoms, and impatience, for example, were associated with poorer control. Stepwise multiple regression retained six predictors but the small sample (20) renders those results rather questionable.

Peyrot and McMurry discussed "enabling/blocking" factors as indirect determinants of diabetes control. In their model, these factors reflect resources (e.g., information, health care services) whose loss would hinder health care behavior. Glasgow et al. (1986) studied impediments to the insulin injection, glucose monitoring, dietary, and exercise components of IDDM treatment. Subjects did not report very high frequencies of barriers to adherence, but reported barriers did relate to reported adherence, including later diary reports of glucose testing and dietary adherence.

In summary, the physiology of diabetes mellitus and the nature of its treatment certainly invite the idea that stress is a significant contributor to this group of disorders. There are plausible mechanisms, and there is some research directly suggesting stress-diabetes links. However, the results are not terribly consistent, and too many of the studies have avoidable methodologic problems.

CANCER

The possibility that psychologic factors affect malignant neoplasia has been much discussed (e.g., Baltrusch et al., 1988; Cooper, 1984; Fox, 1978, 1988; Fox & Newberry, 1984; Justice, 1985; Levy, 1982; Morrison & Paffenbarger, 1981; Newberry, 1981; Newberry et al., 1985; Riley, 1981; Sklar & Anisman, 1981; Stoll, 1979) and researched. In one respect, the importance of psychologic influences is undoubted. Any variables which alter behavioral exposure to carcinogens can alter cancer risk. The most obvious of these external loops involves tobacco use, and as we have noted, evidence suggests a role for stressors (e.g, Leventhal & Cleary, 1980). Evidence for internal loop effects is almost necessarily less persuasive than that for external loops, especially where human cancer is concerned. We shall emphasize internal loop possibilities in our discussion, but the reader must remember that in most studies there are possible confounds with external loops.

Pathologic Processes in Malignancies

Cancers constitute a large group of disorders in which uncontrolled (perhaps better, poorly controlled) cell proliferation is a chief feature. Some disorders of cell proliferation are not considered cancers, however. Benign tumors lack two of the major characteristics of malignancies, namely the capacity for *invasion* and *metastasis*. Invasion is the infiltration of adjacent tissues. Metastasis is the development of new tumors distant from the primary tumor. The primary sheds cells, some survive transport to distant sites in lymph and blood, and some of those are able to leave the circulation and establish tumors in new tissues.

There may be no absolute way to determine how malignant a neoplasm is. If invasion, and especially metastasis, can be demonstrated at diagnosis, the disorder is clearly malignant. Certain cellular characteristics, such as anaplasia (primitiveness, lack of differentiation) along with size diversity and nuclear abnormalities are also taken as indicating malignancy (Robbins et al., 1984).

Oncogenesis, the process of cancer development, is complex and in many respects remains poorly understood after decades of intensive research. Cancers involve disorders at fundamental levels of cell function. (In fact, the attempts to understand cancer have elucidated many aspects of normal cell biology.)

Oncogenesis has several stages, though it is unclear how many. The first event (or first few events) is often called *initiation* or *transformation*. This appears to require certain changes in gene activity. *Oncogenes* (e.g., Bishop, 1987) were discovered through the study of oncogenic viruses. Viral oncogenes (v-*onc* genes) often have cellular counterparts (c-*onc*s), but such homologs are seldom if ever identical. Retroviral *onc* genes have been captured from host cell genomes, and are thus variants of normal cellular oncogenes. Normal cellular oncogenes are often called *protooncogenes* because they are not likely to cause cancer unless mutated or brought under abnormal regulatory control. Protooncogenes are numerous, and they do have normal functions (e.g., Schmid et al., 1989).

Cancer can result from qualitative or quantitative changes at the genetic level. In the first case, abnormal gene products arise due to mutations in c-*onc*s or to the presence of variant viral genes. Quantitative changes involve variations in the amounts of gene products. These may result from *gene amplification* (an increase in the numbers of oncogenes), from translocations which put oncogenes near active control sites on chromosomes, or from the introduction of viral control sequences into the cell genome (e.g., Bishop, 1987; Weinberg, 1985; Yunis, 1983).

Since cancers involve disorders of cell growth, it is not surprising that oncogenes often code for proteins which function in cell multiplication. Oncogenes may produce growth factors with autocrine effects, abnormal cell membrane growth factor receptors, or interior proteins which function in the growth-signalling process (Weinberg, 1985).

Anti-oncogenes are genes whose activation can block the cancer process (Klein, 1987). Normal alleles producing normal products can dominate the effects of mutant oncogenes. Cancers typically arise from undifferentiated or partly differentiated cells (cells that have not yet developed a final commitment to a single function). Some anti-*onc* products stimulate differentiation and can move cells beyond the point at which they are susceptible to oncogenesis. They can even switch already-transformed cells back to seeming normality.

Later changes during the development of malignancies are sometimes put under the rubric of *progression*, which Peyton Rous (cited by Klein, 1987, p. 1541) termed, "the process whereby tumors go from bad to worse." These additional steps are rather poorly understood. They involve additional derangements in the cells and the acquisition of the potential for more aggressive behavior. It is probable that multiple insults (more than one genetic abnormality, chemically induced lesion, etc.) are necessary for the full development of cancer cells' many regrettable characteristics (Nowell, 1990). It may be later in progression that the capacities for invasion and metastasis develop.

With cancer growth and progression comes a variety of effects upon the host—effects which depend not merely upon the mass of the cancer, but also upon the specific actions of its cells (see Robbins et al., 1984; Shapot, 1979). Tumor cells can secrete numerous compounds, including traditional peptide hormones, growth and growth-inhibiting factors, and immunomodulators. There is evidence, for example, that Kaposi's sarcoma cells from AIDS patients secrete certain forms of interleukin-1 and fibroblast growth factor (Ensoli et al., 1989).

Tumor cells' actions and the host's responses alter many bodily processes (e.g., lipid regulation, glucose metabolism, protein synthesis, electrolyte balance, neural function). Among the best known outcomes of these host-tumor interactions is the syndrome of wasting and anorexia called *cachexia*. Cachexia may result when tumors stimulate the production of tumor necrosis factor (Tracey et al., 1986). The term *paraneoplastic syndrome* is applied to some of the effects of cancers on hosts; Robbins et al. (1984, p. 256) list many of these (e.g., hypercalcemia, venous thrombosis). Paraneoplastic symptoms can be presenting symptoms. Since neural disorders can occur and the latent period of the disease can be decades long, psychologic predictors of cancer could conceivably reflect the early effects of undetectable disease rather than effects of psychologic factors upon the disease.

Stress and Cancer

POSSIBLE MECHANISMS

Among the plausible internal loop mechanisms for stress effects on neoplasia, the most discussed is immunodepression. Writers often assume that immunodepression under stress or accompanying stress-related individual differences will broadly enhance cancer development.

However, for several reasons, we would argue against accepting a general stress-immunodepression-cancer hypothesis at present. First, as discussed in Chapter 2, the literature includes instances of immuno-enhancement accompanying stress. There are other problems as well (see Newberry et al., 1984 and references therein). It is not clear how strong and general immune system control over cancers is. Cancer cells are often immunogenic, but they are not always so or necessarily strongly so. Even if cancers express strong antigens, they may lose the histocompatibility molecules which allow T-lymphocytes to attack them (Goodenow, et al. 1985). Nor are all tumors significantly susceptible to natural immunity. There is even evidence that the immune system can protect cancer cells, suggesting that tumorigenesis may sometimes be inhibited by stress-induced immunodepression and stimulated by stress-induced immunoenhancement (e.g., Kimball, 1986). Further, research does not suggest large, general increases in cancer incidence among people who are given immunosuppressive medical treatment.

Finally, there is, so far as we know, no instance in which stress effects on experimental tumors have been unequivocally demonstrated to be due to immunomodulation. The work of Greenberg et al. (1984) comes close. However their experiments dealt with only the first 72 hours after tumor cell transplantation, not with the final development of malignancies.

Immunodepression is very probably important in stress-induced modulation of cancer, but the available evidence does not support it as the only mechanism to consider or as a process which can have only detrimental results. Pettingale (1985) has also warned against over-emphasizing immune function as a link between psychologic variables and cancer.

There are quite a few other means by which internal loop effects on cancer might occur (e.g., Newberry et al., 1984; Pettingale, 1985). These vary with the type of cancer and its stage of development. They have received much less attention than immunomodulation, and there-fore can claim little empirical support. However, they illustrate the range of questions which need consideration.

With regard to cancer initiation, there are several possible mech-anisms. Since hormones can modulate gene expression, oncogenes (normal or abnormal) located near hormone-regulated sites may be turned on or off by stress hormones. Hormones (e.g., somatomedins) affect cell division, and cell division may stabilize mutations, rendering them less susceptible to repair. Pettingale (1985) noted that glucocorticoids inhibit the synthesis of somatomedins. We have already mentioned the fact that DNA repair systems may be disrupted by stress (see Kiecolt-Glaser & Glaser, 1987), making it more likely that genetic abnormalities would become permanent. Given that there are many possible mechanisms for psychobiologic stimulation and inhibition of cancer initiation, it is interesting that glucocorticoids frequently inhibit carcinogenesis (Slaga, 1980).

There are also multiple possibilities for stress influences on later stages of tumorigenesis. Hormones and local growth factors can directly stimulate or inhibit the proliferation of a cancer clone. Glucocorticoids inhibit *angiogenesis* (the growth of new blood vessels) in some experimental systems, and stress might slow the development of solid tumors in this way. Glucocorticoids also inhibit the breakdown of collagen by tumors, thus potentially reducing their invasiveness. Tumor cell nutrition may be affected by circulatory redistribution, by changes in energy substrate levels, and by glucocorticoid-induced reduction in the transport of nutrients out of blood vessels. Any factor which affects the susceptibility of vascular walls to penetration by circulating tumor cells might affect metastasis. Pettingale (1985) cited evidence that several steroids can inhibit the release of vitamin A from the liver and thereby perhaps reduce host control over cancers.

There is presently no way to tell which of the plausible-sounding stress mechanisms are actually significant in tipping the host-tumor balance one way or the other. The outcome ought to depend upon the type of cancer, the type of stressor, the timing of the stressor in relation to stage of cancer development, and the biologic and psychologic characteristics of the host. In light of the research we shall discuss, it is important to keep in mind that there are potential ways for stress to inhibit as well as stimulate cancer development.

FINDINGS

Animal Studies

There has been much research on stress and experimental tumor models (for discussions, Justice, 1985; LaBarba, 1970; Newberry, 1981; Newberry et al., 1984; Newberry et al., 1985; Peters & Mason, 1979; Riley, 1981; Sklar & Anisman, 1981). The outstanding feature of the findings is that stress is clearly capable of stimulating and inhibiting experimental cancers. No general principles have yet been able to account fully for the divergent findings. Tumor system, stressor, and background variables all appear important. We can do no more than mention some work which illustrates the nature of this literature.

Sklar and Anisman (e.g., 1981) emphasized the stressor characteristics of chronicity (or opportunity for adaptation) and controllability in determining whether stress should stimulate, inhibit, or fail to affect cancer development. In their view, acute, uncontrollable stressors are most likely to stimulate tumorigenesis, whereas chronic and/or controllable stress should have either no effect or an inhibitory one. This hypothesis reflects, at least approximately, a more general "functional intensity" view (Newberry et al., 1984), namely that stressors eliciting mild stress responses will tend to inhibit tumor development and more severe stressors will tend to stimulate it. Other versions of this idea have emphasized the physical severity or the predictability of stressors. (This general hypothesis implies that at some intermediate degree of stress, tumor development should not differ from control levels.)

Some of the data are consistent with a functional intensity idea. Inescapable but not escapable shock has been found to stimulate the development of P815 mouse mastocytoma (Sklar & Anisman, 1979) and rat Walker 256 tumors (Visintainer et al., 1982). Sklar and Anisman (1979; Sklar et al., 1980) also reported that increasing stress chronicity eliminated the shock-induced enhancement of P815.

Studies varying the timing of stressor exposure relative to tumor induction are also relevant to the functional intensity notion. If tumor induction and stressor exposure commence together, then tumorigenesis begins in the context of full-blown stress responses. However, if tumor induction begins after stressor exposure it might be occurring in the context of attenuated (adapted) stress responses. Virus-induced sarcomas were inhibited by three days of shock applied prior to virus inoculation, but were enhanced if the stressor exposure was begun after virus inoculation (Amkraut & Solomon, 1972). Dexamethasone (a synthetic glucocorticoid) given before transplantation of lymphoma cells inhibited tumor development, whereas it had a tumor-enhancing effect if given later (Riley et al., 1982).

Unfortunately, a substantial number of findings contradict the functional intensity notion. Sklar and Anisman (1979) found equal P815 enhancement with a range of different shock intensities. In some studies the timing of stressor exposure vis-a-vis tumor induction has not mattered (e.g., Burchfield, et al., 1978; Matthes, 1963) or post-induction stress has had tumor-inhibiting effects (Newberry, 1978).

A study by Deuster et al. (1985) illustrates another aspect of the timing question and also extends the literature in this area by looking at cachexia as well as tumor development. An exercise regimen slowed the growth of rat Walker 256 tumors through the third week after tumor transplantation, but after that the exercised animals' tumors tended to catch up to controls'. (The inhibition of tumor by exercise had been found in several older studies as well, although Madden et al. [1988] found that 33 days of graded exercise had no effect on the development of a chemically induced rat mammary tumor.)

Muscle mass and measures of body protein were taken as indices of cachexia by Deuster et al. The results suggested a biphasic effect of exercise. Early on, exercise protected against cachexia, probably because it reduced tumor growth. However this was followed by higher muscle protein degradation in the exercise condition.

Steplewski et al. (1985) suggested a variation on the functional intensity theme in which recovery from stress inhibits cancer. They studied the development of transplanted mammary adenocarcinoma, comparing 11 days of restraint to a regimen in which 11 restraint days were followed by 12 days without stress. At the end of the eleven days of restraint, stress and control animals did not differ in tumor weight; following 12 days of post-restraint recovery, tumors were smaller in the formerly stressed animals. These data were interpreted to mean that recovery from restraint inhibited tumorigenesis. However, no comparison group was restrained for the entire 23-day period; thus the results may have reflected only a delayed effect of the initial 11-day restraint treatment (cf. Newberry, 1978).

Stressor characteristics can account only partially for the divergent findings in the experimental tumor literature. Other factors such as tumor system variables must be considered. Logically, there is little reason to expect all tumor systems to respond to stress in the same way. Even a cursory look at what is known of tumor biology reveals a wide range of biologic charcteristics and responsivities among cancers (see Newberry et al., 1984, for examples).

One thing that must be taken into consideration is the method of tumor induction. Experimental tumors are induced by a variety of means, and that variety almost certainly contributes to the diversity of stress findings in the literature. Transplanted tumors are frequently employed, for example, but in investigations using such tumors the early stages of cancer development do not take place in the host that is being studied. Therefore stress effects upon those early stages cannot be investigated; transplanted tumor models are relevant only to later stages of disease. In addition, the reaction of the immune system to the sudden appearance of large numbers of tumor cells may be different than its reaction to a slowly developing (and changing) cancer clone.

Cancers induced by chemical carcinogens and exogenous viruses are *autochthonous*—i.e., they develop from the outset in the host under study. However, these methods also have problems, in particular that large doses of oncogenic agents are given to especially susceptible organisms in order to get tumor yields great enough to study. The use of viruses brings with it the possibility that stress-induced modulation of host anti-viral defenses may be critical to the outcome. However, this possibility could reduce those studies' relevance to the human situation because few human cancers appear to derive from exogenous viruses. The study of truly "spontaneous" animal cancers (those in which the researcher does nothing to induce or speed tumor development) is rare because such cancers are themselves relatively rare and because many of their characteristics are almost by definition unknown.

There have been few direct comparisons between tumor systems in response to stress manipulations, but there is some evidence for the importance of the tumor system variable (Justice, 1985; Newberry et al., 1985). One dramatic demonstration was by Albert (1967), who found that crowding inhibited the development of mammary tumors in mice but promoted mesenchymal cancers in the same animals. Greenberg et al. (1984) reported that early host defense against the YAC-1.3 and SLC-5 lymphomas was compromised by a 15-minute shock session, but this did not occur with P815 mastocytoma. Newberry and Mactutus (unpublished) found that both predictable restraint and a varied, unpredictable stress regimen inhibited the development of chemically induced rat mammary tumors. However, spontaneous (viral) mouse mammary tumors responded differently; they were not affected by predictable restraint and were stimulated by the unpredictable regimen. Riley and colleagues used infection with lactate dehydrogenase-elevating virus as a stressor in several experiments. This infection stimulated development of a transplanted lymphoma and a partially histoincompatible B-16 melanoma, had no effect on a histocompatible B-16 (Riley et al., 1982), and inhibited development of mammary tumors (Riley, 1966). Recent research seems to suggest that the development of chemically induced tumors tends to be inhibited by stress, whereas transplanted tumors and experimental metastases tend to be stimulated by stress (Newberry et al., in press).

Human Research

The experimental model work prepares one for a variety of outcomes in the human studies relating psychologic factors to cancer.

Several reviews and discussions are available (e.g., Bieliauskas, 1984; Fox, 1978, 1988; Morrison & Paffenbarger, 1981; Temoshok & Heller, 1984). These authors have been mindful of the problems of getting good data in this area and the seeming inconsistencies in the findings.

Hypotheses about stress-relevant individual differences have been at least as prominent as a general stress-cancer hypothesis. Two ideas stand out in this personality-based theorizing. One is the rather simple hypothesis that depression (not necessarily of pathologic severity) or hopelessness predicts unfavorable outcomes. Bieliauskas (1984) and Bieliauskas and Garron (1982) have discussed depression and cancer. They concluded that the evidence favors depression as a predictor and they would see a depression-cancer link as reflecting a stress-cancer link.

The second individual differences hypothesis, which might be termed a repression/compliance view, is more complex and seems to have several variants. Temoshok & Heller (1984, p. 255) stated themes which they see in the research findings and which illustrate this idea. As they put it, cancer may be associated with, "difficulty in expressing emotions or even feeling them," and with "niceness, industriousness, perfectionism, sociability, conventionality, and more rigid controls of defensiveness." Eysenck (1984) said something similar in suggesting that emotionality (his neuroticism variable) and/or strong emotions are associated with reduced cancer development.

The repression/compliance idea can be hard to differentiate from the possibility that stress has a protective role. It seems to predict that surface signs of distress should be *negatively* associated with cancer, but encourages one to think that underneath, the cancer-prone are really in greater distress than others. Selective interpretation of the data becomes a potential problem. If a study finds worse outcomes predicted by greater disturbance, dysphoria, psychic pain, or life adversity, then distress is associated with cancer. If, on the other hand, the bad outcomes are predicted by less disturbance, pain, or adversity, then the cancer subjects may be said to be defending and, though not expressing it, still the more distressed. Hypotheses which are not refutable are illegitimate, and this one could come close to being non-refutable unless handled gingerly.

Because the results are diverse and because we see cancer as a microcosm of the problems and potentials of a psychobiologic approach to disease, we shall take the space to describe several individual studies rather than summarizing reviews.

Quite a few investigations have used variables relevant to both the depression and the repression/compliance hypotheses, and thus we cannot group them on that basis. Instead, we shall organize this presentation in terms of whether the research was intended to account for the initial development of the disease or the post-diagnosis course of the disease. Psychologic factors might sometimes influence earlier and later disease differently. The pathologic processes themselves are likely to be changing over time. Also, the involvement of the medical system brings new factors into play, factors such as knowledge of diagnosis, others' reactions to the patients, and the often great rigors of medical therapy.

We shall discuss the implications of the research with the aid of Table 5 (below). That table lists variables that did and did not predict cancer outcomes in studies we mention.

Research on Prediagnosis Psychologic Factors —

These studies attempt to identify psychologic precursors of cancer, or at least of the diagnosis. Some of the studies are retrospective, but still attempt to focus on premorbid factors. Several reports have dealt with cancer in general rather than with single types. Since different types of neoplasia might well relate differently to psychologic conditions, such studies may be difficult to interpret.

An oft-cited investigation of depression and cancer was reported by Persky et al. (1987). They did a 20-year follow-up of 2018 men from the Western Electric Health Study. The subjects were given both the Minnesota Multiphasic Personality Inventory (MMPI) and the 16 Personality Factor Questionnaire (16 PF) in 1957-59. MMPI depression clearly predicted cancer. The association was stronger for mortality than for incidence, was stronger in the 10 years immediately following depression assessment than in the next 10 years, and persisted after adjustment for several extraneous variables. Neither incidence nor mortality was predicted by any of the other psychologic variables (Table 5). Depression was also associated with non-cancer mortality. (A 17-year follow-up of these subjects was reported by Shekelle et al., 1981.)

In a prospective archival study, Tirrell (1987) looked at hopelessness from the standpoint of stressful events. She hypothesized that if hopelessness is important, events which portend longer exposures to uncontrollable aversive conditions should predict cancer development. The specific hypothesis was that prisoners who were diagnosed with cancer between 6 months and 5 years after incarceration would have received longer sentences than controls. A search of a state's prison records located 39 cases. Two controls were matched to each case, as well as prison records would permit, on demographics, incarceration history, alcohol and tobacco use, and family history of cancer. The cases had in fact received significantly longer sentences than the controls (about twice as long). Thus the Tirrell study supports the general idea that hopelessness/depression may predict cancer.

A different picture regarding depression comes from Kaplan and Reynolds (1988). They did a 17-year prospective analysis of cancer incidence and mortality in a representative sample (n = 6848) from a California county. There was no evidence that depression predicted cancer, though it predicted non-cancer mortality. A subsample of 1010 employed men was selected to allow a better comparison to be made with the Western Electric sample (Persky et al., 1987) but no significant depression-cancer association was found. Kaplan and Reynolds suggested that the difference between the Western Electric findings and theirs might reflect the fact that their depression measure had no items referring to physical symptoms.

A report by Dattore et al., (1980) suggested an inverse relationship between cancer and depression, although the statistical analyses presented are not as complete as one would wish. This archival study compared MMPI scores of 75 cancer cases with those of non-cancer controls. The controls included five subgroups—four with non-cancer diagnoses and one with no diagnoses. Subjects had been given the MMPI at least one year before any known diagnosis. By discriminant analysis, the cancer cases were lower on pre-diagnosis depression and higher on repressive tendencies than were the controls. The cancer group was older, but age seemed not to account for the personality-cancer relationship.

A long-term prospective study of 972 medical school graduates (Shaffer et al., 1987) used cluster analysis to form personality groups which could be compared for cancer incidence. Five clusters resulted from 14 personality scores; they were labeled bland-normal, healthy-sensitive, acting out-emotional, loner, and interpersonal conflicts. The overall difference among the groups in cancer incidence was significant. The acting out-emotional group had the lowest rate (0.7%) and the loner group the highest (11.1%) over 30 years. By our calculations each of those extreme groups differed significantly from one of the two "normal" groups. Tests on the individual personality variables were not reported. As Shaffer et al. pointed out, their findings support a general repression/compliance hypothesis. (Other analyses of cancer in this sample have been reported [e.g., Thomas et al., 1979].)

Several studies have looked at prediagnosis psychologic factors and breast cancer. In one of the best known, Greer and Morris (1975) studied 160 patients the day before biopsy, when the final diagnosis of breast cancer or benign disease was still unknown. Such designs, in which psychologic data are collected when cancer is only suspected, prevent treatment, knowledge of having disease, and others' responses to those factors from biasing results. However, the effects of the disease itself or suspicion of diagnosis can still bias the results.

Patients subsequently diagnosed with malignancies were more likely to have been judged as extreme in anger expression, expressing it either unusually seldom or unusually often. The tendency toward extreme anger suppression was stronger than that for extreme expression. The cancer cases were also more likely to be judged as extreme suppressors of other emotions. The strength of the tendencies toward abnormal expression of emotions in the cancer patients varied with age. The cancer and benign groups did not differ on a number of other variables (Table 5).

A similar investigation (Morris et al., 1981) compared 17 breast cancer and 32 benign cases. Overall, the cancer cases were slightly but significantly less anger expressive on an interview-derived measure, but when age was accounted for the difference was not significant. The youngest cancer group was lower on trait anxiety and neuroticism than the similar-age benign group. Cancer and benign patients did not differ on questionnaire measures of "psychoticism" (overt hostility, low desire for human contact), state anxiety, introversion-extraversion, or social desirability.

Scherg (1987) addressed the question of how patients' suspicions or fears regarding breast cancer might relate to responses on psychologic measures. The study was a reanalysis of data (Scherg et al., 1981) on women who had come to a German clinic for breast examination. The earlier analyses had not controlled for subjects' reasons for having the examination or for their fear of breast cancer, and only one psychosocial measure (Type A behavior pattern) had been related to cancer diagnosis. In the 1987 reanalysis, the responses of 75 newly diagnosed cancer cases were compared to those of benign breast disease cases matched on age and reason for having the exam. Fear of breast cancer was controlled by including it in regression analyses along with 14 psychosocial measures. The direction of relationship between each psychosocial variable and cancer was hypothesized from what we would term a repression/compliance viewpoint.

Anxiety was negatively related to cancer diagnosis. Adverse war experiences as a child (WW II), commitment to traditional values, and social desirability (tendency to respond in ways that make one look good) were positively associated with cancer. The variables which were not related to cancer are given in Table 5. Scherg emphasized that more relationships between psychosocial factors and cancer were found when reason for consultation and fear of breast cancer were controlled. Patients' suspicions and fears about disease in short-term prospective studies may actually obscure relationships between psychologic factors and cancer, making cases act more like healthy individuals.

Scherg and Blohmke (1988) studied selected life events in what is apparently the same sample used by Scherg (1987). They compared four groups: newly detected breast cancers, for whom the psychologic measures were presumably taken before the diagnoses were known (Scherg, 1987); previously diagnosed breast cancers; previously diagnosed cancers of other sites; and patients (controls) for whom there was no evidence of cancer. Four stressors were studied, namely early death of father or mother, marital separation (including bereavement), and exposure to traumatic war events. The cancer groups did not differ significantly on these variables and were combined for comparison to controls. The analyses tested the significance of age-adjusted relative risks. Early death of the father did not differentiate cases from controls, but the other stressors were positively associated with cancer. Further, relative cancer risk increased with the number of traumatic war events. Adding a measure of denial and repression did not improve discrimination between the groups.

A retrospective study by Jansen & Muenz (1984) compared patients with breast cancer to women with fibrocystic breast disease and healthy controls (total n = 222). (Fibrocystic disorders involve hyperplasia of breast connective tissue or ductal epithelium; the epithelial hyperplasia may be precancerous.) Comparisons were made on a total of 58 scales. Covariance analyses were used to attempt to correct for some, but not all, of the many demographic differences among the groups. Cancer subjects were significantly low on the "understanding" scale of the Personality Research Form. Ten of 28 individual items from an adjective check list discriminated the groups, and by our calculations, the cancer group was significantly different from one of the others on several of them (see Table 5). When significant check list items were added to a logistic regression after a subset of the demographic variables, four helped account for group membership.

Blohmke et al. (1984) did a short-term prospective study of lung cancer. All subjects were smokers. Carcinoma patients (n = 419) were compared with 419 healthy controls and 162 nonmalignant lung disease cases. The predictor variables were apparently quite similar to those employed by Scherg (1987) (cf. Bahnson & Bahnson, 1979). The predictors were grouped into 18 vaguely specified "complexes." In discriminant analyses, 8 complexes significantly differentiated the cancer and healthy groups. As far as we can determine from the presentation, cancer cases were assessed as less nervous, more conforming, more externally controlled, less prone to admit anger, higher in life change, higher in "subjective complaints" (somatic arousal symptoms), more depressed, and higher in "excessive sensitivity" (probably paranoid sensitivity [Scherg, 1987]). When the cancer cases were compared to the nonmalignant disease cases, the findings on nervousness, conformity, and life change were similar to those in the cancer-healthy comparison. The description of methods and results leaves us uncertain about what variables failed to relate to cancer diagnosis.

At least two relatively recent investigations have dealt with stress-relevant factors in leukocytic malignancies. Jacobs and Charles (1980) utilized the Holmes/Rahe life events measure and interviews of parents in a retrospective study of childhood cancers (mostly leukemias and lymphomas). The comparison group were clinic patients matched with cancer cases on sex, age, and socioeconomic status. The cancer cases had more reported psychosocial and somatic problems associated with their births and their mothers' pregnancies. The parents also reported greater overall life change in the family during the two years preceding the cancer diagnosis. Several specific life events also differentiated the groups (Table 5).

A study by Smith et al. (1984) is of particular interest because genetic factors were controlled. They investigated life stress in 22 bone marrow transplant patients and their healthy identical twins. Patients' twins were serving as donors. Both members of the twin pairs reported life events for the period prior to the diagnosis of the malignancies. Some pairs were assessed before the transplant was done and others after. Among twin pairs responding to the questionnaire before the transplant, the donors and recipients did not differ in stress scores. Among those assessed after the transplant, the healthy twins recalled significantly *more* stressful events than did their co-twins.

Goodkin et al. (1986) utilized a quasi-prospective design to investigate a number of psychologic and social factors in five patient groups (total n = 73) undergoing biopsy of the uterine cervix. The biopsies were scored for degree of neoplastic promotion/progression. Degree of tumor promotion appeared to be related to demographic variables, but test statistics on those relationships were not reported. Life stress for six months before the biopsy was correlated significantly ($+.25$) with level of tumor promotion. Neither stress scores for earlier periods nor hopelessness was related to the outcome measure.

Goodkin et al. used 12 of 20 scales from the Millon Behavioral Health Inventory in an attempt to identify variables moderating the stress-neoplasia association. That association was more positive for patients higher on "premorbid pessimism," "life threat reactivity," and "somatic anxiety," and for those low on "cooperative coping style."

There is some evidence that exercise is associated with reduced cancer risk. Vena et al. (1985) compared 486 colon and rectal cancer patients to 1431 patients with other disorders. A history of work in occupations requiring little or no exercise was associated with colon cancer, but not with rectal. These findings suggest that the relationship between exercise and cancer depends upon cancer site. Since the controls in this study were patients, the data also imply that colon cancer and non-malignant disease have different relationships to exercise.

Prediction of Post-Diagnosis Course —

It would be useful for practical purposes to know whether psychologic factors can predict the eventual outcomes for cancer patients. In addition, to the extent that the pathologic processes of pre-diagnosis and post-diagnosis disease are the same, post-diagnosis studies bear on the pre-diagnosis question. This is important because it is easier to do prospective research on post-diagnosis disease course.

Most of these studies have focused on a single type of cancer, something that is more feasible in this context than in pre-diagnosis research. An exception is an investigation by Cassileth et al. (1985). They studied two groups. One consisted of 204 patients with disease (5 sites) so advanced that average survival time would be brief. These patients were followed for length of survival. For the second group, 155 melanoma or breast cancer cases with somewhat better outlooks, time until recurrence was assessed. The psychosocial predictors were social ties and marital history, general life satisfaction, job satisfaction, use of drugs for anxiety or depression, subjective judgments of health before the cancer, hopelessness/helplessness, and perceived degree of adjustment needed in coping with the malignancy. A total psychosocial score was also employed. Several analyses were done, the upshot being that the psychosocial factors failed to predict outcomes for either of the patient groups (e.g., correlations between total psychosocial score and time to death or relapse of -0.02 and -0.01). Cassileth et al. did not report separate analyses for different cancer sites.

Breast cancer is well represented among studies of psychologic factors and disease course. Marshall and Funch (1983) used major life events (for the 5 years before diagnosis) and social involvement in an attempt to account for survival time in 268 patients. They did not give bivariate test statistics, but several multiple regressions were computed. In the youngest patient group, involvement was associated with longer survival when stress was the only other predictor. When disease state and cancer history were included, neither stress nor involvement was related to survival time.

Greer et al. (1979) used several psychologic measures to predict status after 5 years. The only psychologic predictor associated with outcome was patient response to the cancer as coded from an interview. Patients classified as showing either optimism plus instrumental coping ("fighting spirit") or denial were less likely to have suffered recurrence or death than were patients showing "stoic acceptance" or "helplessness/hopelessness." Among the most interesting failures to predict were emotional expressiveness (which did predict in Greer and Morris, 1975), depression (cf. Persky et al. 1987), and social adjustment (cf. Marshall & Funch, 1983). (See Table 5 for other variables that did not predict.)

Derogatis et al. (1979) compared 22 metastatic breast carcinoma patients who survived for at least a year with 13 who did not. The two groups did not differ on several medical variables, but the short-term survivors had had more chemotherapy. The long-term survivors had expressed greater distress at the beginning of the study. They were higher on hostility, psychoticism, depression, guilt, and two summary indices of negative affect. They were also rated as having less positive attitudes toward their illness and treatment. As usual, several variables did not predict (Table 5). Derogatis et al. took survivors' reports of greater distress to mean less use of repressive coping, though the data provided no test of that interpretation.

Disregulation theory (e.g., Schwartz, 1984) provided the context for a study of breast cancer by M. Jensen (1987). The major hypothesis was that cancer progression would be associated with a repressive style of coping—operationalized as simultaneous high social desirability and low reported anxiety, and presumably indicating cerebral inattention to internal signals about host-tumor balance. Jensen studied two breast cancer groups. At the beginning of the study, one (n = 25) had had disease recurrence following initial treatment and the other (n = 27) had not. Subjects responded to several questionnaires in addition to the social desirability and anxiety measures. Psychological testing was done about 3 years after diagnosis and so patients with truly rapidly advancing disease could not have been included. Final disease outcome data were gathered after a variable follow-up period (around 2 years) or at death. The major outcome variable was the arithmetic product of a final clinical staging score and a 5-point rating of growth rate. The two patient groups were combined in statistical analyses. Final status was worse in patients classed as repressors.

Several psychologic variables were significant predictors of outcome when entered into hierarchical multiple regressions last, after a set of biomedical variables and the other psychologic measures. Jensen noted that interrelationships among the predictor variables complicated interpretation of the results. (This may happen in many multivariate studies, but go undetected.) The clearest findings were associations of poor outcome with repression and positive daydreaming. Other relationships were less clear, but still significant in at least one test (see Table 5).

Levy et al. (1985) investigated correlates of a prognostic indicator, lymph node involvement. They also assessed natural killer (NK) cell activity. The psychosocial variables used included general psychologic symptomatology, mood, adjustment to illness, and an interview dealing with social relationships and support. NK and psychosocial measures were taken 5-7 days after surgery, before any radiotherapy or chemotherapy had begun. Low NK activity was significantly associated with degree of nodal involvement. Good rated adjustment to illness, less perceived social support, and fatigue predicted NK activity in a stepwise regression. Fatigue predicted nodal status when NK activity was not controlled, but none of the psychologic variables predicted when NK was controlled.

In a later study Levy and her colleagues (Levy et al., 1988) looked at post-recurrence survival. Thirty-six patients took the Affect Balance Scale (ABS) before treatment for the recurrence commenced. Two ABS variables apparently predicted whether patients would be above or below the median on survival time. Longer survivors had higher scores on a joy scale and on overall positive mood. In multivariate analyses to predict cancer death, joy was significant when entered after length of the disease-free interval preceding recurrence. Joy was negatively related to number of metastatic sites detected at recurrence.

Spiegel et al. (1989) reported a very interesting outcome in which a psychologic intervention was associated with breast cancer survival.

Patients with advanced disease were randomly assigned either to a control condition in which they received only regular oncology treatment or to a behavioral intervention intended to assist them in coping with their disease. Although the treatment was intended to improve quality, not quantity of life, the intervention group survived significantly longer than the controls. This effect held when several other variables were controlled for one at a time. An unspecified battery of psychologic tests was given at the beginning of the study but those tests did not predict survival time.

The Spiegel et al. results are encouraging. The authors were appropriately cautious in considering what might have mediated their effect, but if this finding can be replicated it could lead to real improvements in understanding how and when psychologic factors will affect cancer.

We can give three examples of post-diagnosis studies on malignant melanoma. Rogentine et al. (1979) reported that self-reported response to melanoma predicted freedom from disease one year post-surgery. Patients responded to several questionnaires, and responses to a question, on "the amount of personal adjustment needed to handle or cope with" melanoma and the surgery, predicted recurrence. The relapsing patients had reported less need for adjustment. Rogentine et al. emphasized the possibility that those destined to relapse were denying or repressing the shock of the disease. Number of positive lymph nodes at surgery also predicted relapse, and this was uncorrelated with the adjustment score. Adjustment score seemed to predict recurrence only for cases with fewer than 7 positive nodes, something consistent with the failure of Cassileth et al. (1985) to find psychosocial factors predicting outcome in advanced malignancies. Fox (Temoshok & Fox, 1984) did not find the melanoma adjustment variable to predict later relapses in this sample.

Temoshok et al. (1985) were interested in part in the associations of a "Type C" behavior pattern. Type C is even more divergent from the hostile, competitive, time urgent characteristics of Type A than is Type B. C's try to please others; they avoid conflict and the expression of negative feelings. Temoshok et al. studied the relationship of several psychologic factors to the seriousness of the tumor (tumor thickness and invasion) in 59 recently diagnosed melanoma patients. Thus the study was, like Levy et al. (1985), a retrospective study of possible prognostic features of the cancer. By simple correlations, greater tumor thickness and/or depth were associated with several behavioral factors—lower occupational status, less knowledge of melanoma and its treatment, higher faith (in God and physicians), less self-involvement (less narcissism), a less histrionic (less self-dramatizing) style, and greater nonverbal Type C characteristics. However these variables were not significant when entered in a multiple regression after age and skin pigmentation. Delay in seeking treatment was significant in regression analysis.

In a later paper (Temoshok et al., 1988), this group reported a follow-up for remission of melanoma. Subjects who had died or had developed metastases were compared with a group who were still free of disease 3-4 years after the psychologic measures were taken. It was not clear how well-matched the final groups were. Though the sample was small (25) there were clear differences between relapsed and non-relapsed patients. On seven measures, the relapsers were more distressed or dysphoric (Table 5). On several of these variables (e.g., manifest anxiety, MMPI distress, and depression-dejection and anger-hostility from the Profile of Mood States) relapsers' scores had been over twice those of the non-relapsers.

Edwards et al. (1985) considered survival of testicular cancer. Patients were given self-report inventories after surgery and prior to the initiation of any chemotherapy. Comparisons were made between 7 patients who died within a year and 19 patients who survived for at least 7 years. The groups did not differ significantly on stage or histologic type of disease, or on three demographic variables. Short-term survivors had been less introverted. They also had higher levels of self-regard, and less distress on a summary index of dysfunctional emotions. Like others, Edwards et al. attributed these differences to short-term survivors' inability to express distress rather than to their actually being less distressed.

STRESS-CANCER CONCLUSIONS

What can we make of the research on stress-related factors and human cancer? Not as much as we would like, it seems. Table 5 is intended to illustrate the problem. It summarizes the variables that did and did not relate to cancer outcome in all but two of the studies we discussed. (The reports by Blohmke et al. [1984] and Spiegel et al. [1989] do not provide enough information on variables which failed to predict outcome.) For variables which did predict, the wording in the table reflects what was associated with poorer outcomes for subjects (greater incidence, shorter survival times, etc.) The note at the end of Table 5 describes the way we grouped the predictor variables. This arrangement should be taken only as an attempt to help readers locate

Table 5. Variables Associated and Not Associated with Cancer Outcome Measures in Some Human Studies

Associated with (Poorer) Outcome	Not Associated with Cancer Outcome

PRE-DIAGNOSIS STUDIES

PERSKY ET AL., 1987 (Multiple Cancers)

[3]: Greater depression.	[2]: Repression. [3]: Psychasthenia. [5]: Assertiveness. Self sufficiency. Tendermindedness/dependency. [6]: Paranoia. Shrewdness vs. artlessness. Social introversion. Suspiciousness. [7]: Conscientiousness vs. expedience. Conservatism vs. free thinking. Psychopathic deviance. Prudence/soberness vs. enthusiasm. Reserve. Shyness vs. venturesomness. Social carelessness. [8]: Apprehension vs. placidness. Emotional stability vs. upset. Hypomania. Tenseness vs. drivenness. [9]: Hypochondriasis. [10]: Intelligence. [12]: Hysteria. Imaginativeness vs. practicality. Masculinity vs. femininity. Schizophrenia.

TIRRELL, 1987 (Multiple Cancers)

[1]: Longer prison sentences.	----------------------

KAPLAN & REYNOLDS, 1988 (Multiple Cancers)

----------------------	[3]: Depression.

DATTORE ET AL., 1980 (Multiple Cancers)

[2]: Greater tendency to repression. [3]: Lower depression. [12]: Less denial of hysteria.	[3]: Psychasthenia. [6]: Social introversion. [7]: Psychopathic deviance. [8]: Hypomania. [9]: Hypochondriasis. [12]: Schizophrenia.

SHAFFER ET AL., 1987 (Multiple Cancers)

[4]: Less acting out emotionally. [6]: Greater likelihood of being classed as a loner.	[1]: Interpersonal conflict.

GREER & MORRIS, 1975 (Breast)

[4]: Extreme suppression of anger. Extreme expression of anger. Extreme suppression of other emotions.	[1]: Life stress. [2]: Denial in response to stress. Social desirability. [3]: Depression. [6]: Introversion. Social adjustment (marital, sexual, interpersonal, work). [8]: Hostility. Neuroticism. [10]: Intelligence. [12]: Psychiatric illness in response to stress.

Table 5 (continued)

Associated with (Poorer) Outcome	*Not Associated with Cancer Outcome*

MORRIS ET AL., 1981 (Breast)

[8]: Low anxiety. Low neuroticism.

[2]: Social desirability. **[4]**: Expression of anger. **[6]**: Introversion. Psychoticism.

SCHERG, 1987 (Breast)

[1]: More adverse war experiences. **[2]**: Higher social desirability. **[7]**: High commitment. **[8]**: Low anxiety.

[1]: Adverse childhood. Recent life events. **[3]**: Depression. **[4]**: Suppression of anger. **[5]**: Authoritarianism. Dependence. External control (tendency to adapt to outside world). **[6]**: Paranoid sensitivity (to others' opinions). Type A. **[9]**: Somatization.

SCHERG & BLOHMKE, 1988 (Breast)

[1]: More likely early death of mother. More likely separated/widowed. More likely traumatic war experiences.

[1]: Early death of father.

JANSEN & MUENZ, 1984 (Breast)

[4]: Less expression of anger. **[5]**: Less assertiveness. Less demandingness. More timidity. Less strong will. **[6]**: Low understanding. **[8]**: Less restlessness. **[10]**: Less competitiveness. Less striving.

[1]: Pressure. **[3]**: Apathy. Depression. Locus of control. **[5]**: Autonomy. Confidence. Dependence. Dominance. Passivity. **[6]**: Affiliation. Nurturance. Type A. **[7]**: Caution. Impulsivity. Irresponsibility. Order. **[8]**: Aggression. Anxiety. Being low keyed. Ease of upset. Happiness. Harm-avoidance. Hostility. Irritability. Joyousness. Play. Sensitivity. Tension. Worry. **[10]**: Achievement. Ambition. Industriousness. Social recognition. **[12]**: Endurance. Energy. Exhibition.

JACOBS & CHARLES, 1980 (Childhood Cancers)

[1]: Greater overall life stress. Difficult birth. More maternal somatic or emotional problems during pregnancy. More health/behavior change in family. More change in residence. Pregnancy (with patient) less likely to have been planned.

[1]: Change in schools. Change in social activities. Change in spousal arguments. Change in wife's working. Child leaving home. Death in family. Financial change in family. Frequency of childhood infectious illnesses. Gain of new family member. Injury/illness to family member. Parental marital separation.

Table 5 (Continued)

Associated with (Poorer) Outcome	*Not Associated with Cancer Outcome*

SMITH ET AL., 1984 (Hematologic)

----------------------- | [1]: Overall life stress.

GOODKIN ET AL., 1986 (Uterine Cervix)

[1]: High life stress. | [3]: Hopelessness.

VENA ET AL., 1985 (Colon)

[1]: Low occupational exercise. | -----------------------

VENA ET AL., 1985 (Rectal)

----------------------- | [1]: Occupational exercise.

POST-DIAGNOSIS STUDIES

CASSILETH ET AL., 1985 (Multiple Cancers)

----------------------- | [1]: Job satisfaction. [3]: Hopelessness/helplessness. [6]: Social ties & marital status. [8]: General life satisfaction. Use of psychotropic drugs for anxiety or depression. [9]: Subjective view of adult health. [11]: Amount of adjustment required to cope with the cancer.

MARSHALL & FUNCH, 1983 (Breast)

[6]: Low social involvement. | [1]: Life stress.

GREER ET AL., 1979 (Breast)

[11]: Psychologic response to disease (less denial/fighting spirit; more helplessness/stoic acceptance). | [1]: Life stress. [3]: Depression. [4]: Expression/suppression of anger. [6]: Extraversion. Social adjustment (marital, sexual, interpersonal, work). [8]: Habitual reaction to stressful events. Hostility. Neuroticism.

DEROGATIS ET AL., 1979 (Breast)

[3]: Low depression. Low guilt. [6]: Low psychoticism. [8]: Low hostility. Low negative affect total. High (positive) affect balance. [11]: More positive attitude toward illness and treatment. | [3]: Depression. [6]: Affection. Interpersonal sensitivity. [7]: Obsessive-compulsiveness. [8]: Anxiety. Contentment. Joy. Hostility. Phobic anxiety. Positive symptom total. Vigor. [9]: Somatization. [11]: Global adjustment to illness. [12]: General (psychologic) symptom severity.

Table 5 (Continued)

Associated with (Poorer) Outcome	*Not Associated with Cancer Outcome*
JENSEN, 1987 (Breast)	
[1]: Greater chronic stress. [2]: Greater repressive defensiveness. [3]: Greater helplessness/hopelessness. [4]: Low expression of negative affect. [8]: More positive daydreaming.	[1]: Recent stress and social support. [2]: Absorption. Attentional control. Self-deception. [3]: Guilt/failure daydreaming. [6]: Interactive style. Other-deception. [7]: Self-presentation (as a serious person). [8]: Emotionality.
LEVY ET AL., 1985 (Breast)	
[3]: Greater fatigue (apathy, listlessness).	[6]: Interpersonal sensitivity. Paranoid ideation. [7]: Obsessive-compulsiveness. [8]: Anxiety. Hostility. Phobic anxiety. Summary distress scores. [9]: Somatic concern. [11]: Global adjustment to illness.
LEVY ET AL., 1988 (Breast)	
[8]: Lower joy. Lower overall positive mood.	[3]: Depression. Guilt. [6]: Affection. [8]: Anxiety. Contentment. Hostility. Overall negative affect. Vigor.
ROGENTINE ET AL., 1979 (Melanoma)	
[11]: Less adjustment required to cope with the cancer.	[3]: Depression. Locus of control. [6]: Interpersonal sensitivity. Paranoid ideation. Psychoticism. [7]: Obsessive-compulsiveness. [8]: Anxiety. Hostility. Overall distress score. Phobic anxiety. Positive symptom total. [9]: Somatization. [12]: General (psychologic) symptom severity.
TEMOSHOK ET AL., 1985 (Melanoma)	
[4]: Less histrionic style. [5]: Greater non-verbal Type C. Higher faith. [8]: Lower narcissism. [10]: Lower occupational status. [11]: Less knowledge of melanoma and its treatment.	[1]: Life stress. [4]: Emotional expressiveness. [5]: Type C. [6]: Type A. [8]: Psychologic distress. [11]: Catastrophic reaction to cancer. Coping with cancer by avoidance. Coping with cancer by changing attitudes. Coping with cancer by denial. Coping with cancer by optimism. Coping with cancer by strength. Minimizing seriousness of cancer.

Table 5 (Continued)

Associated with (Poorer) Outcome	*Not Associated with Cancer Outcome*

TEMOSHOK ET AL., 1988 (Melanoma)

[3]: Greater depression. Greater depression-dejection. Greater fatigue-inertia. **[8]**: Greater anger-hostility. Greater anxiety. Greater distress. Greater tension-anxiety.	**[2]**: Social desirability. **[8]**: Vigor-activity. **[12]**: Confusion.

EDWARDS ET AL., 1985 (Testicular)

[6]: Lower social introversion. **[8]**: Higher self-regard. Lower overall distress.	**[3]**: Depression. Guilt. Psychasthenia. **[4]**: Acceptance of aggression. **[5]**: Independence. Sensitivity to values & principles. **[6]**: Affection. Capacity for intimate relationships. Interpersonal sensitivity. Paranoia. Paranoid ideation. Psychoticism. **[7]**: Living in the present. Obsessive-compulsiveness. Psychopathic deviance. Spontaneity. **[8]**: Anxiety. Contentment. Hostility. Hypomania. Joy. Phobic anxiety. Vigor. **[9]**: Hypochondriasis. Somatization. **[12]**: Hysteria. Masculinity-femininity. Perspectives on masculinity-femininity. Relationship of opposites to life. Schizophrenia. Sexual attitudes. Sexual drive. Sexual experience. Sexual information.

Note: The numbers in brackets refer to a rough classification of variables as follows: [1]: Stressful circumstances. [2]: Denial or repressive tendencies. [3]: Depression-related variables. [4]: Expression of emotion. [5]: Social complaisance vs. independence. [6]: Other interpersonal variables or tendencies. [7]: Impulsivity and related variables. [8]: Emotion and self-perception. [9]: Somatization. [10]: Achievement-related variables. [11]: Response to cancer and/or treatment. [12]: Miscellaneous. When a predictor variable was related to cancer outcome, the wording in the table reflects the characteristic associated with poorer outcome.

particular types of variables, and not as a technically valid classification. What Table 5 makes clear is that little is clear.

Of the reports we mentioned, six presented significant positive associations between stressors and cancer outcomes, but six others did not find such a relationship. Jacobs and Charles (1980), Scherg (1987), and Scherg and Blohmke (1988) found that some stressors predicted while others did not. Depression or hopelessness may be associated with poorer outcomes (at least 2 studies), with better outcomes (2 studies) or may fail to relate to outcome (4 studies). Indices of emotional expression were significantly related to cancer outcome variables in at least 4 studies, but were not in at least 3 others.

The same sort of thing holds for social style. Being a loner, low assertiveness and competitiveness, low social involvement, and low introversion (perhaps indicating high sociability) were associated with worse outcomes in studies we discussed. In other studies introversion, assertiveness and numbers of other relevant variables (e.g., affiliation, autonomy, capacity for intimate relationships, dependence, dominance, interpersonal sensitivity, irresponsibility, shyness, social adjustment, Type A) were not related significantly to cancer dependent variables.

As still another example, consider persons' reactions to the disease. In two reports, reactions to cancer predicted outcomes, but in 4 others they did not.

Even though defensiveness has tended to be associated with the idea of social complaisance, it actually cuts across other issues; one can be defensive about nearly anything. If defensiveness is crucial, many other variables are nearly useless because they can have two nearly opposite meanings. This problem is made worse by the fact that defensiveness is difficult to operationalize with confidence. Though several authors have suggested that defensiveness/denial/repression is a critical variable, only three of the studies we discussed (Dattore et al., 1980; Greer et al., 1979; M. Jensen, 1987) have dealt with it explicitly and found it to predict. And Greer et al. (1979) found denial to be associated with *better* outcome. We cannot even guess whether any of the discrepancies in the psychooncology literature reflect unmeasured effects of defensiveness. (Note that the defensiveness question is not limited to cancer, even though it has been most emphasized in discussions of this class of disorder.)

Differences among studies in assessment instruments, sample sizes, statistical analyses, types and stages of malignancy, and temporal factors also contribute to the confusion in the stress-cancer area. The trouble is that there are not enough data to sort these things out.

Fox (1988, p. 50) summarized the evidence on "internal psycho-social factors" and cancer by saying, "We are in no position to identify any such factor as presenting more than a stimulating hypothesis. No firm position can be taken in regard to an association between any such factor and cancer incidence, mortality, or progression." The human research is indeed stimulating. With animal studies clearly demonstrating stimulation and inhibition of cancers by stress, there is good reason to believe that something is happening. We just don't know yet what it is.

OTHER DISORDERS

A stress perspective has been considered in many medical problems beyond those we have already mentioned. Space permits us to mention only a few. Even with those we must limit ourselves to brief descriptions and citations of a few studies or discussions.

Arthritis

"Arthritis" means joint inflammation, but there are several types (e.g., Robbins et al., 1984). Literal inflammation may not always be present. Temporary arthritis may be produced by a variety of conditions, including infections in the joints. The common types of chronic arthritis are *osteoarthritis* (OA) and *rheumatoid arthritis* (RA). OA, or degenerative joint disease, is characterized by relatively straightforward injury to joint cartilage. It is associated with obesity and aging, suggesting that wear exceeding chondrocytes' (cartilage-forming cells') ability to respond is an important mechanism. Joint disease earlier in life seems to predispose to OA. Cartilage destruction results in damage to the underlying bone, the development of bone spurs, pain, and gradually increasing disability.

RA, with which most stress-relevant research has dealt, is quite a different thing (Anderson et al., 1985; Robbins et al., 1984). It has systemic as well as articular manifestations, and it involves autoimmunity. In joints, RA seems to begin with a leukocyte infiltration of the synovia (the fluid which lubricates and cushions joints) and with inflammation of the synovium (the membrane which encloses the synovia). Inflammation of blood vessels often occurs. As the disease progresses, the joint cartilage, bone, and ligaments are damaged. Joint spaces can become filled with fibrous or bony tissue. Eventually joints can deform and even fuse. Systemic aspects of RA include pulmonary fibrosis, inflammation of the heart, and rheumatoid nodules in a variety of organs.

The synovial inflammation in RA is apparently an autoimmune phenomenon. *Rheumatoid factor*, an antibody to the Fc portion of immunoglobulin, is very frequently present. Immune complexes (antibody bound to antigen), complement activation, and the attraction of leukocytes (particularly neutrophils) then participate in the inflammation. The trigger for this autoimmune response is still apparently unknown, however. *Juvenile RA* may differ in pathogenesis from adult-onset RA, as indicated by the fact that rheumatoid factor is less often present.

Internal loop effects of stress-related variables might occur on the development of the autoimmune response, on the inflammatory process (whether or not it reflects autoimmunity), or conceivably on the responsiveness of cartilage and bone to immune and inflammatory attack. Stress-induced muscle tension has also been considered as it may put extra strain on joints. However, that does not accord well with current views of RA etiology (Koehler, 1985) and seems more plausible for OA.

Anderson et al. (1985) are among those who have discussed the relationship of psychologic factors to RA. They suggested that the literature on a possible arthritis-prone personality is too confusing and poor for conclusions to be drawn (cf. Solomon, 1981). Anderson et al. did indicate that stressful situations seem to precede the appearance of RA, although they noted that the research has often had methodologic problems. Koehler (1985) was not so optimistic about stress associations with RA, noting a general inconsistency in the findings and the fact that two large early studies found no relationship. He also pointed out that animal model studies have produced inconsistent results.

Among Koehler's suggestions was the idea that different types of RA should be considered separately. In a study supporting that view Vollhardt et al. (1982) compared three groups of arthritics on measures of mood and psychologic symptoms. The group with the worst disease (i.e., rheumatoid factor-positive and with demonstrable joint erosion) was rather clearly less disturbed than the other groups. Vollhardt et al. suggested defensiveness as the reason for the relative psychologic tranquility of those worse off physically.

Keltikangas-Järvinen et al. (1988) reported a relationship between arthritis and life stress in children with juvenile and temporary arthritis. Control data were taken from an earlier large study of stress in healthy children. The two arthritis groups did not differ in life stress, but both were significantly higher in stress than expected from the healthy children's data. In this study, then, subjects with different types of arthritis were similar on the psychologic predictor, and being physically worse was associated with the presumably greater distress.

There has been some research using behavioral interventions in arthritis. Weinberger et al. (1986) attempted to improve the status of OA patients by giving them social support via telephone interviews. Questionnaires on stressors, social support and arthritis-related disability were given at the beginning of the study and at the end, 6 months later. Patients' reported disability and pain diminished over the study, but as there was neither a control group nor a final medical examination, the meaning of that change is obscure at best. When entered into multiple regression analyses after initial disability or pain scores, hassles reported at the beginning of the study were not significantly related to the level of physical disability or pain reported at 6 months.

O'Leary et al. (1988) compared RA patients given a 5-week cognitive behavioral treatment with controls matched on pain level and medication. At the end of the study period, joint disability—as assessed by physicians blind to patients' group assignments—was apparently less in the intervention group.

Pain Disorders

Pain accompanies many diseases, but there are disorders in which pain itself—pain without obvious organic damage—is the major problem. Common types of headache, chronic back pain (CBP), and temporomandibular pain disorder (TMD) are among medical problems which fall under this heading. Pain involves particular neural pathways (e.g., Guyton, 1986), beginning with pain receptors (free nerve endings) and extending through the dorsal horns of the spinal gray and the thalamus. Mechanical damage, heat, ischemia, and certain chemical messengers such as prostaglandins can stimulate pain receptors. The psychologic severity of the pain depends upon the type of pathway activated. Central neural processes such as opioid systems can modify this input and alter the experience of pain. Cognitive variables are relevant to the totality of pain experience and thus psychologic interventions may be useful (Turk et al., 1983).

When pain occurs in the absence of clear tissue pathology, looking for functional explanations is a fruitful strategy. Muscle tension is the most frequently invoked process (e.g., Blanchard & Andrasik, 1982; Flor & Turk, 1989; Haber et al., 1983). Ischemia and mechanical deformation of nerve endings may contribute to such pain. Anyone who has suffered a charley horse knows that muscle spasm can be painful.

Skeletal muscle tension is a favored explanation for "tension" headache, CBP and TMD. Psychophysiologists have long recognized muscle tension as an index of arousal, and stress influences are therefore quite plausible. Feuerstein et al. (1985) found that some negative aspects of work situations and stress outside of work were associated with greater CBP, but job pressure was inversely related to pain. Speculand et al. (1984) studied recalled pre-symptom life events in TMD patients using age- and sex-matched pain-free dental patients as controls. Life stress was significantly greater for the TMD group. A prospective study of TMD improvement (Salter et al., 1986) found that the most improved patients were intermediate in initial psychologic disturbance, suggesting that moderate distress might be beneficial.

Theories of migraine headache focus on vascular smooth muscle. Constriction of intracranial vessels has been thought to occur prior to the onset of the headache, with the pain accompanying a rebound dilation (Blanchard & Andrasik, 1982). However, Feuerstein et al. (1983) did not find such a simple pattern. There were no overall differences in temporal artery blood volume pulse over 5-day periods ending with attacks, though several subjects showed significant dilation three days prior to the attack. Interestingly, the right temporal artery was more involved than the left. State anxiety did not change over the 5-day period, suggesting that psychologic distress was unrelated to headache occurrence.

Evidence that stress may be important in migraine was provided by Levor et al. (1986). Migraine sufferers kept diaries in which they recorded headaches and a number of other variables. Stressful events were more frequent on days preceding migraines than before non-headache target days. In addition, severity of hassles, assessed prior to the beginning of diary-keeping, was positively correlated with number of migraine days reported in the diaries.

Flor and Turk (1989) have done an excellent review of psycho-physiologic research on pain disorder subjects. They were critical of the methodology of many studies, but did draw some tentative conclusions. Headache sufferers and controls do not differ under baseline conditions, but headache-prone individuals often respond to stressors with more cranial muscle tension. Flor and Turk were less satisfied with the number of good studies on skeletal muscle tension in TMD and CBP and on vascular reactivity in migraine, but there are data suggesting high reactivity to stressors in those persons. Of course, one can always ask whether muscle tension arises in response to pain rather than (or in addition to) causing it.

There is an interesting contrast between the idea that stress participates in functional pain disorders and the phenomenon of stress analgesia (e.g., Watkins & Mayer, 1982). To the extent that stress/distress activates endogenous analgesic mechanisms, it should be associated with less pain, not more. Thus we might expect that when stressors induce the afferent pain signals to begin with, a positive association of stress with pain will be found. However, in other situations stress and pain could be inversely related.

Asthma

Bronchial asthma is difficult to define (Creer, 1988); its signs and symptoms can be shared with other disorders. A key characteristic, however, is obstruction of the airways in the lungs due to one or another sort of bronchial hyperresponsiveness (see Creer, 1988; Robbins et al., 1984). The obstructions are intermittent, of variable severity from attack to attack, and unlike the lesions of something like emphysema, are not permanent. The clinical picture includes dyspnea (labored breathing) with wheezing, mucous plugs in the airways, hyperinflation of the lungs due to difficulty in expelling air, and thickening and inflammation of the bronchial walls. *Status asthmaticus* is persistent attack, potentially fatal.

Robbins et al. classified types of asthma by what triggers attacks and how the airway blockage is mediated. The most common form is *atopic* asthma. This is a form of allergic reaction—that is, an immediate hypersensitivity response to inhaled allergens. Allergen binds to IgE on mucosal and submucosal mast cells, with numerous results. They include parasympathetic reflex bronchoconstriction, direct histamine bronchconstriction, increased vascular permeability, increases in bronchial secretions, the attraction of polymorphonuclear leukocytes, the release of leukotrienes and prostaglandin D_2, and the release of platelet activating factor with subsequent platelet aggregation and additional histamine release.

In non-atopic asthma, the second most common form, respiratory infections (particularly viral infections) precipitate attacks, probably through stimulation of bronchoconstriction reflexes. The most interesting of the rarer asthmas is aspirin-sensitive asthma. Aspirin inhibits the biosynthetic pathway leading from arachidonic acid to the prostaglandin family of compounds; in sensitive persons the blockage of this pathway strongly favors an alternate pathway to leukotriene synthesis. Increased leukotrienes will then trigger bronchoconstriction and vascular permeability.

Asthma is a bit of a paradox in relation to stress. Both gluco-corticoids and epinephrine are anti-asthmatic, enough so to be used in asthma treatment. Yet asthma attacks are universally acknowledged to be inducible by stress (e.g., by emotional situations and exercise). This seeming contradiction presumably means that the glucocorticoid and epinephrine levels reached under stress are not high enough to block the processes producing airway obstruction. (This illustrates a broader quantitative question: how often are the biologic changes produced under stress great enough to affect pathology?)

Creer (1988) dismissed a traditional psychosomatic view of asthma and instead emphasized the *behavior* which occurs in emotional situations. Laughing, crying, shouting, and intense locomotor activity are all emotional responses capable of precipitating asthma attacks. Cluss and Fireman (1985) have taken a wider view. They cited studies seeming to demonstrate that suggestion can alter bronchial reactivity and even trigger attacks, and studies indicating that asthmatics show greater bronchial responses to stressors. In a study by Strunk et al. (1985) conflicts between parents and medical personnel over the care of asthmatic children predicted their deaths after they left the hospital.

Recovery

Something which cuts across disease categories is recovery from acute medical events. The event may be a sudden illness such as stroke or myocardial infarction, or a medical procedure such as surgery. We have touched on related questions in earlier sections, as when we mentioned post-diagnosis interventions or discussed psychologic predictors of post-diagnosis disease course. Since there is considerable interest in the topic of recovery and it is often taken as a separate topic, we treat it briefly here. Our concern is chiefly with medical rather than psychologic outcomes, but these cannot always be differentiated very well. As ever, there are multiple mechanisms, both internal and external loops, through which stress-related variables might act.

One question of interest is whether psychologic interventions can affect recovery from medical procedures. The answer is relevant to practical matters of patient management as well as our basic understanding of stress. Psychotherapy, modeling, and the provision of information are among the procedures that have been studied. A review by

Anderson and Masur (1983) indicates that psychologic interventions can indeed improve patient status. However, as one would expect there are studies in which effects were not obtained and methodologic flaws in much of the research.

As one example of a recent study of preparation for a medical procedure, we cite Pinto and Hollandsworth (1989). Children were randomly assigned to view or not to view a videotape of a child model successfully coping with the surgery experience. Those who saw the tape recovered better than did controls. The recovery index combined ratings of vomiting, crying, fluid intake, ambulation, and pain. Ratings were made by nurses who did not know which children saw the tape.

Subtle variations in hospital environment may also affect recovery. Recovery from coronary bypass surgery was related to the type of hospital roommate the patient had prior to the operation (Kulik & Mahler, 1987). Patients did better post-operatively if their preoperative roommates were themselves post-operative. They reported more post-op walking and were discharged more quickly. The authors suggested that the post-op roommates provided information about the surgery/recovery experience and thus reduced threat. We would expect modeling effects as well. Perhaps even more subtle is an effect suggested by Ulrich (1984). Patients undergoing cholecystectomy (gall bladder removal) spent less post-operative time in the hospital, had fewer negative nursing notes, and took fewer doses of potent analgesics if their rooms looked out on trees rather than a brick wall.

If unobvious hospital variables are related to recovery, then nonhospital factors should be as well. Linn et al. (1988) found that life stress and cardiovascular response to a cold pressor test predicted postsurgical complications and narcotic use in otherwise healthy men who were undergoing hernia repair. Stress and stress responsiveness were associated with reduced lymphocyte mitogen response as well.

Social support has also been investigated in the recovery context. Fontana et al. (1989) studied recovery from MI and bypass surgery over 12 months. They used a rather complex structural equation model to evaluate social support (taken as the inverse of loneliness), appraised threat from the illness, and general psychologic distress. We cannot detail the results, but basically the analyses suggested that social support reduced angina and dyspnea by reducing threat.

Unlike many who study social support, Stephens et al. (1987) investigated both positive and negative social interactions. The subjects were stroke patients with adequate speech who were assessed over the year following hospital discharge. Multiple regressions indicated that higher frequencies of negative social interaction were associated with lower morale and greater psychologic symptomatology. The authors also analyzed cognitive functioning at follow-up, something that might be considered a very relevant medical outcome in stroke. Those results indicated that more frequent positive social interaction was associated with less confusion and disorientation. The Stephens et al. findings remind us that social networks need not have only positive effects.

Psychologic factors have been suggested as participating in many other medical disorders and problems. Among those that we lack the space to discuss, the most prominent are gastrointestinal disorders such as ulcers, irritable bowel syndrome, and esophageal spasm (see, e.g., discussions by Winer, 1977; Whitehead & Bosmajian, 1982). A large animal literature on stress-induced stomach lesions suggests that stress effects on the GI system are complex (e.g., Overmier et al., 1985; Paré, 1986). (The rodent lesions are not comparable to typical human ulcers, but may be more like the rarer lesions which accompany severe physical trauma in humans.)

Birth complications (Istvan, 1986), renal failure (Burton et al., 1986), psoriasis (Arnetz et al., 1985), uticaria (Teshima et al., 1982), eating disorders (Heilbrun & Harris, 1986), and epilepsy (Temkin & Davis, 1984) have also been mentioned. The idea that stress-related factors affect medical disorders seems to have left scarcely a disease unexamined.

CONCLUSION

The reader may join us in our pleasure at nearing the end of this monograph. We need endure only the ritual of summing up.

We have had two major goals. The first has been to illustrate the complexity of the stress-disease question. The number of variables involved, the intricacy of their interactions, and the near-ubiquitousness of reciprocal influences present formidable obstacles to understanding these phenomena. Our second object has been to give readers enough specific information that they can pursue particular topics in more detail without being too perplexed by the terminology and the amount of information or too easily swayed by seductively simple hypotheses.

Although we hope that we have been able to represent the main themes of the area fairly well, we must reiterate that we have not done a comprehensive literature review. Hordes of studies and a substantial number of ideas have gone uncited. Readers who came to this volume with a good knowledge of any of the topics we touched upon will know how much we have had to leave out or simplify in their areas of expertise. Many details are missing from our accounts (and in many areas things are changing so rapidly that only those immersed in a topic can keep up).

Comments on the Stress-Disease Literature

No one can have read everything written on stress and disease. We have read a fair amount of it, however, and have developed some opinions about its character and quality. At this point we wish to comment on the way things are done and written; our views on what it adds up to substantively will be summarized below.

Early in the book, we considered conceptual and methodologic problems. Those problems will not go away, and they bear importantly on how one evaluates the stress-disease data. The term "stress" stands for so many variables that we might well despair of giving it a precise yet useful definition, but the term is probably too firmly entrenched to be abandoned.

There are other unavoidable problems as well. A critical one is the correlational nature of many types of human studies; this necessary limitation creates great difficulties in drawing cause-effect conclusions. Also unavoidable is the fact that animal and in vitro experiments, even though necessary, will rarely be exact models of the human situation.

Many of the limitations encountered in research on stress and disease are avoidable, however. Occasionally, studies are needlessly confounded; independent variables which could have been separated were not, and the data therefore cannot address the questions that the authors ask. One version of this is the needless failure to get information on extraneous variables in correlational studies. For anyone to take seriously the idea that depression contributes to the development of some disease, for example, there should be some sort of evidence that demographic variables and differences in disease status itself are not responsible for any observed association. Naturally, not all relevant variables can be controlled, but a study that does not make a reasonable attempt must be considered as very preliminary.

Related to the issue of extraneous variables is the quality of statistical analysis. Many are the studies that would have benefitted from more appropriate data analyses. The underutilization of multivariate methods stands out. Such methods are highly desirable for controlling the effects of extraneous variables or reducing the inflation in statistical significance level that accompanies the use of multiple dependent variables. There are few good reasons to avoid their use. Among the other statistical deficiencies to be found are the use of multiple pairwise tests instead of factorial analyses, the failure to use appropriate subsequent tests following analysis of variance, and the practice of analyzing different dependent variables with different techniques when that is not required by the nature of the data.

Something else which struck us about the research in this area is the scarcity of replications. Replication is fundamental to scientific work; nothing is quite acceptable until it has been found several times, and preferably by several investigators. (Witness the rush to replicate high-temperature superconductivity and cold fusion.) In a field such as stress and disease where there are multitudes of variables and few of them are well understood, the need for replication is even greater than in the physical sciences, but we have not noticed many scrambles to repeat intriguing observations. It is likely that some frequently cited findings are flukes, but there is no way to tell which ones. Investigators need to see replication as one of their primary obligations. Without it, knowledge simply is not cumulative; we get more data without more confidence.

The way in which methods and results are reported also affects the value of a piece of research. Too often, authors provide too little information. One reasonably common example is the human study in which readers are not told much about the conditions under which the subjects operated. If subjects know, for example, that the research is designed to determine whether stress affects disease, that knowledge might well affect their resposes. The reader needs to know rather precisely what the subjects are told. If subjects take several questionnaires, the reader needs to know in what order, since responding to one questionnaire may alter responses to subsequent ones.

Incomplete statistical reporting is particularly maddening. Authors will fail to report analyses of some variables (did the two patient groups differ significantly in age?); give only a part of a correlation matrix (A and B are both related to Y but how are they related to each other?); not mention some statistical tests (was that interaction significant or not?); fail to report all of the relevant information in multiple regressions (the overall model was significant, but what individual predictors were?); or describe their analysis protocols in ways which leave the reader guessing about what was actually done (were the factors in that combined index also tested separately?).

Incomplete reporting means that readers cannot make independent judgments about what results mean, or sometimes about what they really were. One can get the impression that authors sometimes do not want readers to discover certain things about their methods or results. Hopefully, that will always be a mistaken impression, but in any case inadequate reporting slows progress. If Smith cannot tell what Jones actually did or found, Smith is going to have a hard time building on Jones' work.

Relationship(s) Between Stress and Disease

Our carping about the literature largely done, we can ask what general conclusions are warranted about stress and disease. We offer the following as summations.

Stressors (and stress-relevant individual differences) can have a wide variety of effects on behavior and "normal" internal processes. This seems too obvious to need restating, but its implications are too important for it to be left out. Directly or indirectly, stress affects nearly all aspects of normal function. Moreover, stress effects appear from the evidence to be diverse; they depend significantly on the precise nature of the situation and the organism. Much of this diversity may stem from homeostatic and longer-term adaptational processes—i.e., from changes in stress responses with time and experience. However, not all of the variation in stress response patterns derives from such temporal changes, and even if it did, the implication would be much the same, namely that stress effects on disease should be non-uniform.

Different diseases can respond differently to the biologic processes that stress influences. The extent to which this is so is not clear, but it is certainly so to a significant degree. It is well known that the more or less routine action of the immune system can contribute to pathology as well as protect against pathology. Cancers definitely differ in their responses to stress-labile hormones. Exercise is rather clearly health-threatening in some ways and health-promoting in others. With regard to exogenous agents and potential external loop effects the same thing obtains. Aspirin, for instance, may protect against myocardial infarction but increase the risk of hemorrhagic stroke. There are many pathologies in which the plausible effects of stress will vary with the stage of the disease.

Another way to put this is to say host resistance to disease is not a unitary thing. To be sure, the idea of general resistance is not wholly useless; a catastrophic failure in any major homeostatic system is clearly capable of undermining others, and there are surely less dramatic manifestations of general resistance as well. But we are wise not to rely too much on this idea, particularly since we do not yet know how common the exceptions are.

Stress can influence disease. Some seem to doubt that psychologic factors, including stress, can affect disease. Angell (1985), for instance, questioned the quality and quantity of the evidence for direct (i.e., internal loop) effects of "mental state" on disease. We heartily endorse most of what Angell said about methodologic problems in much of the research, about interpretive biases on the part of authors, and about jumping from questionable (or nonexistent) data to the prescription of psychologic interventions.

However disease *is* in part a "reflection of the psyche" (Angell, p. 1570). Angell accepted the influence of health behaviors, but as such behaviors themselves reflect the psyche, so must the health or illness they engender. Even with regard to internal loop influences, the data are better than Angell's commentary might lead one to believe. Animal model studies have shown unambiguously that stressful conditions affect disease. In these studies food and water are typically the only exogenous agents free to vary, and while some stress effects may be due to changes in nutrient intake, it is vanishingly unlikely that all are.

It goes almost without saying that our understanding of stress and *human* disease is limited. Methodologic problems make definitive conclusions difficult to come by. It is even conceivable that there are no internal loop stress effects on human disease, but we doubt it. We do not see how the situation with animal models could be so vastly different from the human situation, and moreover the human data are certainly consistent with a role for stress. In any case the basic question, "Can stress affect disease?" has been answered quite clearly and in the affirmative.

Relationships between stress and disease are quite variable. It seems not to be true that stress is magically constrained only to stimulate disease processes. Stress-relevant variables have often failed to relate significantly to disease outcomes, and this has occurred with just about every type of disorder on which there is a literature of any size. The reader may recall the many cases described earlier in which seemingly similar studies produced different results. It has been acknowledged that there are circumstances under which stressful conditions will be unrelated to disease. The emphasis on stressor uncontrollability as disease-promoting is one such acknowledgement. The idea that certain personalities are relatively stress- and disease-resistant is another. Both of these general ideas have significant empirical support.

However, there is an even more troublesome difficulty for a general stress-promotes-disease hypothesis: *under some conditions stress should, and does, protect against disease.* This seems foreign to many. Even in conversations with knowledgeable researchers, a not untypical response to the idea is a look of apparent disbelief followed by some variant of, "I never heard of such a thing." The common hypothesis, that if stress is going to have an influence that influence must be detrimental, seems deeply ingrained.

It would be useful to contemplate the data, however. Again, the animal model findings are the clearest. The largest group of studies is probably that on experimental tumors. It has been over 20 years since LaBarba (1970) noted the disparities in this literature, and they have been noted many times since. Dozens of experiments have shown tumor inhibition by stressors. Although there are fewer studies, similar discrepancies exist in the data on animal models of infectious disease. There are scattered examples with other models as well.

Things are muddier in the human research, but there are also cases there. Cardiovascular disease, cancer, diabetes, and arthritis are among the disorders for which there is some evidence for a possible protective effect of stress-associated variables. We have no idea how important such findings are, one of the reasons for our ignorance being researchers' distaste for replicating studies.

We hasten to make it clear that, overall, there are more findings of stress-associated disease exacerbation than of the opposite. But in this particular discussion that is not the main point. The point is that the simple rule, "Stress promotes disease," will not suffice. More is going on than that, and once there is wide acceptance of the possibility that stress is able to promote pathology, a logical next step is to focus on understanding the exceptions.

Indeed, why should we ever have expected stress only to promote disease? At every stage of the present inquiry, we have found disparate effects—apparent inconsistencies among the ways variables operate in different contexts. One could take a cue from the venerable criterion of refutability and ask what could be guaranteed *not* to happen according to our present understanding of stress. The answer would have to be, "Very little." If stress can have a wide variety of different effects on organisms, and if diseases vary in their responses to internal conditions, then divergent disease outcomes ought to be possible. The data only confirm what could have been anticipated.

A holistic conceptualization of stress and disease may be the best basis for proceeding to a more thorough understanding. We assume, and the data suggest, that stress stimulates pathology under numerous conditions, fails to affect it significantly under other numerous conditions, and inhibits it under still other, seemingly less common, circumstances. If we are correct in thinking that the second possibility has been underemphasized and the last has gone largely unremarked, then something is amiss in the way researchers have dealt with this subject matter. Some of the data and logical possibilities have tended to be ignored.

Writers adopting systems viewpoints have repeatedly emphasized the need to consider disease at a number of levels of analysis and to keep in mind the complex nature of the causal networks which affect organismic functioning. These admonitions have not produced much thinking about possible beneficial effects of stress, however.

Perhaps a more thoroughgoing "holism" is needed. Much of the systems-oriented thinking seems to us to encourage the idea of a single optimal kind of functioning, a single "state of harmonious and dynamic equilibrium that may be characterized as a state of health" (Seeman, 1989, p. 1101). Such a viewpoint might be a good first approximation to a biopsychosocial perspective on health and disease, but we must seemingly go beyond it to recognize more possibilities. Indeed, if there is only one truly optimal way for an organismic system to function, or if systems malfunction purely as totalities, then much of the need for a systems view disappears. One or a few indices of a system's function would be sufficient to assess its status; the whole of its complexity could be ignored.

It seems, though, that one cannot ignore the parts which make up the whole. Organismic states which are optimal in some respects need not be so in others. Our version of holism begins with the assumption that complex interactive systems can produce a great diversity of states not only in the system "as a whole" but also in the parts. We assume that causal influences really are interactive (in the statistical sense). We assume that in organismic functioning there is something akin to the sensitive dependence on initial conditions which characterizes many nonlinear physical systems (see Gleick, 1987, for a nontechnical discussion), and that therefore rather small changes in conditions can alter the response of pathophysiologic processes to stress.

In short, although we do not believe that all possible influences are actually significant for all disease outcomes, we assume that the data, with all of their intricacies, give us a reasonable idea of how living things function and interact with their environments. From this perspective, attempting to understand the relationships among psychologic factors and disease must rely as much on the details of organismic processes as on global principles. The whole is more than the sum of its parts. It is also more complex than we tend to give it credit for, and studying the parts can help us understand how that is so.

References

Note: The numbers in brackets [ ] following references are the page numbers in this book on which the references are cited.

Aagaard, J. (1982). Social factors and life events as predictors for children's health: A one-year prospective study after discharge from hospital. *Scandinavian Journal of Social Medicine, 10,* 87-93. [174]

Abbott, B.B., & Badia, P. (1986). Predictable vs unpredictable shock conditions and physiological measures of stress: A reply to Arthur. *Psychological Bulletin, 100,* 384-387. [127]

Abbott, B.B., Schoen, L.S., & Badia, P. (1984). Predictable and unpredictable shock: Behavioral measures of aversion and physiological measures of stress. *Psychological Bulletin, 96,* 45-71. [20, 127]

Abruzzo, L.V., & Rowley, D.A. (1983). Homeostasis of the antibody response: Immunoregulation by NK cells. *Science, 222,* 581-585. [86]

Ader, R. (1980). Psychosomatic and psychoimmunological research. Presidential address. *Psychosomatic Medicine, 42,* 307-321. [14]

Ader, R. (Ed.). (1981). *Psychoneuroimmunology.* New York: Academic Press. [86]

Ader, R., & Cohen, N. (1984). Behavior and the immune system. In W.D. Gentry (Ed.), *Handbook of behavioral medicine* (pp. 117-173). New York: Guilford Press. [93, 152]

Ahadi, S., & Diener, E. (1989). Multiple determinants and effect size. *Journal of Personality and Social Psychology, 56,* 398-406. [165]

Albert, Z. (1967). Effect of number of animals per cage on the development of spontaneous neoplasms. In M.L. Conalty (Ed.), *Husbandry of laboratory animals* (pp. 275-282). New York: Academic Press. [215]

Aldwin, C.M., Levenson, M.R., Spiro, A., III, & Bossé, R. (1989). Does emotionality predict stress? Findings from the Normative Aging Study. *Journal of Personality and Social Psychology, 56,* 618-624. [108]

Alqvist, J. (1981). Hormonal influences on immunologic and related phenomena. In R. Ader (Ed.), *Psychoneuroimmunology* (pp. 355-403). New York: Academic Press. [86, 87, 88]

Altura, B.M., Altura, B.T., & Carella, A. (1983). Magnesium deficiency-induced spasms of umbilical vessels: Relation to preeclampsia, hypertension, growth retardation. *Science, 221,* 376-378. [146]

American Psychiatric Association (1980). *Diagnostic and statistical manual of mental disorders* (3rd ed.). Washington, DC: Author. [23, 113]

Ames, B.N. (1983). Dietary carcinogens and anticarcinogens: Oxygen radicals and degenerative diseases. *Science, 221,* 1256-1263. [134, 139, 146]

Amkraut, A.A., & Solomon, G.F. (1972). Stress and murine sarcoma virus (Moloney)-induced tumors. *Cancer Research, 32,* 1428-1433. [213]

Amsterdam, J.D., Henle, W., Winokur, A., Wolkowitz, O.M., Pickar, D., & Paul, S.M. (1986). Serum antibodies to Epstein-Barr virus in patients with major depressive disorder. *American Journal of Psychiatry, 143,* 1593-1596. [199]

Anderson, K.O., Bradley, L.A., Young, L.D., McDaniel, L.K., & Wise, C.M. (1985). Rheumatoid arthritis: Review of psychological factors related to etiology, effects, and treatment. *Psychological Bulletin, 98,* 358-387. [233, 234]

Anderson, K.O., & Masur, F.T., III. (1983). Psychological preparation for invasive medical and dental procedures. *Journal of Behavioral Medicine, 6*, 1-40. [239]

Andreev, B.V., Ignatov, Yu.D., Nikitina, Z.S., & Sytinski, I.A. (1983). The antistress role of the GABAergic system of the brain. *Neuroscience and Behavioral Physiology, 13*, 434-441. [56]

Angell, M. (1985). Disease as a reflection of the psyche. *New England Journal of Medicine, 312*, 1570-1572. [244]

Anisman, H., Kokkinidis, L., & Sklar, L.S. (1985). Neurochemical consequences of stress: Contribution of adaptive processes. In S.R. Burchfield (Ed.), *Stress: Psychological and physiological interactions* (pp. 67-97). Washington, D.C.: Hemisphere. [22, 56]

Antonovsky, A. (1979). *Health, stress, and coping.* San Francisco: Jossey-Bass. [127]

Arkin, R.M., Kolditz, T.A., & Kolditz, K.K. (1983). Attributions of the test-anxious student: Self-assessment in the classroom. *Personality and Social Psychology Bulletin, 9*, 271-280. [118]

Arnetz, B.B., Fjellner, B., Eneroth, P., & Kallner, A. (1985). Stress and psoriasis: Psychoendocrine and metabolic reactions in psoriatic patients during standardized stressor exposure. *Psychosomatic Medicine, 47*, 528-541. [240]

Arnetz, B.B., Wasserman, J., Petrini, B., Brenner, S.-O., Levi, L., Eneroth, P., Salovaara, H., Hjelm, R., Salovaara, L., Therrell, T., & Petterson, I.-L. (1987). Immune function in unemployed women. *Psychosomatic Medicine, 49*, 3-12. [96]

Arthur, A.Z. (1986). Stress of predictable and unpredictable shock. *Psychological Bulletin, 100*, 379-383. [127]

Asterita, M.F. (1985). *The physiology of stress.* New York: Human Sciences Press. [65, 73, 75, 76]

Axelrod, J., & Reisine, T.D. (1984). Stress hormones: Their interaction and regulation. *Science, 224*, 452-459. [64, 71]

Bahnson, M.B., & Bahnson, C.B. (1979). Development of a psychosocial screening questionnaire for cancer. *Cancer Detection and Prevention, 2*, 295-305. [221]

Baker, L.J., Dearborn, M., Hastings, J.E., & Hamberger, K. (1984). Type A behavior in women: A review. *Health Psychology, 3*, 477-497. [187]

Baltrusch, H.-J. F., Seidel, J., Stangel, W., & Waltz, M.E. (1988). Psychosocial stress, aging, and cancer. *Annals of the New York Academy of Sciences, 521*, 1-15. [208]

Bammer, K. (1981). Stress, spread and cancer. In K. Bammer & B.H. Newberry (Eds.), *Stress and cancer* (pp. 137-163). Toronto: C.J. Hogrefe. [150]

Bandura, A. (1982). Self-efficacy mechanism in human agency. *American Psychologist, 37*, 122-147. [104, 126]

Bandura, A., Cioffi, D., Taylor, C.B., & Brouillard, M.E. (1988). Perceived self-efficacy in coping with cognitive stressors and opioid activation. *Journal of Personality and Social Psychology, 55*, 479-488. [124]

Bandura, A., Taylor, C.B., Williams, S.L., Mefford, I.N., & Barchas, J.D. (1985). Catecholamine secretion as a function of perceived coping self-efficacy. *Journal of Consulting and Clinical Psychology, 53*, 406-414. [115]

Barnes, D.M. (1986). AIDS research in new phase. *Science, 233*, 282-283. [195]

Barnes, D.M. (1987). Cytokines alter AIDS virus production. *Science, 236*, 1627. [197]

Barnes, D.M. (1988). Another glitch for AIDS vaccines? *Science, 241*, 533-534. [197]

Barr, B.P., & Benson, H. (1984). The relaxation response and cardiovascular disorders. *Behavioral Medicine Update, 6*(4), 28-30. [192]

Barrett, D.E., & Radke-Yarrow, M. (1985). Effects of nutritional supplementation on children's responses to novel, frustrating, and competitive situations. *American Journal of Clinical Nutrition, 42*, 102-120. [146]

Barrett, J.T. (1983). *Textbook of immunology* (4th ed.). St. Louis: C.V. Mosby. [77, 86, 137, 146]

Barton, S., & Hicks, R.A. (1985). Type A-B behavior and incidence of infectious mononucleosis in college students. *Psychological Reports, 56*, 545-546. [199]

Baruch, G.K., Biener, L., & Barnett, R.C. (1987). Women and gender in research on work and family stress. *American Psychologist, 42,* 130-136. [123]

Baum, A., Aiello, J.R., & Calesnick, L.E. (1978). Crowding and personal control: Social density and the development of learned helplessness. *Journal of Personality and Social Psychology, 36,* 1000-1011. [119, 125]

Baum, A., Schaeffer, M.A., Lake, C.R., Fleming, R., & Collins, D.L. (1985). Psychological and endocrinological correlates of chronic stress at Three Mile Island. In R.B. Williams, Jr. (Ed.), *Perspectives on behavioral medicine. Vol. 2. Neuroendocrine control and behavior* (pp. 201-217). New York: Academic Press. [67, 73]

Baum, A., Singer, J.E., & Baum, C.S. (1981). Stress and the environment. *Journal of Social Issues, 37,* 4-35. [22, 163]

Baumgardner, A.H., & Brownlee, E.A. (1987). Strategic failure in social interaction: Evidence for expectancy disconfirmation processes. *Journal of Personality and Social Psychology, 52,* 525-535. [117, 118]

Becker, M.H. (1986). The tyranny of health promotion. *Public Health Reviews, 14,* 15-23. [120]

Bendtzen, K., Mandrup-Poulsen, T., Nerup, J., Nielsen, J.H., Dinarello, C.A., & Svenson, M. (1986). Cytotoxicity of human pI 7 interleukin-1 for pancreatic islets of Langerhans. *Science, 232,* 1545-1547. [92, 204]

Berczi, I. (Ed.). (1986a). *Pituitary function and immunity.* Boca Raton, FL: CRC Press. [36, 86, 89]

Berczi, I. (1986b). The influence of pituitary-adrenal axis on the immune system. In I. Berczi (Ed.), *Pituitary function and immunity* (pp. 49-132). Boca Raton, FL: CRC Press. [87, 88]

Berczi, I. (1986c). Gonadotropins and sex hormones. In I. Berczi (Ed.), *Pituitary function and immunity* (pp. 185-211). Boca Raton, FL: CRC Press. [88]

Berczi, I. (1986d). Immunoregulation by pituitary hormones. In I. Berczi (Ed.), *Pituitary function and immunity* (pp. 227-240). Boca Raton, FL: CRC Press. [88, 89]

Berczi, I. (1986e). The effects of growth hormone and related hormones on the immune system. In I. Berczi (Ed.), *Pituitary function and immunity* (pp. 133-159). Boca Raton, FL: CRC Press. [89]

Berczi, I., & Nagy, E. (1986). Prolactin and other lactogenic hormones. In I. Berczi (Ed.), *Pituitary function and immunity* (pp. 161-183). Boca Raton, FL: CRC Press. [89]

Berkanovic, E., Hurwicz, M.-L., & Landsverk, J. (1988). Psychological distress and the decision to seek medical care. *Social Science & Medicine, 27,* 1215-1221. [159]

Berkowitz, A.D., & Perkins, H.W. (1985). Correlates of psychosomatic stress symptoms among farm women: A research note on farm and family functioning. *Journal of Human Stress, 11,* 76-81. [128]

Berkowitz, L. (1962). *Aggression: A social psychological analysis.* New York: McGraw-Hill. [113]

Berkowitz, L. (1990). On the formation and regulation of anger and aggression. *American Psychologist, 45,* 494-503. [113]

Bertell, R. (1977). X-ray exposure and premature aging. *Journal of Surgical Oncology, 9,* 379-391. [147]

Besedovsky, H., del Rey, A., & Sorkin, E. (1986). Regulatory immune-neuroendocrine feedback signals. In I. Berczi (Ed.), *Pituitary function and immunity* (pp. 241-249). Boca Raton, FL: CRC Press. [86, 90]

Beutler, B., & Cerami, A. (1988). The common mediator of shock, cachexia, and tumor necrosis. *Advances in Immunology, 42,* 213-231. [183]

Bieliauskas, L.A. (1980). Life events, 17-OHCS measures, and psychological defensiveness in relation to aid-seeking. *Journal of Human Stress, 6,* 28-36. [174]

Bieliauskas, L.A. (1984). Depression, stress, and cancer. In C.L. Cooper (Ed.), *Psychosocial stress and cancer* (pp. 37-48). Chichester, U.K.: Wiley. [216]

Bieliauskas, L.A., & Garron, D.C. (1982). Psychological depression and cancer. *General Hospital Psychiatry, 4,* 187-195. [216]

Bielinski, R., Schutz, Y., & Jéquier, E. (1985). Energy metabolism during the postexercise recovery in man. *American Journal of Clinical Nutrition, 42,* 69-82. [149]

Billings, A.G., & Moos, R.H. (1981). The role of coping resources and social resources in attenuating the stress of life events. *Journal of Behavioral Medicine, 4,* 139-158. [110]

Bishop, G.D. (1984). Gender, role, and illness behavior in a military population. *Health Psychology, 3,* 519-534. [168]

Bishop, J.M. (1987). The molecular genetics of cancer. *Science, 235,* 305-311. [209]

Blalock, J.E., Harbour-McMenamin, D., & Smith, E.M. (1985). Peptide hormones secreted by the neuroendocrine and immunologic systems. *Journal of Immunology, 135,* 858s-861s. [91]

Blanchard, E.B., & Andrasik, F. (1982). Psychological assessment and treatment of headache: Recent developments and emerging issues. *Journal of Consulting and Clinical Psychology, 50,* 859-879. [235, 236]

Blattner, W., Gallo, R.C., & Temin, H.M. (1988). HIV causes AIDS. *Science, 241,* 514, 515, 517. [195]

Blohmke, M., von Engelhardt, B., & Stelzer, O. (1984). Psychosocial factors and smoking as risk factors in lung carcinoma. *Journal of Psychosomatic Research, 28,* 221-229. [221, 226]

Bloom, B.L., Asher, S.J., & White, S.W. (1978). Marital disruption as a stressor: A review and analysis. *Psychological Bulletin, 85,* 867-894. [122]

Blumenthal, J.A., & Levenson, R.M. (1987). Behavioral approaches to secondary prevention of coronary heart disease. *Circulation, 76* (No. 1, Part 2, Suppl. 1), 130-137. [192]

Bondy, P.K. (1985). Disorders of the adrenal cortex. In J.D. Wilson & D.W. Foster (Eds.), *Williams textbook of endocrinology* (7th ed.) (pp. 816-890). Philadelphia: Saunders. [61, 63, 146, 151]

Booth-Kewley, S., & Friedman, H.S. (1987). Psychological predictors of heart disease: A quantitative review. *Psychological Bulletin, 101,* 343-362. [187, 189, 191]

Borkovec, T.D. (1982). Insomnia. *Journal of Consulting and Clinical Psychology, 50,* 880-895. [154]

Borysenko, M. (1987). The immune system: An overview. *Annals of Behavioral Medicine, 9* (2), 3-10. [77]

Borysenko, M., & Borysenko, J. (1982). Stress, behavior, and immunity: Animal models and mediating mechanisms. *General Hospital Psychiatry, 4,* 59-67. [93]

Brady, J.V. (1975). Toward a behavioral biology of emotion. In L. Levi (Ed.), *Emotions: Their parameters and measurement* (pp. 17-45). New York: Raven Press. [71, 121]

Brand, A.H., Johnson, J.H., & Johnson, S.B. (1986). Life stress and diabetic control in children and adolescents with insulin-dependent diabetes. *Journal of Pediatric Psychology, 11,* 481-495. [206]

Brett, J.F., Brief, A.P., Burke, M.J., George, J.M., & Webster, J. (1990). Negative affectivity and the reporting of stressful life events. *Health Psychology, 9,* 57-68. [166]

Brewin, C.R. (1985). Depression and causal attributions: What is their relation? *Psychological Bulletin, 98,* 297-309. [113, 126]

Broadbent, D.E. (1978). The current state of noise research: Reply to Poulton. *Psychological Bulletin, 85,* 1052-1067. [117, 118]

Brownell, K.D. (1982). Obesity: Understanding and treating a serious, prevalent, and refractory disorder. *Journal of Consulting and Clinical Psychology, 50*, 820-840. [149, 155, 156]

Brush, F.R. (Ed.). (1971). *Aversive conditioning and learning.* New York: Academic Press. [121]

Bukstel, L.H., & Kilman, P.R. (1980). Psychological effects of imprisonment on confined individuals. *Psychological Bulletin, 88*, 469-493. [114]

Bullinger, M., Naber, D., Pickar, D., Cohen, R.M., Kalin, N.H., Pert, A., & Bunney, Jr., W.E. (1984). Endocrine effects of the cold pressor test: Relationships to subjective pain appraisal and coping. *Psychiatry Research, 12*, 227-233. [74]

Bunney, W., Jr., Shapiro, A., Ader, R., Davis, J., Herd, A., Kopin, I.J., Jr., Krieger, D., Matthysse, S., Stunkard, A., Weissman, M., & Wyatt, R.J. (1982). Panel report on stress and illness. In G.R. Elliott, & C. Eisdorfer (Eds.), *Stress and human health: Analysis and implications of research* (pp. 255-337). New York: Springer. [162]

Burchfield, S.R. (1979). The stress response: A new perspective. *Psychosomatic Medicine, 41*, 661-672. [22, 66, 111]

Burchfield, S.R., Woods, S.C., & Elich, M.S. (1978). Effects of cold stress on tumor growth. *Physiology and Behavior, 21*, 537-540. [213]

Burger, J.M., & Arkin, R.M. (1980). Prediction, control and learned helplessness. *Journal of Personality and Social Psychology, 38*, 482-491. [127]

Burish, T.G., & Carey, M.P. (1984). Conditioned responses to cancer chemotherapy: Etiology and treatment. In B.H. Fox, & B.H. Newberry (Eds.), *Impact of psychoendocrine systems in cancer and immunity* (pp. 147-178). Lewiston, NY: Hogrefe. [147]

Burton, H.J., Kline, S.A., Lindsay, R.M., & Heidenheim, A.P. (1986). The relationship of depression to survival in chronic renal failure. *Psychosomatic Medicine, 48*, 261-269. [240]

Byrne, D.G. (1981). Type A behavior, life events, and myocardial infarction: Independent or related risk factors? *British Journal of Medical Psychology, 54*, 371-377. [188]

Byrne, D.G., & Rosenman, R.H. (1986). The Type A behavior pattern as a precursor to stressful life events: A confluence of coronary risk. *British Journal of Medical Psychology, 59*, 75-82. [108, 154, 188]

Byrne, D.G., & Whyte, H.M. (1980). Life events and myocardial infarction revisited: The role of measures of individual impact. *Psychosomatic Medicine, 42*, 1-10. [185]

Calabresi, P., & Parks, Jr., R.E. (1975). Alkylating agents, antimetabolites, hormones, and other antiproliferative agents. In L.S. Goodman & A. Gilman (Eds.), *The pharmacological basis of therapeutics* (5th ed.) (pp. 1254-1307). New York: Macmillan. [140]

Caldwell, R.A., Pearson, J.L., & Chin, R.J. (1987). Stress-moderating effects: Social support in the context of gender and locus of control. *Personality and Social Psychology Bulletin, 13*, 5-17. [129]

Campbell, D.T., & Stanley, J.C. (1966). *Experimental and quasi-experimental designs for research.* Chicago: Rand McNally. [29]

Cannon, J.G., & Kluger, M.J. (1983). Endogenous pyrogen activity in human plasma after exercise. *Science, 220*, 617-619. [149]

Carmelli, D., Chesney, M.A., Ward, M.M., & Rosenman, R.H. (1985). Twin similarity in cardiovascular stress response. *Health Psychology, 4*, 413-423. [141]

Caroff, S., Winokur, A., Snyder, P.J., & Amsterdam, J. (1984). Diurnal variation of growth hormone secretion following thyrotropin-releasing hormone infusion in normal men. *Psychosomatic Medicine, 46*, 59-66. [62]

Carver, C.S., Blaney, P.H., & Scheier, M.F. (1979). Focus of attention, chronic expectancy, and responses to a feared stimulus. *Journal of Personality and Social Psychology, 37*, 1186-1195. [120]

Cassileth, B.R., Lusk, E.J., Miller, D.S., Brown, L.L., & Miller, C. (1985). Psychosocial correlates of survival in advanced malignant disease? *New England Journal of Medicine, 312*, 1551-1555. [222, 225, 229]

Cheng-Mayer, C., Seto, D., Tateno, M., & Levy, J.A. (1988). Biologic features of HIV-1 that correlate with virulence in the host. *Science, 240*, 80-82. [195]

Chesney, M.A., Agras, W.S., Benson, H., Blumenthal, J.A., Engel, B.T., Foreyt, J.P., Kaufman, P.G., Levenson, R.M., Pickering, T.G., Randall, W.C., & Schwartz, P.J. (1987). Task Force 5: Nonpharmacologic approaches to the treatment of hypertension. *Circulation, 76* (No. 1, Part 2, Suppl. 1), 104-109. [180, 182]

Chesney, M.A., Eagleston, J.R., & Rosenman, R.H. (1981). Type A behavior: Assessment and intervention. In C.K. Prokop & L.A. Bradley (Eds.), *Medical psychology: Contributions to behavioral medicine* (pp. 19-36). New York: Academic Press. [187]

Chirigos, M.A., Mitchell, M., Mastrangelo, M.J., & Krim, M. (Eds.). (1981). *Mediation of cellular immunity in cancer by immune modifiers.* New York: Raven Press. [80]

Ciaranello, R. Lipton, M., Barchas, J., Barchas, P.R., Bonica, J., Ferrario, C., Levine, S., & Stein, M. (1982). Panel report on biological substrates of stress. In G.R. Elliot & C. Eisdorfer (Eds.), *Stress and human health: Analysis and implications of research* (pp. 189-254). New York: Springer. [47, 66, 141]

Clark, J.H., Schrader, W.T., & O'Malley, B.W. (1985). Mechanisms of steroid hormone action. In J.D. Wilson & D.W. Foster (Eds.), *Williams textbook of endocrinology* (7th ed.) (pp. 33-75). Philadelphia: Saunders. [49, 60]

Clark, S.C., & Kamen, R. (1987). The human hematopoietic colony-stimulating factors. *Science, 236*, 1229-1237. [58, 85]

Clarkson, T.B., Weingand, K.W., Kaplan, J.R., & Adams, M.R. (1987). Mechanisms of atherogenesis. *Circulation, 76* (No. 1, Part 2, Suppl. 1), 20-28. [178]

Cluss, P.A., & Fireman, P. (1985). Recent trends in asthma research. *Annals of Behavioral Medicine, 7*(4), 11-16. [238]

Coates, T.J., Stall, R., Mandel, J.S., Boccellari, A., Sorensen, J.L., Morales, E.F., Morin, S.F., Wiley, J.A., & McKusick, L. (1987). AIDS: A psychosocial research agenda. *Annals of Behavioral Medicine, 9*(2), 21-28. [195]

Cobb, S., & Rose, R.M. (1973). Hypertension, peptic ulcer, and diabetes in air traffic controllers. *Journal of the American Medical Association, 224*, 489-492. [181]

Coe, C.L., Stanton, M.E., & Levine, S. (1983). Adrenal responses to reinforcement and extinction: Role of expectancy versus instrumental responding. *Behavioral Neuroscience, 97*, 654-657. [66]

Cohen, F. (1981). Stress and bodily illness. *Psychiatric Clinics of North America, 4*, 269-285. [162]

Cohen, F., Horowitz, M.J., Lazarus, R.S., Moos, R.H., Robins, L.N., Rose, R.M., & Rutter, M. (1982). Panel report on psychosocial assets and modifiers of stress. In G.R. Elliott & C. Eisdorfer (Eds.), *Stress and human health: Analysis and implications of research* (pp. 147-188). New York: Springer. [121, 161]

Cohen, M.R., Pickar, D., & Dubois, M. (1983). The role of the endogenous opioid system in the human response to stress. *Psychiatric Clinics of North America, 6*, 457-471. [76]

Cohen, S. (1980). Aftereffects of stress on human performance and social behavior: A review of research and theory. *Psychological Bulletin, 88*, 82-108. [115, 116, 117, 119, 125, 129]

Cohen, S., & Williamson, G.M. (1991). Stress and infectious disease in humans. *Psychological Bulletin, 109*, 5-24. [198]

Cohen, S., & Wills, T.A. (1985). Stress, social support, and the buffering hypothesis. *Psychological Bulletin, 98*, 310-357. [128, 171]

Committee on Diet, Nutrition, and Cancer. (1982). *Diet, nutrition, and cancer.* Washington, D.C.: National Academy Press. [146]

Contrada, R.J., & Krantz, D.S. (1988). Stress, reactivity, and Type A behavior: Current status and future directions. *Annals of Behavioral Medicine, 10* (2), 64-70. [187]

Cook, J.R. (1985). Repression-sensitization and approach-avoidance as predictors of response to a laboratory stressor. *Journal of Personality and Social Psychology, 49*, 759-773. [107, 115]

Cook, W.W., & Medley, D.M. (1954). Proposed hostility and pharisaic virtue scales for the MMPI. *Journal of Applied Psychology, 38*, 414-418. [190, 191]

Coombs, W.N., & Schroeder, H.E. (1988). Generalized locus of control: An analysis of factor analytic data. *Personality and Individual Differences, 9*, 79-85. [105]

Cooper, C.L. (Ed.). (1984). *Psychosocial stress and cancer.* Chichester, U.K.: Wiley. [208]

Cooper, C.L., & Melhuish, A. (1984). Executive stress and health: Differences between men and women. *Journal of Occupational Medicine, 26*, 99-104. [168, 181]

Coover, G.D., Sutton, B.R., & Heybach, J.B. (1977). Conditioning decreases in plasma corticosterone level in rats by pairing stimuli with daily feedings. *Journal of Comparative and Physiological Psychology, 91*, 716-726. [66]

Costa, P.T., & McCrae, R.R. (1985). Hypochondriasis, neuroticism, and aging: When are somatic complaints unfounded? *American Psychologist, 40*, 19-28. [24, 166]

Cottington, E.M., Matthews, K.A., Talbott, E., & Kuller, L.H. (1980). Environmental events preceding sudden death in women. *Psychosomatic Medicine, 42*, 567-574. [186]

Cottington, E.M., Matthews, K.A., Talbott, E., & Kuller, L.H. (1986). Occupational stress, suppressed anger, and hypertension. *Psychosomatic Medicine, 48*, 249-259. [182]

Cox, R.H., Hubbard, J.W., Lawler, J.E., Sanders, B.J., & Mitchell, V.P. (1985). Exercise training attenuates stress-induced hypertension in the rat. *Hypertension, 7*, 747-751. [180]

Creer, T.L. (1988). The synthesis of medical and behavioral sciences with respect to bronchial asthma. In R. Ader, H. Weiner, & A. Baum (Eds.), *Experimental foundations of behavioral medicine: Conditioning approaches* (pp. 111-158). Hillsdale, NJ: Erlbaum. [237, 238]

Crocker, J., & Major, B. (1989). Social stigma and self-esteem: The self-protective properties of stigma. *Psychological Review, 96*, 608-630. [106]

Cronkite, R.C., & Moos, R.H. (1984). The role of predisposing and moderating factors in the stress-illness relationship. *Journal of Health and Social Behavior, 25*, 372-393. [163, 165, 174]

Cryer, P.E. (1985). Glucose homeostasis and hypoglycemia. In J.D. Wilson & D.W. Foster (Eds.), *Williams textbook of endocrinology* (7th ed.) (pp. 989-1017). Philadelphia: Saunders. [59]

Curtis, G.C. (1979). Psychoendocrine stress response: Steroid and peptide hormones. In B.A. Stoll (Ed.), *Mind and cancer prognosis* (pp. 61-72). Chichester, U.K.: Wiley. [73, 74, 75]

Dattore, P.J., Shontz, F.C., & Coyne, L. (1980). Premorbid personality differentiation of cancer and noncancer groups: A test of the hypothesis of cancer proneness. *Journal of Consulting and Clinical Psychology, 48*, 388-394. [218, 227, 232]

Davidson, J.M., Smith, E.R., & Levine, S. (1978). Testosterone. In H. Ursin, E. Baade, & S. Levine (Eds.), *Psychobiology of stress: A study of coping men.* (pp. 57-62). New York: Academic Press. [75]

De Bold, A.J. (1985). Atrial natriuretic factor: A hormone produced by the heart. *Science, 230*, 767-770. [58]

Dechambre, R.-P. (1981). Psychosocial stress and cancer in mice. In K. Bammer & B.H. Newberry (Eds.), *Stress and cancer* (pp. 43-58). Toronto: Hogrefe. [135]

DeLongis, A., Coyne, J.C., Dakof, G., Folkman, S., & Lazarus, R.S. (1982). Relationship of daily hassles, uplifts, and major life events to health status. *Health Psychology, 1,* 119-136. [167]

Del Rosario, M.W., Brines, J.L., & Coleman, W.R. (1984). Emotional response patterns to body weight-related cues: Influence of body weight image. *Personality and Social Psychology Bulletin, 10,* 369-373. [120]

Dembroski, T.M. (1984). Stress and substance interaction effects on risk factors and reactivity. *Behavioral Medicine Update, 6*(3), 16-20. [184]

Dembroski, T.M., & Costa, P.T. (1988). Assessment of coronary-prone behavior: A current overview. *Annals of Behavioral Medicine, 10*(2), 60-63. [187]

Dembroski, T.M., MacDougall, J.M., Cardozo, S.R., Ireland, S.K., & Krug-Fite, J. (1985). Selective cardiovascular effects of stress and cigarette smoking in young women. *Health Psychology, 4,* 153-167. [155]

Denenberg, V.H. (1967). Stimulation in infancy, emotional reactivity, and exploratory behavior. In D.C. Glass (Ed.), *Neurophysiology and emotion* (pp. 161-190). New York: Rockefeler University Press and Russell Sage Foundation. [23]

Depue, R.A., & Monroe, S.M. (1986). Conceptualization and measurement of human disorder in life stress research: The problem of chronic disturbance. *Psychological Bulletin, 99,* 36-51. [176]

De Quattro, V., Loo, R., & Foti, A. (1985). Sympathoadrenal response to stress: The linking of Type A behavior pattern to ischemic heart disease. *Clinical and Experimental Theory and Practice, A7,* 469-481. [187]

Derogatis, L.R., Abeloff, M.D., & Melisaratos, N. (1979). Psychological coping mechanisms and survival time in metastatic breast cancer. *Journal of the American Medical Association, 242,* 1504-1508. [223, 229]

Dess, N.K., Linwick, D., Patterson, J., Overmier, J.B., & Levine, S. (1983). Immediate and proactive effects of controllability and predictability on plasma cortisol responses to shock in dogs. *Behavioral Neuroscience, 97,* 1005-1016. [127]

Deuster, P.A., Morrison, S.D., & Ahrens, R.A. (1985). Endurance exercise modifies cachexia of tumor growth in rats. *Medicine and Science in Sports and Exercise, 17,* 385-392. [213]

De Wied, D. (1980) Hormonal influences on motivation, learning, memory, and psychosis. In D.T. Krieger & J.C. Hughes (Eds.), *Neuroendocrinology* (pp. 194-204). Sunderland, MA: Sinauer. [53]

Diamond, E.L. (1982). The role of anger and hostility in essential hypertension and coronary heart disease. *Psychological Bulletin, 92,* 410-433. [182]

Diamond, T., Stiel, D., Lunzer, M., Wilkinson, M., & Posen, S. (1989). Ethanol reduces bone formation and may cause osteoporosis. *American Journal of Medicine, 86,* 282-288. [144]

Dienstbier, R.A. (1989). Arousal and physiological toughness: Implications for mental and physical health. *Psychological Review, 96,* 84-100. [22, 66]

Dimsdale, J.E. (1988). A perspective on Type A behavior and coronary disease. *New England Journal of Medicine, 318,* 110-112. [190]

Dimsdale, J.E., Hartley, L.H., Guiney, T., Ruskin, J.N., & Greenblat, D. (1984). Postexercise peril: Plasma catecholamines and exercise. *Journal of the American Medical Association, 251,* 630-632. [149]

Dinarello, C.A. (1985). An update on human interleukin-1: From molecular biology to clinical relevance. *Journal of Clinical Immunology, 5,* 287-297. [90]

Ditto, P.H., Jemmott, J.B., III, & Darley, J.M. (1988). Appraising the threat of illness: A mental representational approach. *Health Psychology, 7,* 183-201. [106]

Dobkin, P.L., & Morrow, G.R. (1985/86). Long-term side effects in patients who have been treated successfully for cancer. *Journal of Psychosocial Oncology, 3*(4), 23-51. [152]

Doherty, W.J., Schrott, H.G., Metcalf, L., & Iasiello-Vailas, L. (1983). Effect of spouse support and health beliefs on medication adherence. *Journal of Family Practice*, *17*, 837-841. [128]

Dohrenwend, B.P., & Shrout, P.E. (1985). "Hassles" in the conceptualization and measurement of life stress variables. *American Psychologist*, *40*, 780-785. [15]

Dohrenwend, B.S., Krasnoff, L., Askenasy, A.R., & Dohrenwend, B.P. (1982). The Psychiatric Epidemiology Research Interview Life Events Scale. In L. Goldberger & S. Breznitz (Eds.), *Handbook of stress: Theoretical and clinical aspects* (pp. 332-363). New York: The Free Press. [121, 122, 165]

Drudge, O.W., Rosen, J.C., Peyser, J.M., & Pieniadz, J. (1986). Behavioral and emotional problems and treatment in chronically brain-impaired adults. *Annals of Behavioral Medicine*, *8*(1), 9-14. [152]

Dunkel-Schetter, C., Folkman, S., & Lazarus, R.S. (1987). Correlates of social support receipt. *Journal of Personality and Social Psychology*, *53*, 71-80. [129]

Durel, L.A., Krantz, D.S., Eisold, J.F., & Lazar, J.D. (1985). Behavioral effects of beta blockers: Reduction of anxiety, acute stress, and Type A behavior. *Journal of Cardiopulmonary Rehabilitation*, *5*, 267-273. [143]

Du Ruisseau, P., Taché, Y., Brazeau, P., & Collu, R. (1978). Pattern of adeno-hypophyseal hormone changes induced by various stressors in female and male rats. *Neuroendocrinology*, *27*, 257-271. [75]

Durum, S.K., Schmidt, J.A., & Oppenheim, J.J. (1985). Interleukin-1: An immunological perspective. *Annual Review of Immunology*, *3*, 263-287. [85]

Dustan, H.P. (1987). Biobehavioral factors in hypertension: Overview. *Circulation*, *76* (No. 1, Part 2, Suppl. 1), 57-59. [179]

Edelstein, J., & Linn, M.W. (1985). The influence of the family on control of diabetes. *Social Science & Medicine*, *21*, 541-544. [206]

Edwards, J., DiClemente, C., & Samuels, M.L. (1985). Psychological characteristics: A pretreatment survival marker of patients with testicular cancer. *Journal of Psychosocial Oncology*, *3*, 79-94. [226, 231]

Eichner, E.R. (1983). Exercise and heart disease: Epidemiology of the "exercise hypothesis." *American Journal of Medicine*, *75*, 1008-1023. [186]

Eliasz, A., & Wrześniewski, K. (1988). *Rizyo chorób psychosomatycznych: Środowisko i temperament a wzór Zachowania A*. (Psychosomatic disease risk: Environment, temperament, and Type A behavior.) Wroclaw, Poland: Zaklad Narodowy imenia Ossolińskich Wydawnictwo Polskiej Akademii Nauk. [114]

Eliot, R.S. (1979). *Stress and the major cardiovascular disorders*. Mount Kisco, NY: Futura. [176]

Ellis, A. (1978). What people can do for themselves to cope with stress. In C.L. Cooper & R. Payne (Eds.), *Stress at work* (pp. 209-222). Chichester, U.K.: Wiley. [104, 120]

Endler, N.S., & Magnusson, D. (1976). Toward an interactional psychology of personality. *Psychological Bulletin*, *83*, 956-974. [107]

Ensoli, B., Nakamura, S., Salahuddin, S.Z., Biberfeld, P., Larsson, L., Beaver, B., Wong-Staal, F., & Gallo, R.C. (1989). AIDS-Kaposi's sarcoma-derived cells express cytokines with autocrine and paracrine growth effects. *Science*, *243*, 223-226. [210]

Eskay, R., Zukowska-Grojec, Z., Haass, M., Dave, J.R., & Zamir, N. (1986). Circulating atrial natriuretic peptides in conscious rats: Regulation of release by multiple factors. *Science*, *232*, 636-639. [58]

Euker, J.S., Meites, J., & Riegle, G.D. (1975). Effects of acute stress on serum LH and prolactin in intact, castrate and dexamethasone-treated male rats. *Endocrinology*, *96*, 85-92. [75]

Eysenck, H.J. (1984). Lung cancer and the stress-personality inventory. In C.L. Cooper (Ed.), *Psychosocial stress and cancer* (pp. 231-260). Chichester, U.K.: Wiley. [216]

Eysenck, M.W. (1976). Arousal, learning, and memory. *Psychological Bulletin, 83*, 389-404. [116]

Fajzi, K., Reinhardt, V., & Smith, M.D. (1989). A review of environmental enrichment strategies for singly caged primates. *Lab Animal, 18*(2), 23-29, 31. [129]

Fauci, A.S. (1988). The human immunodeficiency virus: Infectivity and mechanisms of pathogenesis. *Science, 239*, 617-622. [194, 195]

Felton, B.J., & Revenson, T.A. (1984). Coping with chronic illness: A study of illness controllability and the influences of coping strategies on psychological adjustment. *Journal of Consulting and Clinical Psychology, 52*, 343-353. [125]

Fertig, J.B., Pomerleau, O.F., & Sanders, B. (1986). Nicotine-produced antinociception in minimally deprived smokers and ex-smokers. *Addictive Behaviors, 11*, 239-248. [144]

Feuerstein, M., Bortolussi, L., Houle, M., & Labbé, E. (1983). Stress, temporal artery activity, and pain in migraine headache: A prospective analysis. *Headache, 23*, 296-304. [236]

Feuerstein, M., Sult, S., & Houle, M. (1985). Environmental stressors and chronic low back pain: Life events, family and work environment. *Pain, 22*, 295-307. [236]

Fish Oil for the Heart (1987). *The Medical Letter, 29*, 7-9. [145]

Flier, J.S., Cook, K.S., Usher, P., & Spiegelman, B.M. (1987). Severely impaired adipsin expression in genetic and acquired obesity. *Science, 237*, 405-408. [156]

Flor, H., & Turk, D.C. (1989). Psychophysiology of chronic pain: Do chronic pain patients exhibit symptom-specific psychophysiological responses? *Psychological Bulletin, 105*, 215-259. [235, 236]

Foa, E.B., & Kozak, M.J. (1986). Emotional processing of fear: Exposure to corrective information. *Psychological Bulletin, 99*, 20-35. [111]

Foldes, A., Maxwell, C.A., Hinks, N.T., Hoskinson, R.M., & Scaramuzzi, R.J. (1982). Effects of steroids on ß-adrenergic binding sites in sheep pineal glands. *Biochemical Pharmacology, 31*, 1369-1374. [70]

Folkins, C.H., & Sime, W.E. (1981). Physical fitness training and mental health. *American Psychologist, 36*, 373-389. [149]

Folkman, J., & Klagsbrun, M. (1987). Angiogenic factors. *Science, 235*, 442-447. [90]

Folkman, S., & Lazarus, R.S. (1985). If it changes it must be a process: Study of emotion and coping during three stages of a college examination. *Journal of Personality and Social Psychology, 48*, 150-170. [112]

Folkman, S., Lazarus, R.S., Dunkel-Schetter, C., DeLongis, A., & Gruen, R.J. (1986a). Dynamics of a stressful encounter: Cognitive appraisal, coping, and encounter outcomes. *Journal of Personality and Social Psychology, 50*, 992-1003. [111, 113]

Folkman, S., Lazarus, R.S., Gruen, R.J., & DeLongis, A. (1986b). Appraisal, coping, health status, and psychological symptoms. *Journal of Personality and Social Psychology, 50*, 571-579. [163, 175]

Folkow, B. (1987). Psychosocial and central nervous influences in primary hypertension. *Circulation, 76* (No. 1, Part 2, Suppl. 1), 10-19. [177. 179, 180, 181]

Folks, T.M., Justement, J., Kinter, A., Dinarello, C.A., & Fauci, A.S. (1987). Cytokine-induced expression of HIV-1 in a chronically infected promonocyte cell line. *Science, 238*, 800-802. [197]

Folsom, A.R., Hughes, J.R., Buehler, J.F., Mittlemark, M.B., Jacobs, D.R., Jr., & Grimm, R.H., Jr. (1985). Do Type A men drink more frequently than Type B Men? Findings in the Multiple Risk Factor Intervention Trial (MRFIT). *Journal of Behavioral Medicine, 8*, 227-235. [188]

Fontana, A.F., Kerns, R.D., Rosenberg, R.L., & Colonese, K.L. (1989). Support, stress, and recovery from coronary heart disease: A longitudinal causal model. *Health Psychology, 8*, 175-193. [239]

Fox, B.H. (1978). Premorbid psychological factors as related to cancer incidence. *Journal of Behavioral Medicine, 1*, 45-133. [208, 216]

Fox, B.H. (1982). Endogenous psychosocial factors in cross-national cancer incidence. In J.R. Eiser (Ed.), *Social psychology and behavioral medicine* (pp. 101-141). New York: Wiley. [161]

Fox, B.H. (1988). Psychogenic factors in cancer, especially its incidence. In S. Maes, C.D. Spielberger, P.B. Defares, & I.G. Sarason (Eds.), *Topics in health psychology* (pp. 37-55). New York: Wiley. [208, 216, 233]

Fox, B.H., & Newberry, B.H. (Eds.). (1984). *Impact of psychoendocrine systems in cancer and immunity*. Lewiston, NY: Hogrefe. [208]

Frankel, A.I., & Ryan, E.L. (1981). Testicular innervation is necessary for the response of plasma testosterone levels to acute stress. *Biology of Reproduction, 24*, 491-495. [75]

Frankenhaeuser, M. (1975). Experimental approaches to the study of catecholamines and emotion. In L. Levi (Ed.), *Emotions: Their parameters and measurement* (pp. 209-234). New York: Raven Press. [72, 118]

Frasure-Smith, N., & Prince, R. (1985). The Ischemic Heart Disease Life Stress Monitoring Program: Impact on mortality. *Psychosomatic Medicine, 47*, 431-445. [192]

Fredrikson, M., & Engel, B.T. (1985). Cardiovascular and electrodermal adjustments during a vigilance task in patients with borderline and established hypertension. *Journal of Psychosomatic Research, 29*, 235-246. [72]

Freifelder, D. (1983). *Molecular biology*. Boston: Jones and Bartlett. [140]

Friedman, H.S., & Booth-Kewley, S. (1987). The "disease-prone personality": A meta-analytic view of the construct. *American Psychologist, 42*, 539-555. [162, 163, 164, 171, 172]

Friedman, M., & Rosenman, R.H. (1959). Association of specific overt behavior pattern with blood and cardiovascular findings. *Journal of the American Medical Association, 169*, 1286-1296. [187]

Friedman, M., Thoreson, C.D., Gill, J.J., Powell, L.H., Ulmer, D., Thompson, L., Price, V.A., Rabin, D.D., Breall, W.S., Dixon, T., Levy, R., & Bourg, E. (1984). Alteration of Type A behavior and reduction in cardiac recurrences in postmyocardial infarction patients. *American Heart Journal, 108*, 237-248. [192]

Friedman, S.B., Ader, R., Grota, L.J., & Larson, T. (1967). Plasma corticosterone response to parameters of electric shock stimulation in the rat. *Psychosomatic Medicine, 29*, 323-328. [20, 21]

Funk, S.C., & Houston, B.K. (1987). A critical analysis of the hardiness scale's validity and utility. *Journal of Personality and Social Psychology, 53*, 572-578. [169, 175]

Furth, J. (1975). Hormones as etiological agents in neoplasia. In F.F. Becker (Ed.), *Cancer: A comprehensive treatise* (pp. 75-120). New York: Plenum. [142]

Ganong, W.F. (1985). Changing concepts of neuroendocrine control. In R.B. Williams, Jr. (Ed.), *Perspectives on behavioral medicine*. Vol. 2. Neuroendocrine control and behavior (pp. 25-38). New York: Academic Press. [39, 54]

Gartner, S., Markovits, P., Markovits, D.M., Kaplan, M.H., Gallo, R.C., & Popovic, M. (1986). The role of mononuclear phagocytes in HTLV-III/LAV infection. *Science, 233*, 215-218. [195]

Gatchel, R.J., & Baum, A. (1983). *An introduction to health psychology*. Reading, MA: Addison-Wesley. [24]

Georgas, J., & Giakoumaki, E. (1984). Psychosocial stress, symptoms, and anxiety of male and female teachers in Greece. *Journal of Human Stress, 10*, 191-197. [168]

Gilbert, D.G. (1979). Paradoxical tranquilizing and emotion-reducing effects of nicotine. *Psychological Bulletin, 86*, 643-661. [144]

Gilman, A.G., Goodman, L.S., & Gilman, A. (Eds.). (1980). *Goodman and Gilman's the pharmacological basis of therapeutics* (6th ed.). New York: Macmillan. [142]

Gilman, A.G., Goodman, L.S., Rall, T.W., & Murad, F. (Eds.). (1985). *Goodman and Gilman's the pharmacological basis of therapeutics* (7th ed.). New York: Macmillan. [142]

Glaser, R., Kiecolt-Glaser, J.K., Speicher, C.E., & Holliday, J.E. (1985). Stress, loneliness, and changes in herpesvirus latency. *Journal of Behavioral Medicine, 8,* 249-260. [198, 199]

Glaser, R., Rice, J., Speicher, C.E., Stout, J.C., & Kiecolt-Glaser, J.K. (1986). Stress depresses interferon production by leukocytes concomitant with a decrease in natural killer cell activity. *Behavioral Neuroscience, 100,* 675-678. [98]

Glasgow, R.E., McCaul, K.D., & Schafer, L.C. (1986). Barriers to regimen adherence among persons with insulin-dependent diabetes. *Journal of Behavioral Medicine, 9,* 65-77. [207]

Glass, D.C. (1977). Stress, behavior patterns, and coronary disease. *American Scientist, 65,* 177-187. [114, 119, 154, 187]

Glass, D.C. (1985). Type A behavior: Mechanisms linking behavioral and pathophysiological processes. In R.B. Williams, Jr. (Ed.), *Perspectives on behavioral medicine: Volume 2. Neuroendocrine control and behavior* (pp. 189-199). New York: Academic Press. [30]

Gleick, J. (1987). *Chaos.* New York: Viking. [5, 246]

Glorioso, N., Atlas, S.A., Laragh, J.H., Jewelewicz, R., & Sealey, J.E. (1986). Prorenin in high concentrations in human ovarian follicular fluid. *Science, 233,* 1422-1424. [58]

Godkin, M.A., & Rice, C.A. (1981). Psychosocial stress and its relationship to illness behavior and illnesses encountered commonly by family practitioners. *Social Science and Medicine, 15,* 155-159. [167]

Goldman, L., Coover, G.D., & Levine, S. (1973). Bidirectional effects of reinforcement shifts on pituitary adrenal activity. *Physiology and Behavior, 10,* 209-214. [120]

Gonder-Frederick, L.A., Carter, W.R., Cox, D.J., & Clarke, W.L. (1990). Environmental stress and blood glucose change in insulin-dependent diabetes mellitus. *Health Psychology, 9,* 503-515. [206]

Goodenough, D.R. (1976). The role of individual differences in field dependence as a factor in learning and memory. *Psychological Bulletin, 83,* 675-694. [118]

Goodenow, R.S., Vogel, J.M., & Linsk, R.L. (1985). Histocompatibility antigens on murine tumors. *Science, 230,* 777-783. [211]

Goodkin, K., Antoni, M.H., & Blaney, P.H. (1986). Stress and hopelessness in the promotion of cervical intraepithelial neoplasia to invasive squamous cell carcinoma of the cervix. *Journal of Psychosomatic Research, 30,* 67-76. [221, 229]

Gordon, J.S. (1980). The paradigm of holistic medicine. In A.C. Hastings, J. Fadiman, & J.S. Gordon (Eds.), *Health for the whole person* (pp. 3-27). Boulder, CO: Westview. [12, 13, 24]

Graham, N.M.H., Douglas, R.M., & Ryan, P. (1986). Stress and acute respiratory infection. *American Journal of Epidemiology, 124,* 389-401. [200]

Greenberg, A.H., Dyck, D.G., & Sandler, L.S. (1984). Opponent processes, neurohormones and natural resistance. In B.H. Fox & B.H. Newberry (Eds.), *Impact of psychoendocrine systems in cancer and immunity* (pp. 225-257). Lewiston, NY: Hogrefe. [93, 211, 215]

Greenberg, J., & Pyszczynski, T. (1986). Persistent high self-focus after failure and low self-focus after success: The depressive self-focusing style. *Journal of Personality and Social Psycholology, 50,* 1039-1044. [114]

Greene, J.W., Walker, L.S., Hickson, G., & Thompson, J. (1985). Stressful life events and somatic complaints in adolescents. *Pediatrics, 75,* 19-22. [175]

Greer, S., & Morris, T. (1975). Psychological attributes of women who develop breast cancer: A controlled study. *Journal of Psychosomatic Research, 19,* 147-153. [219, 223, 227]

Greer, S., Morris, T., & Pettingale, K.W. (1979). Psychological response to breast cancer: Effect on outcome. *Lancet, ii,* 785-787. [223, 229, 232]

Gristina, A.G. (1987). Biomaterial-centered infection: Microbial adhesion versus tissue integration. *Science, 237,* 1588-1595. [197]

Grossman, C.J. (1984). Regulation of the immune system by sex steroids. *Endocrine Reviews*, 5, 435-455. [88, 91]

Gurney, M.E., Apatoff, B.R., Spear, G.T., Baumel, M.J., Antel, J.P., Bania, M.B., & Reder, A.T. (1986). Neuroleukin: A lymphokine product of lectin-stimulated T cells. *Science*, 234, 574-581. [91]

Guyton, A.C. (1986). *Textbook of medical physiology* (7th ed.). Philadelphia: Saunders. [58, 176, 177, 235]

Haber, J.D., Moss, R.A., Kuczmierczyk, A.R., & Garrett, J.C. (1983). Assessment and treatment of stress in myofascial pain dysfunction syndrome: A model for analysis. *Journal of Oral Rehabilitation*, 10, 187-196. [235]

Hadley, M.E. (1984). *Endocrinology*. Englewood Cliffs, N.J.: Prentice-Hall. [47, 51, 52, 53, 55, 57, 58, 59, 60, 61, 68, 89]

Halford, W.K., Cuddihy, S., & Mortimer, R.H. (1990). Psychological stress and blood glucose regulation in Type 1 diabetic patients. *Health Psychology*, 9, 516-528. [206]

Hall, G.S., & Lindzey, G. (1978). *Theories of personality* (3rd ed.). New York: Wiley. [8]

Halstead, S.B. (1988). Pathogenesis of dengue: Challenges to molecular biology. *Science*, 239, 476-481. [197]

Hamburg, D.A., Hamburg, B.A., & Barchas, J.D. (1975). Anger and depression in perspective of behavioral biology. In L. Levi (Ed.), *Emotions: Their parameters and measurement* (pp. 235-278). New York: Raven Press. [141, 142]

Hancock, P.A. (1986). Sustained attention under thermal stress. *Psychological Bulletin*, 99, 263-281. [118]

Hand, R.P. (1990). What's behind the L-tryptophan ban? *Medical Sciences Bulletin*, 12(9), 1-2. [146]

Hansell, S., Sparacino, J., & Ronchi, D. (1982). Physical attractiveness and blood pressure: Sex and age differences. *Personality and Social Psychology Bulletin*, 8, 113-121. [120]

Hansen, J.R., Støa, K.F., Blix, A.S., & Ursin, H. (1978). Urinary levels of epinephrine and norepinephrine in parachutist trainees. In H. Ursin, E. Baade, & L. Levine (Eds.), *Psychobiology of stress: A study of coping men* (pp. 63-74). New York: Academic Press. [72]

Hanson, C.L., Henggeler, S.W., & Burghen, G.A. (1987). Social competence and parental support as mediators of the link between stress and metabolic control in adolescents with insulin-dependent diabetes mellitus. *Journal of Consulting and Clinical Psychology*, 55, 529-533. [206]

Hansson, R.O., Noulles, D., & Bellovich, S.J. (1982). Social comparison and urban-environmental stress. *Personality and Social Psychology Bulletin*, 8, 68-73. [119]

Harrison, D.E. (1982). Experience with developing assays of physiological age. In M.E. Reff & E.L. Schneider (Eds.), *Biological markers of aging* (NIH Publication No. 82-2221. pp. 2-12). Washington, D.C.: U.S. Department of Health and Human Services. [145]

Hastings, A.C., Fadiman, J., & Gordon, J.S. (Eds.). (1980). *Health for the whole person*. Boulder, CO: Westview. [13]

Haughey, B.P., Brasure, J., Maloney, M.C., & Graham, S. (1984). The relationship between stressful life events and electrocardiogram abnormalities. *Heart and Lung*, 13, 405-410. [186]

Haynes, Jr., R.C., & Larner, J. (1975). Adrenocorticotropic hormone; adrenocortical steroids and their synthetic analogs; inhibitors of adrenocortical steroid bio-synthesis. In L.S. Goodman & A. Gilman (Eds.), *The pharmacological basis of therapeutics* (5th ed.) (pp. 1472-1506). New York: Macmillan. [63]

Haynes, S.G. (1984). Type A behavior, employment status, and coronary heart disease in women. *Behavioral Medicine Update*, 6(4), 11-15. [185, 189]

Haynes, S.G., & Matthews, K.A. (1988). Review and methodologic critique of recent studies on Type A behavior and cardiovascular disease. *Annals of Behavioral Medicine, 10*(2), 47-59. [189, 190]

Hegsted, D.M. (1986). Serum-cholesterol response to dietary cholesterol: A reevaluation. *American Journal of Clinical Nutrition, 44*, 299-305. [145]

Heide, F.J., & Borkovec, T.D. (1983). Relaxation-induced anxiety: Paradoxical anxiety enhancement due to relaxation training. *Journal of Consulting and Clinical Psychology, 51*, 171-182. [120]

Heilburn, A.B., Jr., & Harris, A. (1986). Psychological defenses in females at-risk for anorexia nervosa: An explanation for excessive stress found in anorexic patients. *International Journal of Eating Disorders, 5*, 503-516. [240]

Henderson, B.E., Ross, R.K., Paganini-Hill, A., & Mack, T.M. (1986). Estrogen use and cardiovascular disease. *American Journal of Obstetrics and Gynecology, 154*, 1181-1186. [142]

Hendrix, W.H. (1985). Factors predictive of stress, organizational effectiveness, and coronary heart disease potential. *Aviation, Space, and Environmental Medicine, 56*, 654-659. [185]

Henry, J.L. (1982). Circulating opioids: Possible physiological roles in central nervous function. *Neuroscience and Biobehavioral Reviews, 6*, 229-245. [53]

Henry, J.P. (1982). The relation of social to biological processes in disease. *Social Science and Medicine, 16*, 369-380. [66, 72, 162]

Henry, J.P., Ely, D.L., Watson, F.M.C., & Stephens, P.M. (1975). Ethological methods as applied to the measurement of emotion. In L. Levi (Ed.), *Emotions: Their parameters and measurement* (pp. 469-497). New York: Raven Press. [16, 73]

Henry, J.P., & Stephens, P.M. (1980). Caffeine as an intensifier of stress-induced hormonal and pathophysiologic changes in mice. *Pharmacology, Biochemistry, and Behavior, 13*, 719-727. [145]

Herberman, R.B., & Ortaldo, J.R. (1981). Natural killer cells: Their role in defense against disease. *Science, 214*, 24-30. [80]

Herd, J.A. (1981). Behavioral factors in the physiological mechanisms of cardiovascular disease. In S.M. Weiss, J.A. Herd, & B.H. Fox (Eds.), *Perspectives on behavioral medicine* (pp. 55- 65). New York: Academic Press. [59, 150, 183]

Herman, C.P., Zanna, M.P., & Higgins, E.T. (Eds.). (1986). *Physical appearance, stigma, and social behavior.* Hillsdale, NJ: Lawrence Erlbaum. [137]

Higgins, E.T. (1987). Self-discrepancy: A theory relating self and affect. *Psychological Review, 94*, 319-340. [105, 112, 120]

Hilton, D.J., & Slugoski, B.R. (1986). Knowledge-based causal attribution: The abnormal conditions focus model. *Psychological Review, 93*, 75-88. [104]

Hines, M. (1982). Prenatal gonadal hormones and sex differences in human behavior. *Psychological Bulletin, 92*, 56-80. [52]

Hobfoll, S.E. (1988). *The ecology of stress.* Washington, D.C.: Hemisphere. [100]

Hogarth, R.M. (1981). Beyond discrete biases: Functional and dysfunctional aspects of judgmental heuristics. *Psychological Bulletin, 90*, 197-217. [105]

Hohmann, E.L., Elde, R.P., Rysavy, J.A., Einzig, S., & Gebhard, R.L. (1986). Innervation of periosteum and bone by sympathetic vasoactive intestinal peptide-containing nerve fibers. *Science, 232*, 868-871. [55, 68]

Hoiberg, A. (1982). Occupational stress and illness incidence. *Journal of Occupational Medicine, 24*, 445-451. [167]

Holahan, C.J., & Moos, R.H. (1985). Life stress and health: Personality, coping, and family support in stress resistance. *Journal of Personality and Social Psychology, 49*, 739-747. [114]

Holahan, C.K., Holahan, C.J., & Belk, S.S. (1984). Adjustment in aging: The roles of life stress, hassles, and self-efficacy. *Health Psychology, 3*, 315-328. [123]

262 *References*

Holland, J.C., & Tross, S. (1985). The psychosocial and neuropsychiatric sequelae of the acquired immunodeficiency syndrome and related disorders. *Annals of Internal Medicine, 103,* 760-764. [152, 195]

Holmes, D.S., & Will, M.J. (1985). Expression of interpersonal aggression by angered and nonangered persons with the Type A and Type B behavior patterns. *Journal of Personality and Social Psychology, 48,* 723-727. [114]

Holmes, T.H., & Rahe, R.H. (1967). The social readjustment rating scale. *Journal of Psychosomatic Research, 11,* 213-218. [20]

Holt, R.R. (1982). Occupational stress. In L. Goldberger & S. Breznitz (Eds.), *Handbook of stress: Theoretical and clinical aspects* (pp. 419-444). New York: The Free Press. [122]

Hull, J.G., & Bond, C.F., Jr. (1986). Social and behavioral consequences of alcohol consumption and expectancy: A meta-analysis. *Psychological Bulletin, 99,* 347-360. [143]

Hull, J.G., Van Treuren, R.R., & Virnelli, S. (1987). Hardiness and health: A critique and alternative approach. *Journal of Personality and Social Psychology, 53,* 518-530. [169]

Hulse, G.K., & Coleman, G.J. (1983). The role of endogenous opioids in the blockade of reproductive function in the rat following exposure to acute stress. *Pharmacology, Biochemistry and Behavior, 19,* 795-799. [75]

Humphreys, M.S., & Revelle, W. (1984). Personality, motivation, and performance: A theory of the relationship between individual differences and information processing. *Psychological Review, 91,* 153-184. [115, 118]

Hymowitz, N. (1979). Suppression of responding during signaled and unsignaled shock. *Psychological Bulletin, 86,* 175-190. [127]

Hyyppa, M.T., Aunda, S., Lahtela, K., Lahti, R., & Marniemi, J. (1983). Psychoneuroendocrine responses to mental load in an achievement-oriented task. *Ergonomics, 26,* 1155-1162. [67]

Immune interferon: A possible role in pulmonary fibrosis. (1987). *Medical Sciences Bulletin, 9*(5), 1. [92]

Ingbar, S.H. (1985). The thyroid gland. In J.D. Wilson & D.W. Foster (Eds.), *Williams textbook of endocrinology* (7th ed.) (pp. 682-815). Philadelphia: Saunders. [146]

Institute of Medicine Study Steering Committee (1982). Conceptual issues in stress research. In G.R. Elliot & C. Eisdorfer (Eds.), *Stress and human health: Analysis and implications of research* (pp. 11-24). New York: Springer. [13]

Istvan, J. (1986). Stress, anxiety, and birth outcomes: A critical review of the evidence. *Psychological Bulletin, 100,* 331-348. [240]

Jacobs, T.J., & Charles, E. (1980). Life events and the occurrence of cancer in children. *Psychosomatic Medicine, 42,* 11-24. [221, 228, 232]

Jacobs, W.J., & Nadel, L. (1985). Stress-induced recovery of fears and phobias. *Psychological Review, 92,* 512-531. [112]

Jacobson, A.M., Rand, L.I., & Hauser, S.T. (1985). Psychologic stress and glycemic control: A comparison of patients with and without proliferative diabetic retinopathy. *Psychosomatic Medicine, 47,* 372-381. [207]

Jaffe, J.H. (1985). Drug addiction and drug abuse. In A.G. Gilman, L.S. Goodman, T.W. Rall, & F. Murad (Eds.), *Goodman and Gilman's the pharmacological basis of therapeutics* (7th ed.) (pp. 532-581). New York: Macmillan. [144]

James, S.A. (1987). Psychosocial precursors of hypertension: A review of the epidemiologic evidence. *Circulation, 76* (No. 1, Part 2, Suppl. 1), 60-66. [181, 182]

Janković, B.D., Marković, B.M., & Spector, N.H. (Eds.). (1987). Neuroimmune interactions: Proceedings of the Second International Workshop on Neuroimmunomodulation. *Annals of the New York Academy of Sciences, 496.* [86]

Jansen, M.A., & Muenz, L.R. (1984). A retrospective study of personality variables associated with fibrocystic disease and breast cancer. *Journal of Psychosomatic Research, 28,* 35-42. [220, 228]

Jeffery, R.W. (1987). Behavioral treatment of obesity. *Annals of Behavioral Medicine, 9*(1), 20-24. [155]

Jemmott, J.B., III, & Locke, S.E. (1984). Psychosocial factors, immunologic mediation, and human susceptibility to infectious diseases: How much do we know? *Psychological Bulletin, 95,* 78-108. [93, 95, 197, 198]

Jensen, M.M. (1981). Emotional stress and susceptibility to infectious diseases. In K. Bammer & B.H. Newberry (Eds.), *Stress and cancer* (pp. 59-70). Toronto: C.J. Hogrefe. [201]

Jensen, M.R. (1987). Psychobiological factors predicting the course of breast cancer. *Journal of Personality, 55,* 317-342. [223, 230, 232]

Jensen, R.V. (1987). Classical chaos. *American Scientist, 75,* 168-181. [5]

Jobin, M., Feland, L., Cote, J., & Labrie, R. (1975). Effect of exposure to cold on hypothalamic TRH and plasma levels of TSH and prolactin in the rat. *Neuroendocrinology, 18,* 204-212. [74]

Johansson, G.G., Laakso, M.-L., Peder, M., & Karonen, S.-L. (1988). Examination stress decreases plasma level of luteinizing hormone in male students. *Psychosomatic Medicine, 50,* 286-294. [76]

Johnson, D.W. (1982). Behavioural treatment in the reduction of coronary risk factors: Type A behaviour and hypertension. *British Journal of Clinical Psychology, 21,* 281-294. [31, 192]

Jones, E.E. (1986). Interpreting interpersonal behavior: The effects of expectancies. *Science, 234,* 41-46. [104]

Jones, W.H., Hobbs, S.A., & Hockenbury, D. (1982). Loneliness and social skill deficits. *Journal of Personality and Social Psychology, 42,* 682-689. [129, 154]

Jordan, R.E., Kilpatrick, J., & Nelson, R.M. (1987). Heparin promotes the inactivation of antithrombin by neutrophil elastase. *Science, 237,* 777-779. [91]

Julius, M., Harburg, E., Cottington, E.M., & Johnson, E.H. (1986). Anger-coping types, blood pressure, and all cause mortality: A follow-up in Tecumseh, Michigan (1971-1983). *American Journal of Epidemiology, 124,* 220-233. [172]

Justice, A. (1985). Review of the effects of stress on cancer in laboratory animals: Importance of time of stress application and type of tumor. *Psychological Bulletin, 98,* 108-138. [208, 212, 215]

Kalin, N.H., & Loevinger, B.L. (1983). The central and peripheral opioid peptides: Their relationships and functions. *Psychiatric Clinics of North America, 6,* 415-428. [53]

Kamarck, T., & Jennings, J.R. (1991). Biobehavioral factors in sudden cardiac death. *Psychological Bulletin, 109,* 42-75. [186]

Kaplan, G.A., & Reynolds, P. (1988). Depression and cancer mortality and morbidity: Prospective evidence from the Alameda County Study. *Journal of Behavioral Medicine, 11,* 1-13. [218, 227]

Kasch, F.W., Wallace, J.P., & VanCamp, S.P. (1985). Effects of 18 years of endurance exercise on the physical work capacity of older men. *Journal of Cardiopulmonary Rehabilitation, 5,* 308-312. [149]

Keinan, G. (1987). Decision making under stress: Scanning of alternatives under controllable and uncontrollable threats. *Journal of Personality and Social Psychology, 52,* 639-644. [116]

Keller, S.E., Stein, M., Camerino, M.S., Schleifer, S.J., & Sherman, J. (1980). Suppression of lymphocyte stimulation by anterior hypothalamic lesions in the guinea pig. *Cellular Immunology, 52,* 334-340. [32]

Keller, S.E., Weiss, J.M., Schleifer, S.J., Miller, N.E., & Stein, M. (1981). Suppression of immunity by stress: Effect of a graded series of stressors on lymphocyte stimulation in the rat. *Science, 213,* 1397-1400. [20]

Keller, S.E., Weiss, J.M., Schleifer, S.J., Miller, N.E., & Stein, M. (1983). Stress-induced suppression of immunity in adrenalectomized rats. *Science, 221,* 1301-1304. [94, 95]

Kellner, R. (1985). Functional somatic symptoms and hypochondriasis: A survey of empirical studies. *Archives of General Psychiatry, 42,* 821-833. [24, 166]

Kelly, K.E., & Houston, B.K. (1985). Type A behavior in employed women: Relation to work, marital, and leisure variables, social support, stress, tension, and health. *Journal of Personality and Social Psychology, 48,* 1067-1079. [129]

Kelly, P.H. (1983). Inhibition of voluntary activity by growth hormone. *Hormones and Behavior, 17,* 163-168. [54]

Kelly, T.L., Gilpin, E., Ahnve, S., Henning, H., & Ross, J., Jr. (1985). Smoking status at the time of acute myocardial infarction and subsequent prognosis. *American Heart Journal, 110,* 535-541. [144]

Keltikangas-Järvinen, L., Pelkonen, P., & Kunnamo, I. (1988). Life changes related to juvenile rheumatoid arthritis. *Psychotherapy and Psychosomatics, 50,* 102-108. [234]

Kemeny, M.E., Cohen, F., Zegans, L.S., & Conant, M.A. (1989). Psychological and immunological predictors of genital herpes recurrence. *Psychosomatic Medicine, 51,* 195-208. [200]

Kernis, M.H., Granneman, B.D., & Barclay, L.C. (1989). Stability and level of self-esteem as predictors of anger arousal and hostility. *Journal of Personality and Social Psychology, 56,* 1013-1022. [113]

Kessler, J.A., Adler, J.E., & Black, I.B. (1983). Substance P and somatostatin regulate sympathetic noradrenergic function. *Science, 221,* 1059-1061. [68]

Khaw, K., & Barrett-Connor, E. (1986). Family history of heart attack: A modifiable risk factor? *Circulation, 74,* 239-244. [155]

Kiecolt-Glaser, J.K., Fisher, L.D., Ogrocki, P., Stout, J.C., Speicher, C.E., & Glaser, R. (1987). Marital quality, marital disruption, and immune function. *Psychosomatic Medicine, 49,* 13-34. [96, 97]

Kiecolt-Glaser, J.K., Garner, W., Speicher, C., Penn, G.M., Holliday, J., & Glaser, R. (1984). Psychosocial modifiers of immunocompetence in medical students. *Psychosomatic Medicine, 46,* 7-14. [97]

Kiecolt-Glaser, J.K., & Glaser, R. (1987). Psychosocial moderators of immune function. *Annals of Behavioral Medicine, 9*(2), 16-20. [93, 96, 140, 212]

Kiecolt-Glaser, J.K., Glaser, R., Williger, D., Stout, J., Messick, G., Sheppard, S., Ricker, D., Romister, S.C., Briner, W., Bonnell, G., & Donnerberg, R. (1985). Psychosocial enhancement of immunocompetence in a geriatric population. *Health Psychology, 4,* 25-41. [97]

Kiecolt-Glaser, J.K., Ricker, D., George, J., Messick, G., Speicher, C.E., Garner, W., & Glaser, R. (1984). Urinary cortisol levels, cellular immunocompetency, and loneliness in psychiatric inpatients. *Psychosomatic Medicine, 46,* 15-23. [97]

Kiesler, C.A., & Pallack, M.S. (1976). Arousal properties of dissonance manipulations. *Psychological Bulletin, 83,* 1014-1025. [120]

Kimball, J.W. (1986). *Introduction to immunology* (2nd. ed.). New York: Macmillan. [77, 211]

Kirmeyer, S.L., & Biggers, K. (1988). Environmental demand and demand engendering behavior: An observational analysis of the Type A pattern. *Journal of Personality and Social Psychology, 54,* 997-1005. [188]

Kirschbaum, B.B., & Schoolwerth, A.C. (1989). Acute aluminum toxicity associated with oral citrate and aluminum-containing antacids. *American Journal of Medical Sciences, 297,* 9-12. [148]

Klaassen, C.D. (1985). Nonmetalic environmental toxicants: Air pollution, solvents and vapors, and pesticides. In A.G. Gilman, L.S. Goodman, T.W. Rall, & F. Murad (Eds.), *Goodman and Gilman's the pharmacological basis of therapeutics* (7th ed) (pp. 1628-1650). New York: Macmillan. [147, 148]

Klein, G. (1987). The approaching era of the tumor suppressor genes. *Science, 238,* 1539-1545. [209, 210]

Kobasa, S.C. (1979). Stressful life events, personality, and health: An inquiry into hardiness. *Journal of Personality and Social Psychology, 37,* 1-11. [169]

Kobasa, S.C. (1982). *The hardy personality: Toward a social psychology of stress and health.* In G. Sanders & J. Suls (Eds.), *Social psychology of health and illness* (pp. 3-32). Hillsdale, NJ: Lawrence Erlbaum. [114]

Kobasa, S.C., Maddi, S.R., & Courington, S. (1981). Personality and constitution as mediators in the stress-illness relationship. *Journal of Health and Social Behavior, 22,* 368-378. [166]

Kobasa, S.C., Maddi, S.R., & Kahn, S. (1982). Hardiness and health: A prospective study. *Journal of Personality and Social Psychology, 42,* 168-177. [169]

Kobasa, S.C.O., Maddi, S.R., Puccetti, M.C., & Zola, M.A. (1985). Effectiveness of hardiness, exercise and social support as resources against illness. *Journal of Psychosomatic Research, 29,* 525-533. [169, 173]

Kobasa, S.C., Maddi, S.R., & Zola, M.A. (1983). Type A and hardiness. *Journal of Behavioral Medicine, 6,* 41-51. [169]

Koehler, T. (1985). Stress and rheumatoid arthritis: A survey of empirical evidence in human and animal studies. *Journal of Psychosomatic Research, 29,* 655-663. [234]

Kolata, G. (1986). Weight regulation may start in our cells, not psyches. *Smithsonian, 16* (10), 91-97. [156]

Koob, G.F. (1985). Stress, corticotropin-releasing factor, and behavior. In R.B. Williams, Jr. (Ed.), *Perspectives on behavioral medicine: Volume 2. Neuroendocrine control and behavior* (pp. 39-52). New York: Academic Press. [54, 55]

Kosten, T.R., Jacobs, S., Mason, J., Wahby, V., & Atkins, S. (1984). Psychological correlates of growth hormone response to stress. *Psychosomatic Medicine, 46,* 49-58. [74]

Koyanagi, Y., Miles, S., Mitsuyasu, R.T., Merrill, J.E., Vinters, H.V., & Chen, I.S.Y. (1987). Dual infection of the nervous system by AIDS viruses with distinct cellular tropisms. *Science, 236,* 819-822. [195]

Krantz, D.S., & Glass, D.C. (1984). Personality, behavior patterns, and physical illness: Conceptual and methodological issues. In W.D. Gentry (Ed.), *Handbook of behavioral medicine* (pp. 38-86). New York: Guilford Press. [166]

Krantz, D.S., & Manuck, S.B. (1984). Acute physiologic reactivity and risk of cardiovascular disease: A review and methodologic critique. *Psychological Bulletin, 96,* 435-464. [181]

Krieg, N.R. (Ed.). (1984). *Bergey's manual of systematic bacteriology* (vol. 1). Baltimore: Williams & Wilkins. [193]

Krieger, D.T. (1983). Brain peptides: What, where, and why? *Science, 222,* 975-985. [54, 55, 58]

Krulich, L., Hefco, E., Illner, P., & Read, C.B. (1974). The effects of acute stress on the secretion of LH, FSH, prolactin and GH in the normal male rat, with comments on their statistical evaluation. *Neuroendocrinology, 16,* 293-311. [21]

Kulik, J.A., & Mahler, H.I.M. (1987). Effects of preoperative roommate assignment on preoperative anxiety and recovery from coronary-bypass surgery. *Health Psychology, 6,* 525-543. [239]

LaBarba, R.C. (1970). Experiential and environmental factors in cancer: A review of research with animals. *Psychosomatic Medicine, 32,* 259-276. [212, 245]

Lacey, J.I. (1967). Somatic response patterning and stress: Some revisions of activation theory. In M.H. Appley & R. Trumbull (Eds.), *Psychological stress* (pp. 14-37). New York: Appleton-Century-Crofts. [16, 72, 109]

Lacroix, J.M., & Offutt, C. (1988). Type A and genital herpes. *Journal of Psychosomatic Research, 32,* 207-212. [200]

Lahti, R.A., & Barsuhn, C. (1974). The effect of minor tranquilizers on stress-induced increases in rat plasma corticosteroids. *Psychopharmacologia, 35,* 215-220. [143]

Landsberg, L., & Young, J.B. (1985). Catecholamines and the adrenal medulla. In J.D. Wilson & D.W. Foster (Eds.), *Williams textbook of endocrinology* (7th ed.) (pp. 891-965). Philadelphia: Saunders. [52, 53, 68, 69, 70, 71, 148]

Langer, E.J. (1975). The illusion of control. *Journal of Personality and Social Psychology, 32,* 311-328. [124]

Langer, E.J., & Piper, A.I. (1987). The prevention of mindlessness. *Journal of Personality and Social Psychology, 53,* 280-287. [105]

Lansky, S.B., Smith, S.D., Cairns, N.V., & Cairns, G.F., Jr. (1983). Psychological correlates of compliance. *American Journal of Pediatric Hematology/Oncology, 5,* 87-92. [157]

Larsson, K., Einarsson, S., Lundstrom, K., & Hakkarainen, J. (1983). Endocrine effects of heat stress in boars. *Acta Veterinary Scandinavia, 24,* 305-314. [75]

Lau, R.R., Hartman, K.A., & Ware, J.E., Jr. (1986). Health as a value: Methodological and theoretical considerations. *Health Psychology, 5,* 25-43. [159]

Laudenslager, M.L., Ryan, S.M., Drugan, R.C., Hyson, R.L., & Maier, S.F. (1983). Coping and immunosuppression: Inescapable but not escapable shock suppresses lymphocyte proliferation. *Science, 221,* 568-570. [20, 94]

Lazarus, R.S., DeLongis, A., Folkman, S., & Gruen, R. (1985). Stress and adaptational outcomes. *American Psychologist, 40,* 770-779. [15]

Lazarus, R.S., & Folkman, S. (1984). *Stress, appraisal, and coping.* New York: Springer. [16, 18, 19, 20, 21, 66, 99, 100, 101, 108, 110, 117, 121]

Leaverton, D.R., White, C.A., McCormick, C.R., Smith, P., & Sheikholislam, B. (1980). Parental loss antecedent to childhood diabetes mellitus. *Journal of the American Academy of Child Psychiatry, 19,* 678-689. [206]

LeDoux, J.E., Sakaguchi, A., & Reis, D.J. (1983). Strain differences in fear between spontaneously hypertensive and normotensive rats. *Brain Research, 277,* 137-143. [141]

Lefcourt, H.M., Martin, R.A., & Saleh, W.E. (1984). Locus of control and social support: Interactive moderators of stress. *Journal of Personality and Social Psychology, 47,* 378-389. [129]

Lehman, C.D., Rodin, J., McEwen, B., & Brinton, R. (1991). Impact of environmental stress on the expression of insulin-dependent diabetes mellitus. *Behavioral Neuroscience, 105,* 241-245. [98]

Leon, G.R., Finn, S.E., Murray, D., & Bailey, J.M. (1988). Inability to predict cardiovascular disease from hostility scores or MMPI items related to Type A behavior. *Journal of Consulting and Clinical Psychology, 56,* 597-600. [191]

Lerner, M.J., & Miller, D.T. (1978). Just world research and the attribution process: Looking back and ahead. *Psychological Bulletin, 85,* 1030-1051. [106]

Leshner, A.I., Korn, S.J., Mixon, J.F., Rosenthal, C., & Besser, A.K. (1980). Effects of corticosterone on submissiveness in mice: Some temporal and theoretical considerations. *Physiology and Behavior, 24,* 283-288. [53]

Levenkron, J.C., & Moore, L.G. (1988). The Type A behavior pattern: Issues for intervention research. *Annals of Behavioral Medicine, 10*(2), 78-83. [192]

Leventhal, H., & Cleary, P.D. (1980). The smoking problem: A review of research and theory in behavioral risk modification. *Psychological Bulletin, 88,* 370-405. [159, 208]

Levine, S. (1978). Cortisol changes following repeated experience with parachute training. In H. Ursin, E. Baade, & S. Levine (Eds.), *Psychobiology of stress: A study of coping men* (pp. 51-56). New York: Academic Press. [65]

Levine, S., & Saltzman, A. (1987). Nonspecific stress prevents relapses of experimental allergic encephalomyelitis in rats. *Brain, Behavior, and Immunity, 1,* 336-341. [98]

Levor, R.M., Cohen, M.J., Naliboff, B.D., McArthur, D., & Heuser, G. (1986). Psychosocial precursors and correlates of migraine headache. *Journal of Consulting and Clinical Psychology, 54,* 347-353. [236]

Levy, S.M. (Ed.). (1982). *Biological mediators of behavior and disease: Neoplasia.* New York: Elsevier. [208]

Levy, S.M., Herberman, R.B., Maluish, A.M., Schlien, B., & Lippman, M. (1985). Prognostic risk assessment in primary breast cancer by behavioral and immunological parameters. *Health Psychology, 4*, 99-113. [224, 225, 230]

Levy, S.M., Lee, J., Bagley, C., & Lippman, M. (1988). Survival hazards analysis in first recurrent breast cancer patients: Seven-year follow-up. *Psychosomatic Medicine, 50*, 520-528. [224, 230]

Lewis, J.W., Sherman, J.E., & Liebeskind, J.C. (1981). Opioid and non-opioid stress analgesia: Assessment of tolerance and cross tolerance with morphine. *Journal of Neuroscience, 1*, 358-363. [16]

Light, K.C. (1987). Psychosocial precursors of hypertension: Experimental evidence. *Circulation, 76* (No. 1, Part 2, Suppl. 1), 67-76. [179, 181]

Light, K.C., Koepke, J.P., Obrist, P.A., & Willis, P.W., IV. (1983). Psychosocial stress induces sodium and fluid retention in men at high risk for hypertension. *Science, 220*, 429-431. [181]

Linden, W., & Feuerstein, M. (1983). Essential hypertension and social coping behavior: Experimental findings. *Journal of Human Stress, 9*(3), 22-31. [181]

Linn, B.S., Linn, M.W., & Klimas, N.G. (1988). Effects of psychophysical stress on surgical outcome. *Psychosomatic Medicine, 50*, 230-244. [239]

Linville, P.W. (1987). Self-complexity as a cognitive buffer against stress-related illness and depression. *Journal of Personality and Social Psychology, 52*, 663-676. [170]

Lipowski, Z.J., Lipsitt, D.R., & Whybrow, P.C. (Eds.). (1977). *Psychosomatic medicine: Current trends and clinical applications.* New York: Oxford University Press. [8]

Little, R.E., Anderson, K.W., Ervin, C.H., Worthington-Roberts, B., & Clarren, S.K. (1989). Maternal alcohol use during breast-feeding and infant mental and motor development at one year. *New England Journal of Medicine, 321*, 425-430. [144]

Lloyd, R. (1984). Mechanisms of psychoneuroimmunological response. In B.H. Fox & B.H. Newberry (Eds.), *Impact of psychoendocrine systems in cancer and immunity* (pp. 1-57). Lewiston, NY: C.J. Hogrefe. [93]

Locke, S.E., Kraus, L., Leserman, J., Hurst, M.W., Heisel, J.S., & Williams, R.M. (1984). Life change stress, psychiatric symptoms, and natural killer cell activity. *Psychosomatic Medicine, 46*, 441-453. [95]

Lombardo, T., & Carreno, L. (1987). Relationship of Type A behavior pattern in smokers to carbon monoxide exposure and smoking topography. *Health Psychology, 6*, 445-452. [188, 189]

Longo, D.J., Clum, G.A., & Yeager, N.J. (1988). Psychosocial treatment for recurrent genital herpes. *Journal of Consulting and Clinical Psychology, 56*, 61-66. [200]

Loucks, A.B., & Horvath, S.M. (1984). Exercise-induced stress responses of amenorrheic and eumenorrheic runners. *Journal of Clinical Endocrinology and Metabolism, 59*, 1109-1120. [74]

Lown, B. (1987). Sudden cardiac death: Biobehavioral perspective. *Circulation, 76* (No. 1, Part 2, Suppl. 1), 186-196. [184, 186]

Lucas, C.P., Estigarribia, J.A., Darga, L.L., & Reaven, G.M. (1985). Insulin and blood pressure in obesity. *Hypertension, 7*, 702-706. [179]

Lumpkin, M.D., Samson, W.K., & McCann, S.M. (1987). Arginine vasopressin as a thyrotropin-releasing hormone. *Science, 235*, 1070-1073. [62]

Luria, S.E., Darnell, J.E., Jr., Baltimore, D., & Campbell, A. (1978). *General virology* (3rd. ed.). New York: Wiley. [193]

Maas, J.W., & Medniecks, M. (1971). Hydrocortisone-mediated increase of norepinephrine uptake by brain slices. *Science, 171*, 178-179. [53]

MacDougall, J.M., Dembroski, T.M., Dimsdale, J.E., & Hackett, T.P. (1985). Components of Type A, hostility, and anger-in: Further relationships to angiographic findings. *Health Psychology, 4*, 137-152. [190]

MacLennan, A.J., & Maier, S.F. (1983). Coping and stress-induced potentiation of stimulant stereotypy in the rat. *Science, 219*, 1091-1093. [20]

Madden, J.E., Baldwin, D.R., Chu, E., Gerstenberger, T.J., Noorbakhsh, H., Steele, J.H., Stevenson, J.R., & Newberry, B.H. (1988). Stress, mammary tumors, mitogen response and cardiac size. In A. Lobo & A. Tres (Eds.), *Psicosomatica y cancer* (pp. 61-72). Madrid: Ministerio de Sanidad y Consumo. [214]

Magnus, K., Matroos, A.W., & Strackee, J. (1983). The self-employed and the self-driven: Two coronary-prone subpopulations from the Zeist study. *American Journal of Epidemiology, 118*, 799-805. [185]

Maier, S.F., Ryan, S.M., Barksdale, C.M., & Kalin, N.H. (1986). Stressor controllability and the pituitary-adrenal system. *Behavioral Neuroscience, 100*, 669-674. [126]

Maier, S.F., & Seligman, M.E.P. (1976). Learned helplessness: Theory and evidence. *Journal of Experimental Psychology: General, 105*, 3-46. [125]

Majerus, P.W., Connolly, T.M., Deckmyn, H., Ross, T.S., Bross, T.E., Ishii, H., Bansal, V.S., & Wilson, D.B. (1986). The metabolism of phosphoinositide-derived messenger molecules. *Science, 234*, 1519-1526. [49]

Majewska, M.D., Harrison, N.L., Schwartz, R.D., Barker, J.L., & Paul, S.M. (1986). Steroid hormone metabolites are barbiturate-like modulators of the GABA receptor. *Science, 232*, 1004-1007. [53]

Mandler, G. (1975). The search for emotion. In L. Levi (Ed.), *Emotions: Their parameters and measurement* (pp. 1-15). New York: Raven Press. [109]

Marshall, J.R., & Funch, D.P. (1983). Social environment and breast cancer: A cohort analysis of patient survival. *Cancer, 52*, 1546-1550. [223, 229]

Martin, J.E., & Dubbert, P.M. (1982). Exercise applications and promotion in behavioral medicine: Current status and future directions. *Journal of Consulting and Clinical Psychology, 50*, 1004-1017. [149, 186]

Marx, J.L. (1987). Polyphosphoinositide research updated. *Science, 235*, 974-976. [49]

Mason, J.W. (1971). A re-evaluation of the concept of "non-specificity" in stress theory. *Journal of Psychosomatic Research, 8*, 323-333. [120]

Mason, J.W. (1975). Emotion as reflected in patterns of endocrine integration. In L. Levi (Ed.), *Emotions: Their parameters and measurement* (pp. 143-181). New York: Raven Press. [16, 20, 21, 65, 72]

Mason, J.W., Kenion, C.C., Collins, D.R., Mougey, E.H., Jones, J.A., Driver, G.C., Brady, J.V., & Beer, B. (1968). Urinary testosterone response to 72-hr. avoidance sessions in the monkey. *Psychosomatic Medicine, 30*, 721-732. [75]

Matarazzo, J.D. (1980). Behavioral health and behavioral medicine: Frontiers for a new health psychology. *American Psychologist, 35*, 807-817. [109]

Matthes, T. (1963). Experimental contribution to the question of emotional stress reactions on the growth of tumors in animals. *Proceedings of the Eighth Anti-Cancer Congress, 3*, 471-473. [213]

Matthews, K.A. (1982). Psychological perspectives on the Type A behavior pattern. *Psychological Bulletin, 91*, 293-323. [187]

Matthews, K.A., & Carra, J. (1982). Suppression of menstrual distress symptoms: A study of Type A behavior. *Personality and Social Psychology Bulletin, 8*, 146-151. [111]

Matthews, K.A., & Woodall, K.L. (1988). Childhood origins of overt Type A behaviors and cardiovascular reactivity to behavioral stressors. *Annals of Behavioral Medicine, 10*(2), 71-77. [188]

McCann, I.L., & Holmes, D.S. (1984). Influence of aerobic exercise on depression. *Journal of Personality and Social Psychology, 46*, 1142-1147. [149]

McCarron, D.A., Morris, C.D., Henry, H.J., & Stanton, J.L. (1984). Blood pressure and nutrient intake in the United States. *Science, 224*, 1392-1398. [147]

McCaul, K.D., & Malott, J.M. (1984). Distraction and coping with pain. *Psychological Bulletin, 95*, 516-533. [111]

McClelland, D.C. (1989). Motivational factors in health and disease. *American Psychologist, 44*, 675-683. [96, 126]

McCranie, E.W., Watkins, L.O., Brandsma, J.M., & Sisson, B.D. (1986). Hostility, coronary heart disease (CHD) incidence, and total mortality: Lack of association in a 25-year follow-up study of 478 physicians. *Journal of Behavioral Medicine, 9*, 119-125. [191]

McCubbin, H.I., Joy, C.B., Cauble, A.E., Comeau, J.K., Patterson, J.M., & Needle, R.H. (1980). Family stress and coping: A decade review. *Journal of Marriage and the Family, 42*, 855-871. [122]

McCubbin, J.A., Surwit, R.S., & Williams, R.B., Jr. (1985). Endogenous opiate peptides, stress reactivity, and risk for hypertension. *Hypertension, 7*, 808-811. [179]

McGinley, H., LeFevre, R., & McGinley, P. (1975). The influence of a communicator's body position on opinion change in others. *Journal of Personality and Social Psychology, 31*, 686-690. [153]

McGrath, J.E. (1970). A conceptual formulation for research on stress. In J.E. McGrath (Ed.), *Social and psychological factors in stress* (pp. 10-21). New York: Holt, Rinehart and Winston. [16]

McKinney, M.E., Hofschire, P.J., Buell, J.C., & Eliot, R.S. (1984). Hemodynamic and biochemical responses to stress: The necessary link between Type A behavior and cardiovascular disease. *Behavioral Medicine Update, 6*(4), 16-21. [183, 187]

Mechanic, D. (1972). Social psychologic factors affecting the presentation of bodily complaints. *New England Journal of Medicine, 286*, 1132-1139. [24, 166]

Merrill, J.E., Kutsunai, S., Mohlstrom, C., Hofman, F., Groopman, J., & Golde, D.W. (1984). Proliferation of astroglia and oligodendroglia in response to human T cell-derived factors. *Science, 224*, 1428-1430. [91]

Messer, S.B. (1976). Reflection-impulsivity: A review. *Psychological Bulletin, 83*, 1026-1052. [108]

Meyer, D., Leventhal, H., & Gutmann, M. (1985). Common-sense models of illness: The example of hypertension. *Health Psychology, 4*, 115-135. [180]

Meyerhoff, J.L., Kant, G.J., Sessions, G.R., Moughey, E.H., Pennington, L.L., & Lenox, R.H. (1985). Brain and pituitary cyclic nucleotide response to stress. In R.B. Williams, Jr. (Ed.), *Perspectives on behavioral medicine. Vol. 2. Neuroendocrine control and behavior* (pp. 53-70). New York: Academic Press. [56]

Milenković, L., Bogić, L., & Martinović, J.V. (1986). Effects of oestradiol and progesterone on stress-induced secretion of prolactin in ovariectomized and/or adrenalelctomized female rats. *Acta Endocrinologica, 112*, 79-82. [74]

Miles, M.S. (1985). Emotional symptoms and physical health in bereaved parents. *Nursing Research, 34*(2), 76-81. [175]

Miller, I.W., III, & Norman, W.H. (1979). Learned helplessness in humans: A review and attribution theory. *Psychological Bulletin, 86*, 93-118. [125, 126]

Miller, N.E. (1959). Liberalization of basic S-R concepts: Extensions to conflict behavior, motivation, and social learning. In S. Koch (Ed.), *Psychology: A study of a science* (vol. 2) (pp. 196-292). New York: McGraw-Hill. [5]

Miller, N.E. (1981). An overview of behavioral medicine: Opportunities and dangers. In S.M. Weiss, J.A. Herd, & B.H. Fox (Eds.), *Perspectives on behavioral medicine* (pp. 3-22). New York: Academic Press. [3, 35]

Miller, S.M., Brody, D.S., & Summerton, J. (1988). Styles of coping with threat: Implications for health. *Journal of Personality and Social Psychology, 54*, 142-148. [153]

Miller, S.M., Lack, E.R., & Asroff, S. (1985). Preference for control and the coronary-prone behavior pattern: "I'd rather do it myself." *Journal of Personality and Social Psychology, 49*, 492-499. [120]

Mischel, W. (1973). Toward a cognitive social learning reconceptualization of personality. *Psychological Review, 80*, 252-283. [104]

Monden, Y., Koshiyama, K., Tanaka, H., Mizutani, S., Aono, T., Hamanaka, Y., Uozumi, T., & Matsumoto, K. (1972). Influence of major surgical stress on plasma testosterone, plasma LH, and urinary steroids. *Acta Endocrinologica, 69,* 542-552. [75]

Monjan, A.A. (1981). Stress and immunologic competence: Studies in animals. In R. Ader (Ed.), *Psychoneuroimmunology* (pp. 185-228). New York: Academic Press. [93, 94]

Monjan, A.A., & Collector, M.I. (1977). Stress-induced modulation of the immune response. *Science, 196,* 307-308. [93]

Moos, R.H. (1982). Coping with acute health crises. In T. Millon, C. Green, & R. Meagler (Eds.), *Handbook of clinical health psychology* (pp. 129-151). New York: Plenum. [120]

Morris, T., Greer, S., Pettingale, K.W., & Watson, M. (1981). Patterns of expression of anger and their psychological correlates in women with breast cancer. *Journal of Psychosomatic Research, 25,* 111-117. [219, 228]

Morrison, D.C., & Ryan, J.L. (1987). Endotoxins and disease mechanisms. *Annual Review of Medicine, 38,* 417-432. [183]

Morrison, F.R., & Paffenbarger, R.S., Jr. (1981). Epidemiological aspects of biobehavior in the etiology of cancer: A critical review. In S.M. Weiss, J.A. Herd, & B.H. Fox (Eds.), *Perspectives on behavioral medicine* (pp. 135-161). New York: Academic Press. [208, 216]

Murison, R.C. (1983). Time course of plasma corticosterone under immobilization stress in rats. *IRCS Medical Sciences: Psychology and Psychiatry, 11,* 20-21. [65]

Murison, R.C., Isaksen, E., & Ursin, H. (1981). "Coping" and gastric ulceration in rats after prolonged active avoidance performance. *Physiology and Behavior, 27,* 345-348. [127]

Murphy, G. (1947). *Personality: A biosocial approach to origins and structure.* New York: Harper & Brothers. [12]

Murphy, M.T., Richards, D.B., & Lipton, J.M. (1983). Antipyretic potency of centrally administered α-melanocyte stimulating hormone. *Science, 221,* 192-193. [54]

Nakashima, A., Koshiyama, K., Uozumi, T., Monden, Y., Hamanaka, Y., Kurachi, K., Aono, T., Mizutani, S., & Matsumoto, K. (1975). Effects of general anesthesia and severity of surgical stress on serum LH and testosterone in males. *Acta Endocrinologica, 78,* 258-269. [75]

Naliboff, B.D., Cohen, M.J., & Sowers, J.D. (1985). Physiological and metabolic responses to brief stress in non-insulin dependent diabetic and control subjects. *Journal of Psychosomatic Research, 29,* 367-374. [205]

Natelson, B.H. (1983). Stress, predisposition and the onset of serious disease: Implications about psychosomatic etiology. *Neuroscience and Biobehavioral Reviews, 7,* 511-527. [162, 164]

Natelson, B.H., Krasnegor, N., & Holaday, J.W. (1976). Relations between behavioral arousal and plasma cortisol in monkeys performing repeated free-operant avoidance sessions. *Journal of Comparative and Physiological Psychology, 90,* 958-969. [67]

Naughton, J. (1985). Role of physical activity as a secondary intervention for healed myocardial infarction. *American Journal of Cardiology, 55,* 21D-26D. [186]

Newberry, B.H. (1978). Restraint-induced inhibition of 7,12-dimethylbenz(a)-anthracene-induced mammary tumors: Relation to stages of tumor development. *Journal of the National Cancer Institute, 61,* 725-729. [35, 213, 214]

Newberry, B.H. (1981). Effects of presumably stressful stimulation (PSS) on the development of animal tumors: Some issues. In S.M. Weiss, J.A. Herd, & B.H. Fox (Eds.), *Perspectives on behavioral medicine* (pp. 329-349). New York: Academic Press. [208, 212]

Newberry, B.H., Gerstenberger, T.J., Madden, J.E., & Newberry, D.L. (1985). Evidence for tumor system specificity in experimental tumor response to "stress". In O.

Lindfors, R. Lehvonen, M.-J. Vauhkonen, & K. Achté (Eds.), *Psychosomatics of cancer* (Report No. 65, World Psychiatric Association Regional Symposium. pp. 1-20). Helsinki: Psykiatrian Tutkimussäätiö. [32, 208, 212, 215]

Newberry, B.H., Gordon, T.L., & Meehan, S.M. (in press). Animal studies of stress and cancer. In C.L. Cooper & M. Watson (Eds.), *Cancer and stress: Recent research.* Chichester, U.K.: Wiley. [215]

Newberry, B.H., Liebelt, A.G., & Boyle, D.A. (1984). Variables in behavioral oncology: Overview and assessment of current issues. In B.H. Fox & B.H. Newberry (Eds.), *Impact of psychoendocrine systems in cancer and immunity* (pp. 86-146). Lewiston, NY: C.J. Hogrefe. [22, 151, 211, 212, 213, 214]

Newcomb, M.D., & Harlow, L.L. (1986). Life events and substance abuse among adolescents: Mediating effects of perceived loss of control and meaninglessness in life. *Journal of Personality and Social Psychology, 51,* 564-577. [159]

Nisbett, R.E., & Wilson, T.D. (1977). Telling more than we can know: Verbal reports on mental processes. *Psychological Review, 84,* 231-259. [18, 105]

Notarius, C.I., & Levenson, R.W. (1979). Expressive tendencies and physiological response to stress. *Journal of Personality and Social Psychology, 37,* 1204-1210. [115, 139]

Nowell, P.C. (1990). Cytogenetics of tumor progression. *Cancer, 65,* 2172-2177. [210]

Oatley, K., & Bolton, W. (1985). A social-cognitive theory of depression in reaction to life events. *Psychological Review, 92,* 372-388. [114]

Oberman, A. (1985). Exercise and the primary prevention of cardiovascular disease. *American Journal of Cardiology, 55,* 10D-20D. [186]

Ogle, T.F., & Kitay, J.I. (1979). Interactions of prolactin and adrenocorticotropin in the regulation of adrenocortical secretions in female rats. *Endocrinology, 104,* 40-44. [64]

O'Leary, A., Shoor, S., Lorig, K., & Holman, H.R. (1988). A cognitive-behavioral treatment for rheumatoid arthritis. *Health Psychology, 7,* 527-544. [235]

O'Malley, M.N., & Becker, L.A. (1984). Removing the egocentric bias: The relevance of distress cues to evaluation of fairness. *Personality and Social Psychology Bulletin, 10,* 235-242. [106]

Overmier, J.B., Murison, R., Skoglund, E.J., & Ursin, H. (1985). Safety signals can mimic responses in reducing the ulcerogenic effects of prior shock. *Physiological Psychology, 13,* 243-247. [240]

Paffenbarger, R.S., Hyde, R.T., Wing, A.L., & Hsieh, C.-C. (1986). Physical activity, all-cause mortality, and longevity of college alumni. *New England Journal of Medicine, 314,* 605-613. [172]

Page, T., Harris, R.H., & Epstein, S.S. (1976). Drinking water and cancer mortality in Louisiana. *Science, 193,* 55-57. [147]

Palmblad, J. (1981). Stress and immunologic competence: Studies in man. In R. Ader (Ed.), *Psychoneuroimmunology* (pp. 229-257). New York: Academic Press. [93]

Pardine, P., & Napoli, A. (1983). Physiological reactivity and recent life-stress experience. *Journal of Consulting and Clinical Psychology, 51,* 467-469. [73]

Paré, W.P. (1986). Prior stress and susceptibility to stress ulcer. *Physiology & Behavior, 36,* 1155-1159. [240]

Pavlidis, N., & Chirigos, M. (1980). Stress-induced impairment of macrophage tumoricidal function. *Psychosomatic Medicine, 42,* 47-54. [94, 95]

Pennebaker, J.W., Kiecolt-Glaser, J.K., & Glaser, R. (1988). Disclosure of traumas and immune function: Health implications for psychotherapy. *Journal of Consulting and Clinical Psychology, 56,* 239-245. [97]

Perkins, D.P. (1982). The assessment of stress using life events scales. In L. Goldberger & S. Breznitz (Eds.), *Handbook of stress: Theoretical and clinical aspects* (pp. 320-331). New York: The Free Press. [121, 122]

Perkins, K.A. (1985). The synergistic effect of smoking and serum cholesterol on coronary heart disease. *Health Psychology, 4,* 337-360. [144, 148, 184]

Persky, V.W., Kempthorne-Rawson, J., & Shekelle, R.B. (1987). Personality and risk of cancer: 20-year follow-up of the Western Electric study. *Psychosomatic Medicine, 49*, 435-449. [217, 218, 223, 227]

Peters, L.J., & Mason, K.A. (1979). Influence of stress on experimental cancer. In B.A. Stoll (Ed.), *Mind and cancer prognosis* (pp. 103-124). Chichester, U.K.: Wiley. [212]

Peterson, C., & Seligman, M.E.P. (1984). Causal explanations as a risk factor for depression: Theory and evidence. *Psychological Review, 91*, 347-374. [113, 114, 125, 126]

Peterson, C., Seligman, M.E.P., & Vaillant, G.E. (1988). Pessimistic explanatory style is a risk factor for physical illness: A thirty-five-year longitudinal study. *Journal of Personality and Social Psychology, 55*, 23-27. [170]

Pettigrew, T. (1979). The ultimate attribution error: Extending Allport's cognitive analysis of prejudice. *Personality and Social Psychology Bulletin, 5*, 461-476. [106]

Pettingale, K.W. (1985). Towards a psychobiological model of cancer: Biological considerations. *Social Science and Medicine, 20*, 779-787. [211, 212]

Petty, R.E., Wells, G.L., Heesacker, M., Brock, T.C., & Cacioppo, J.T. (1983). The effects of recipient posture on persuasion: A cognitive response analysis. *Personality and Social Psychology Bulletin, 9*, 209-222. [139]

Peyrot, M., & McMurry, J.F., Jr. (1985). Psychosocial factors in diabetes control: Adjustment of insulin-treated adults. *Psychosomatic Medicine, 47*, 542-557. [207]

Pinto, R.P., & Hollandsworth, J.G., Jr. (1989). Using videotape modeling to prepare children for surgery: Influence of parents and costs versus benefits of providing preparation services. *Health Psychology, 8*, 79-85. [239]

Plaut, M. (1987). Lymphocyte hormone receptors. *Annual Review of Immunology, 5*, 621-669. [86, 87, 88, 89]

Plaut, S.M., & Friedman, S.B. (1981). Psychosocial factors in infectious disease. In R. Ader (Ed.), *Psychoneuroimmunology* (pp. 3-30). New York: Academic Press. [164, 201]

Plaut, S.M., & Friedman, S.B. (1982). Stress, coping behavior and resistance to disease. *Psychotherapy and Psychosomatics, 38*, 274-283. [32, 36, 201]

Pontiroli, A.E., Baio, G., Stella, L., Crescenti, A., & Girardi, A.M. (1982). Effects of naloxone on prolactin, luteinizing hormone, and cortisol responses to surgical stress in humans. *Journal of Clinical Endocrinology and Metabolism, 55*, 378-380. [75]

Poulton, E.C. (1978). A new look at the effects of noise: A rejoinder. *Psychological Bulletin, 85*, 1068-1079. [117, 118]

Pozniak, P.C. (1985). The carcinogenicity of caffeine and coffee: A review. *Journal of the American Dietetic Association, 85*, 1127-1133. [145]

Price, R.A. (1987). Genetics of human obesity. *Annals of Behavioral Medicine, 9*(1), 9-14. [155]

Price, R.W., Brew, B., Sidtis, J., Rosenblum, M., Scheck, A.C., & Cleary, P. (1988). The brain in AIDS: Central nervous system HIV-1 infection and AIDS dementia complex. *Science, 239*, 586-592. [152, 195, 198]

Puddey, I.B., Beilin, L.J., Vandongen, R., Rouse, I.L., & Rogers, P. (1985). Evidence for a direct effect of alcohol consumption on blood pressure in normotensive men: A randomized controlled trial. *Hypertension, 7*, 707-713. [143]

Pyszczynski, T., Greenberg, J., & Holt, K. (1985). Maintaining consistency between self-serving beliefs and available data: A bias in information evaluation. *Personality and Social Psychology Bulletin, 11*, 179-190. [106]

Quattrone, G.A. (1985). On the congruity between internal states and action. *Psychological Bulletin, 98*, 3-40. [138]

Rabkin, J.G., & Struening, E.L. (1976). Life events, stress, and illness. *Science, 194*, 1013-1020. [164, 165]

References 273

Ragland, D.R., & Brand, R.J. (1988). Type A behavior and mortality from coronary heart disease. *New England Journal of Medicine, 318*, 65-69. [189]

Rall, T.W. (1985). Central nervous stimulants (continued): The methylxanthines. In A.G. Gilman, L.S. Goodman, T.W. Rall, & F. Murad (Eds.), *Goodman and Gilman's the pharmacological basis of therapeutics* (7th ed.) (pp. 589-603). New York: Macmillan. [145, 148]

Ray, W.A., Griffin, M.R., Schaffner, W., Baugh, D.K., & Melton, L.J. (1987). Psychotropic drug use and risk of hip fracture. *New England Journal of Medicine, 316*, 363-369. [160]

Read, D.A. (1983). Holistic health from the inside. *Journal of School Health, 53*, 382-385. [13]

Reichlin, S. (1985). Neuroendocrinology. In J.D. Wilson & D.W. Foster (Eds.), *Williams textbook of endocrinology* (7th ed.) (pp. 492-567). Philadelphia: Saunders. [51, 52, 53, 55, 61, 62, 63, 74, 149]

Reid, R.L., & Yen, S.C.C. (1981). Premenstrual syndrome. *American Journal of Obstetrics and Gynecology, 135*, 85-104. [53]

Reis, H.T., Wheeler, L., Kernis, M.H., Spiegel, N., & Nezlek, J. (1985). On specificity in the impact of social participation on physical and psychological health. *Journal of Personality and Social Psychology, 48*, 456-471. [172]

Revicki, D.A., & May, H.J. (1985). Occupational stress, social support, and depression. *Health Psychology, 4*, 61-77. [129]

Richardson, R., Riccio, D.C., & Devine, L. (1984). ACTH-induced recovery of extinguished avoidance responding. *Physiological Psychology, 12*, 184-192. [53]

Riley, V. (1966). Spontaneous mammary tumors: Decrease in incidence of mice infected with an enzyme-elevating virus. *Science, 153*, 1657-1658. [215]

Riley, V. (1981). Psychoendocrine influences on immunocompetence and neoplasia. *Science, 212*, 1100-1109. [164, 208, 212]

Riley, V., Fitzmaurice, M.A., & Spackman, D.H. (1982). Immunocompetence and neoplasia: Role of anxiety stress. In S.M. Levy (Ed.), *Biological mediators of behavior and disease: Neoplasia* (pp. 175-218). New York: Elsevier. [213, 215]

Ritchie, J.M. (1985). The aliphatic alcohols. In A.G. Gilman, L.S. Goodman, T.W. Rall, & F. Murad (Eds.), *Goodman and Gilman's the pharmacological basis of therapeutics* (7th ed.) (pp. 372-386). New York: Macmillan. [143, 144, 148]

Robbins, S.L., Cotran, R.S., & Kumar, V. (1984). *The pathologic basis of disease* (3rd ed.). Philadelphia: Saunders. [91, 92, 141, 142, 143, 147, 151, 155, 176, 178, 193, 202, 209, 210, 233, 237]

Rodin, J. (1985). Insulin levels, hunger, and food intake: An example of feedback loops in body weight regulation. *Health Psychology, 4*, 1-24. [156]

Rodin, J. (1986). Aging and health: Effects of the sense of control. *Science, 233*, 1271-1276. [124, 125]

Rodin, J., & Langer, E.J. (1977). Long-term effects of a control-relevant intervention with the institutionalized aged. *Journal of Personality and Social Psychology, 35*, 897-902. [124]

Rodin, J., Solomon, S.K., & Metcalf, J. (1978). Role of control in mediating perceptions of density. *Journal of Personality and Social Psychology, 36*, 988-999. [125]

Rofé, Y. (1984). Stress and affiliation: A utility theory. *Psychological Review, 91*, 235-250. [119]

Rogentine, G.N., Jr., van Kammen, D.P., Fox, B.H., Docherty, J.P., Rosenblatt, J.E., Boyd, S.C., & Bunney, W.E., Jr. (1979). Psychological factors in the prognosis of malignant melanoma: A prospective study. *Psychosomatic Medicine, 41*, 647-655. [225, 230]

Rose, R.M. (1980). Endocrine responses to stressful psychological events. *Psychiatric Clinics of North America, 3*, 251-276. [22, 23, 65, 67, 72, 73, 74, 75, 148]

Rose, R.M. (1985). Psychoendocrinology. In J.D. Wilson & D.W. Foster (Eds.), *Williams textbook of endocrinology* (7th ed.) (pp. 653-681). Philadelphia: Saunders. [52, 53, 54, 65, 73, 74, 75, 76]

Rosellini, R.A., & Seligman, M.E.P. (1978). Role of shock intensity in the learned helplessness paradigm. *Animal Learning and Behavior, 6*, 155-159. [126]

Rosoff, C.B., & Goldman, H. (1968). Effect of the intestinal bacterial flora on acute gastric stress ulceration. *Gastroenterology, 55*, 212-222. [142]

Ross, G.T. (1985). Disorders of the ovary and female reproductive tract. In J.D. Wilson & D.W. Foster (Eds.), *Williams textbook of endocrinology* (7th ed.) (pp. 206-258). Philadelphia: Saunders. [151]

Ross, M., & Olson, J.M. (1982). Placebo effects in medical research and practice. In J.R. Eiser (Ed.), *Social psychology and behavioral medicine* (pp. 441-458). New York: Wiley. [152]

Roth, D.L., & Holmes, D.S. (1985). Influence of physical fitness in determining the impact of stressful life events on physical and psychological health. *Psychosomatic Medicine, 47*, 164-173. [173]

Roth, D.L., Wiebe, D.J., Fillingim, R.B., & Shay, K.A. (1989). Life events, fitness, hardiness, and health: A simultaneous analysis of proposed stress-resistance effects. *Journal of Personality and Social Psychology, 57*, 136-142. [173]

Roth, J., & Grunfeld, C. (1985). Mechanism of action of peptide hormones and catecholamines. In J.D. Wilson & D.W. Foster (Eds.), *Williams textbook of endocrinology* (7th ed.) (pp. 76-122). Philadelphia: Saunders. [48, 49]

Rotter, J.B. (1966). Generalized expectancies for internal versus external control of reinforcement. *Psychological Monographs, 80*(1, whole No. 609). [105]

Rowland, K.F. (1977). Environmental events predicting death for the elderly. *Psychological Bulletin, 84*, 349-372. [162]

Rowland, R.R.R., Chukwuocha, R., & Tokuda, S. (1987). Modulation of the *in vitro* murine immune response by met-enkephalin. *Brain, Behavior, and Immunity, 1*, 342-348. [89]

Rozanski, A., Bairey, C.N., Krantz, D.S., Friedman, J., Resser, K.J., Morell, M., Hilton-Chalfen, S., Hestrin, L., Bietendorf, J., & Berman, D.S. (1988). Mental stress and the induction of silent myocardial ischemia in patients with coronary artery disease. *New England Journal of Medicine, 318*, 1005-1012. [185, 186]

Ruderman, A.J. (1983). Obesity, anxiety, and food consumption. *Addictive Behaviors, 8*, 235-242. [159]

Ruderman, A.J. (1986). Dietary restraint: A theoretical and empirical review. *Psychological Bulletin, 99*, 247-262. [155]

Rule, B.G., & Nesdale, A.R. (1976). Emotional arousal and aggressive behavior. *Psychological Bulletin, 83*, 851-863. [113]

Rushton, J.P., Fulker, D.W., Neale, M.C., Nias, D.K.B., & Eysenck, H.J. (1986). Altruism and aggression: The heritability of individual differences. *Journal of Personality and Social Psychology, 50*, 1192-1198. [141]

Salter, M.W., Brooke, R.L., & Merskey, H. (1986). Temporomandibular pain and dysfunction syndrome: The relationship of clinical and psychological data to outcome. *Journal of Behavioral Medicine, 9*, 97-109. [236]

Santiago, J.V. (1984). Effect of treatment on the long term complications of IDDM. *Behavioral Medicine Update, 6*(1), 26-31. [205]

Sarason, B.R., Sarason, I.G., Hacker, T.A., & Basham, R.B. (1985). Concomitants of social support: Social skills, physical attractiveness, and gender. *Journal of Personality and Social Psychology, 49*, 469-480. [171]

Sarason, I.G., & Sarason, B.R. (1986). Experimentally provided social support. *Journal of Personality and Social Psychology, 50*, 1222-1225. [128]

Sarason, I.G., Sarason, B.R., Potter, E.H., III, & Antoni, M.H. (1985). Life events, social support, and illness. *Psychosomatic Medicine, 47*, 156-163. [171]

Schachter, S. (1959). *The psychology of affiliation: Experimental studies of the sources of gregariousness.* Stanford, CA: Stanford University Press. [119]

Schachter, S., Silverstein, B., & Perlick, D. (1977). Psychological and pharmacological explanations of smoking under stress. *Journal of Experimental Psychology: General, 106,* 31-40. [159]

Scheier, M.F., & Carver, C.S. (1985). Optimism, coping, and health: Assessment and implications of generalized outcome expectancies. *Health Psychology, 4,* 219-247. [169, 170]

Scherg, H. (1987). Psychosocial factors and disease bias in breast cancer patients. *Psychosomatic Medicine, 49,* 302-312. [219, 220, 221, 228, 232]

Scherg, H., & Blohmke, M. (1988). Associations between selected life events and cancer. *Behavioral Medicine, 14,* 119-124. [220, 228, 232]

Scherg, H., Cramer, I., & Blohmke, M. (1981). Psychosocial factors and breast cancer: A critical reevaluation of established hypotheses. *Cancer Detection and Prevention, 4,* 165-171. [219]

Schlegel, R., & Pardee, A.B. (1986). Caffeine-induced uncoupling of mitosis from the completion of DNA replication in mammalian cells. *Science, 232,* 1264-1266. [145]

Schlesier-Stropp, B. (1984). Bulimia: A review of the literature. *Psychological Bulletin, 95,* 247-257. [159]

Schlundt, D.G., & Langford, H.G. (1985). Dietary approaches to the treatment of hypertension. *Annals of Behavioral Medicine, 7(1),* 19-24. [146]

Schmid, P., Schultz, W.A., & Hameister, H. (1989). Dynamic expression pattern of the *myc* protooncogene in midgestation mouse embryos. *Science, 243,* 226-229. [209]

Schmidt, D.D., Zyanski, S., Ellner, J., Kumar, M.L., & Arno, J. (1985). Stress as a precipitating factor in recurrent herpes labialis. *Journal of Family Practice, 20,* 359-366. [199]

Schneiderman, N., & Tapp, J.T. (Eds.). (1985). *Behavioral medicine: The biopsychosocial approach.* Hillsdale, NJ: Lawrence Erlbaum. [8]

Schorr, D., & Rodin, J. (1984). Motivation to control one's environment in individuals with obsessive-compulsive, depressive, and normal personality traits. *Journal of Personality and Social Psychology, 46,* 1148-1161. [124]

Schroeder, D.H., & Costa, P.T., Jr. (1984). Influence of life event stress on physical illness: Substantive effects or methodological flaws? *Journal of Personality and Social Psychology, 46,* 853-863. [166]

Schuckit, M.A. (1985). Genetics and the risk for alcoholism. *Journal of the American Medical Association, 254,* 2614-2617. [141]

Schuit, F.C., & Pipeleers, D.G. (1986). Differences in adrenergic recognition by pancreatic A and B cells. *Science, 232,* 875-877. [59]

Schwartz, G.E. (1982). Testing the biopsychosocial model: The ultimate challenge facing behavioral medicine? *Journal of Consulting and Clinical Psychology, 50,* 1040-1053. [8]

Schwartz, G.E. (1984). Psychobiology of health: A new synthesis. In B.J. Hammonds & C.J. Scheirer (Eds.), *Psychology and health* (Master Lecture Series, vol. 3, pp. 149-193). Washington, D.C.: American Psychological Association. [9, 24, 223]

Sclafani, A., & Springer, D. (1976). Dietary obesity in adult rats: Similarities to hypothalamic and human obesity syndromes. *Physiology and Behavior, 17,* 461-471. [145]

Scroggs, J.R. (1985). *Key ideas in personality theory.* St. Paul, MN: West Publishing. [12]

Sedek, G., & Kofta, M. (1990). When cognitive exertion does not yield cognitive gain: Toward an informational explanation of learned helplessness. *Journal of Personality and Social Psychology, 58,* 729-743. [126]

Seeman, J. (1989). Toward a model of positive health. *American Psychologist, 44,* 1099-1109. [246]

276 *References*

Seligman, M.E.P., Maier, S.F., & Solomon, R.L. (1971). Unpredictable and uncontrollable aversive events. In F.R. Brush (Ed.), *Aversive conditioning and learning* (pp. 347-400). New York: Academic Press. [20, 124, 127]

Selye, H. (1976). *The stress of life* (rev. ed.). New York: McGraw-Hill. [15]

Setlow, R.B. (1983). Variations in DNA repair among humans. In C.H. Curtis & N.A. Herman (Eds.), *Human carcinogenesis* (pp. 231-254). New York: Academic Press. [141]

Shaffer, J.W., Graves, P.L., Swank, R.T., & Pearson, T.A. (1987). Clustering of personality traits in youth and the subsequent development of cancer among physicians. *Journal of Behavioral Medicine, 10,* 441-447. [218, 227]

Shapiro, A.P., Alderman, M.H., Clarkson, T.B., Furberg, C.D., Jesse, M.J., Julius, S., Miller, R.E., & Pitt, B. (1987). Task Force 4: Behavioral consequences of hypertension and antihypertensive therapy. *Circulation, 76* (No. 1, Part 2, Suppl. 1), 101-103. [152, 179]

Shapiro, D., & Goldstein, I.B. (1982). Biobehavioral perspectives on hypertension. *Journal of Consulting and Clinical Psychology, 50,* 841-858. [146, 182]

Shapot, V.S. (1979). On the multiform relationships between the tumor and the host. *Advances in Cancer Research, 30,* 89-150. [210]

Shavit, Y., Lewis, J.W., Terman, G.W., Gale, R.P., & Liebeskind, J.C. (1984). Opioid peptides mediate the suppressive effect of stress on natural killer cell cytotoxicity. *Science, 223,* 188-190. [95]

Shavit, Y., & Martin, F.C. (1987). Opiates, stress, and immunity. *Annals of Behavioral Medicine, 9*(2), 11-15. [89, 93, 95, 179]

Shekelle, R.B., Gale, M., & Norusis, M. (1985). Type A score (Jenkins Activity Survey) and risk of recurrent coronary heart disease in the Aspirin Myocardial Infarction Study. *American Journal of Cardiology, 56,* 221-225. [189]

Shekelle, R.B., Hulley, S.B., Neaton, J.D., Billings, J.H., Borhani, N.O., Gerace, T.A., Jacobs, D.R., Lasser, N.L., Mittlemark, M.B., & Stamler, J. (1985). The MRFIT Behavior Pattern Study. II. Type A behavior and incidence of coronary heart disease. *American Journal of Epidemiology, 122,* 559-570. [189]

Shekelle, R.B., Raynor, W.J., Ostfeld, A.M., Garron, D.C., Bieliauskas, L.A., Liu, S.C., Maliza, C., & Oglesby, P. (1981). Psychological depression and 17-year risk of death from cancer. *Psychosomatic Medicine, 43,* 117-125. [33, 217]

Sher, K. (1984). Alcohol and stress. *Behavioral Medicine Abstracts, 5,* 80-82. [154, 159]

Sherman, S.J., Presson, C.C., Chassin, L., Corty, E., & Olshavsky, R. (1983). The false consensus effect in estimates of smoking prevalence: Underlying mechanisms. *Personality and Social Psychology Bulletin, 9,* 197-207. [106]

Sherwood, G.S. (1981). Self-serving biases in person perception: A reexamination of projection as a mechanism of defense. *Psychological Bulletin, 90,* 445-459. [110]

Siekevitz, M., Josephs, S.F., Dukovich, M., Peffer, N., Wong-Staal, F., & Greene, W.C. (1987). Activation of the HIV-1 LTR by T cell mitogens and the trans-activator protein of HTLV-I. *Science, 238,* 1575-1578. [197]

Skinner, E.A. (1985). Action, control judgments, and the structure of control experience. *Psychological Review, 92,* 39-58. [124]

Sklar, L.S., & Anisman, H. (1979). Stress and coping factors influence tumor growth. *Science, 205,* 513-515. [213]

Sklar, L.S., & Anisman, H. (1981). Stress and cancer. *Psychological Bulletin, 89,* 369-406. [208, 212, 213]

Sklar, L.S., Bruto, V., & Anisman, H. (1981). Adaptation to the tumor enhancing effects of stress. *Psychosomatic Medicine, 43,* 331-342. [213]

Slaga, T.J. (1980). Antiinflammatory steroids: Potent inhibitors of tumor promotion. In T.J. Slaga (Ed.), *Carcinogenesis. Vol. 5: Modifiers of chemical carcinogenesis* (pp. 111-126). New York: Raven Press. [151, 212]

Slusher, M.P., & Anderson, C.A. (1987). When reality monitoring fails: The role of imagination in stereotype maintenance. *Journal of Personality and Social Psychology, 52,* 653-662. [105]

Smith, C.K., Harrison, S.D., Ashworth, C., Montano, D., Davis, A., & Fefer, A. (1984). Life change and onset of cancer in identical twins. *Journal of Psychosomatic Research, 28,* 525-532. [221, 229]

Smith, K.A. (1984). Interleukin-2. *Annual Review of Immunology, 2,* 319-333. [85]

Smith, T.W., & Frohm, K.D. (1985). What's so unhealthy about hostility? Construct validity and psychosocial correlates of the Cook and Medley Ho scale. *Health Psychology, 4,* 503-520. [191]

Smuts, J.C. (1961). *Holism and evolution.* New York: Viking. (Original work published 1923) [7, 8]

Solomon, G.F. (1981). Emotional and personality factors in the onset and course of autoimmune disease, particularly rheumatoid arthritis. In R. Ader (Ed.), *Psychoneuroimmunology* (pp. 159-182). New York: Academic Press. [234]

Sowers, J.R., Raj, R.P., Herschman, J.M., Carlson, H.E., & McCallum, R.W. (1977). The effect of stressful diagnostic studies and surgery on anterior pituitary hormone release in man. *Acta Endocrinologica, 86,* 25-32. [75]

Speculand, B., Hughes, A.O., & Goss, A.N. (1984). Role of recent stressful life events experience in the onset of TMJ dysfunction pain. *Community Dentistry and Oral Epidemiology, 12,* 197-202. [236]

Spettell, C.M., & Liebert, R.M. (1986). Training for safety in automated person-machine systems. *American Psychologist, 41,* 545-550. [116]

Spiegel, D., Bloom, J.R., Kraemer, H.C., & Gottheil, E. (1989). Effect of psychosocial treatment on survival of patients with metastatic breast cancer. *Lancet, ii,* 888-891. [224, 226]

Stanton, M.E., & Levine, S. (1988). Pavlovian conditioning of endocrine responses. In R. Ader, H. Weiner, & A. Baum (Eds.), *Experimental foundations of behavioral medicine: Conditioning approaches* (pp. 25-46). Hillsdale, NJ: Erlbaum. [121]

Stedman's medical dictionary (20th ed.) (1961). Baltimore: Williams & Wilkins. [23]

Steering Committee of the Physicians' Health Study Research Group (1988). Preliminary report: Findings from the aspirin component of the ongoing Physicians' Health Study. *New England Journal of Medicine, 318,* 262-264. [143]

Stephens, M.A.P., Kinney, J.M., Norris, V.K., & Ritchie, S.W. (1987). Social networks as assets and liabilities in recovery from stroke by geriatric patients. *Psychology and Aging, 2,* 125-129. [239]

Steplewski, Z., & Vogel, W.H. (1986). Total leukocytes, T cell subpopulation and natural killer (NK) cell activity in rats exposed to restraint stress. *Life Sciences, 38,* 2419-2427. [93, 94]

Steplewski, Z., Vogel, W.H., Ehya, H., Poropatich, C., & Smith, J.M. (1985). Effect of restraint stress on inoculated tumor growth and immune response in rats. *Cancer Research, 45,* 5128-5133. [214]

Stern, G.S., McCants, T.R., & Pettine, P.W. (1982). Stress and illness: Controllable and uncontrollable life events' relative contributions. *Personality and Social Psychology Bulletin, 8,* 140-145. [167]

Stewart, A.L., Greenfield, S., Hays, R.D., Wells, K., Rogers, W.H., Berry, S.D., McGlynn, E.A., & Ware, J.E., Jr. (1989). Functional status and well-being of patients with chronic conditions. *Journal of the American Medical Association, 262,* 907-913. [152]

Stoll, B.A. (Ed.). (1979). *Mind and cancer prognosis.* Chichester, U.K.: Wiley. [208]

Stone, A.A., Cox, D.S., Valdimarsdottir, H., Jandorf, L., & Neale, J.M. (1987). Evidence that secretory IgA antibody is associated with daily mood. *Journal of Personality and Social Psychology, 52,* 988-993. [96]

Stricker, E.M., & Verbalis, J.G. (1987). Biological bases of hunger and satiety. *Annals of Behavioral Medicine, 9*(1), 3-8. [155, 156]

Stroebe, M.S., & Stroebe, W. (1983). Who suffers more? Sex differences in health risks of the widowed. *Psychological Bulletin, 93,* 279-301. [168]

Strube, M.J. (1985). Attributional style and the Type A coronary-prone behavior pattern. *Journal of Personality and Social Psychology, 49,* 500-509. [112]

Strube, M.J., Berry, J.M., & Moergen, S. (1985). Relinquishment of control and the Type A behavior pattern: The role of performance evaluation. *Journal of Personality and Social Psychology, 49,* 831-842. [120]

Strube, M.J., & Werner, C. (1984). Psychological reactance and the relinquishment of control. *Personality and Social Psychology Bulletin, 10,* 225-234. [119]

Strunk, R.C., Mrazek, D.A., Fuhrman, G.S.W., & La Brecque, J.F. (1985). Physiologic and psychological characteristics associated with deaths due to asthma in childhood: A case-controlled study. *Journal of the American Medical Association, 254,* 1193-1198. [238]

Stuart, J.C., & Brown, B.M. (1981). The relationship of stress and coping ability to incidence of disease and accidents. *Journal of Psychosomatic Research, 25,* 255-260. [172]

Sugarman, B.J., Aggarwal, B.B., Hass, P.E., Figari, I.S., Palladino, M.A., Jr., & Shepard, H.M. (1985). Recombinant human tumor necrosis factor-α: Effects on proliferation of normal and transformed cells in vitro. *Science, 230,* 943-945. [90]

Suls, J., & Fletcher, B. (1985a). The relative efficacy of avoidant and nonavoidant coping strategies: A meta-analysis. *Health Psychology, 4,* 249-288. [110, 114, 163]

Suls, J., & Fletcher, B. (1985b). Self-attention, life stress, and illness: A prospective study. *Psychosomatic Medicine, 47,* 469-481. [170]

Suls, J., & Marco, C.A. (1990). Relationship between JAS- and FTAS-Type A behavior and non-CHD illness: A prospective study controlling for negative affectivity. *Health Psychology, 9,* 479-492. [187]

Surwit, R.S. (1988). Stress, behavior, and glucose control in diabetes mellitus. In R. Ader, H. Weiner, & A. Baum (Eds.), *Experimental foundations of behavioral medicine: Conditioning approaches* (pp. 159-173). Hillsdale, NJ: Erlbaum. [205]

Surwit, R.S., & Feinglos, M.N. (1984). Stress and diabetes. *Behavioral Medicine Update, 6*(1), 8-11. [205, 206]

Swaim, R.C., Oetting, E.R., Edwards, R.W., & Beauvais, F. (1989). Links from emotional distress to adolescent drug use: A path model. *Journal of Consulting and Clinical Psychology, 57,* 227-231. [159]

Swann, W.B., Jr., Griffin, J.J., Jr., Predmore, S.C., & Gaines, B. (1987). The cognitive-affective crossfire: When self-consistency confronts self-enhancement. *Journal of Personality and Social Psychology, 52,* 881-889. [106]

Syme, S.L. (1984). Sociocultural factors in disease etiology. In W.D. Gentry (Ed.), *Handbook of behavioral medicine* (pp. 13-37). New York: Guilford Press. [162]

Taché, Y., Du Ruisseau, P., Ducharme, J.R., & Collu, R. (1978). Pattern of adenohypophyseal hormone changes in male rats following chronic stress. *Neuroendocrinology, 26,* 208-219. [74, 75]

Taché, Y., Du Ruisseau, P., Taché, J., Selye, H., & Collu, R. (1976). Shift in adenohypophyseal activity during chronic intermittent immobilization of rats. *Neuroendocrinology, 22,* 325-336. [75]

Tapp, J.T., & Warner, R. (1985). The multisystems view of health and disease. In N. Schneiderman & J.T. Tapp (Eds.), *Behavioral medicine: The biopsychosocial approach* (pp. 1-23). Hillsdale, NJ: Lawrence Erlbaum. [8]

Tapp, W.N., & Natelson, B.H. (1986). Life extension in heart disease: An animal model. *Lancet, 1,* 238-240. [153]

Targan, S., Britvan, L., & Dorey, F. (1981). Activation of human NKCC by moderate exercise: Increased frequency of NK cells with enhanced capability of effector-target lytic interactions. *Clinical and Experimental Immunology, 45,* 352-360. [149]

Tarter, R.E., Edwards, K.L., & Van Thiel, D.H. (1986). Cerebral dysfunction consequential to medical illness: Neuropsychological perspectives and findings. *Annals of Behavioral Medicine, 8*(1), 3-7. [152]

Taylor, P. (1985a). Ganglionic stimulating and blocking agents. In A.G. Gilman, L.S. Goodman, T.W. Rall, & F. Murad (Eds.), *Goodman and Gilman's the pharmacological basis of therapeutics* (7th ed.) (pp. 215-221). New York: Macmillan. [144]

Taylor, P. (1985b). Anticholinesterase agents. In A.G. Gilman, L.S. Goodman, T.W. Rall, & F. Murad (Eds.), *Goodman and Gilman's the pharmacological basis of therapeutics* (7th. ed.) (pp. 110-129). New York: Macmillan. [147]

Taylor, S.E., Buunk, B.P., & Aspinwall, L.G. (1990). Social comparison, stress, and coping. *Personality and Social Psychology Bulletin, 16,* 74-89. [111]

Taylor, S.P., & Leonard, K.E. (1983). Alcohol and human physical aggression. In R. Geen, & E. Donnerstein (Eds.), *Aggression: Theoretical and empirical review* (Vol. 2) (pp. 77-101). New York: Academic Press. [154]

Telner, J.I., Meralic, Z., & Singhal, R.L. (1982). Stress controllability and plasma prolactin levels in the rat. *Psychoneuroendocrinology, 7,* 361-364. [126]

Temkin, N.R., & Davis, G.R. (1984). Stress as a risk factor for seizures among adults with epilepsy. *Epilepsis, 25,* 450-456. [240]

Temoshok, L., & Fox, B.H. (1984). Coping styles and other psychological factors related to medical status and to prognosis in patients with cutaneous malignant melanoma. In B.H. Fox, & B.H. Newberry (Eds.), *Impact of psychoendocrine systems in cancer and immunity* (pp. 258-287). Lewiston, N.Y.: C.J. Hogrefe. [225]

Temoshok, L., & Heller, B.W. (1984). On comparing apples, oranges and fruit salad: A methodological overview of medical outcome studies in psychosocial oncology. In C.L. Cooper (Ed.), *Psychosocial stress and cancer* (pp. 231-260). Chichester, U.K.: Wiley. [33, 216]

Temoshok, L., Heller, B.W., Sagebiel, R.W., Blois, M.S., Sweet, D.M., DiClemente, R.J., & Gold, M.L. (1985). The relationship of psychosocial factors to prognostic indicators in cutaneous malignant melanoma. *Journal of Psychosomatic Research, 29,* 139-153. [225, 230]

Temoshok, L., Sagebiel, R.W., Blois, M.S., & Sweet, D.M. (1988). Psychological factors related to outcome in cutaneous malignant melanoma: A matched samples design. In A. Lobos, & A. Tres (Eds.), *Psicosomatica y cancer* (pp. 23-32). Madrid: Ministerio de Sanidad y Consumo. [226, 231]

Tennes, K., & Kreye, M. (1985). Children's adrenocortical responses to classroom activities and tests in elementary school. *Psychosomatic Medicine, 47,* 451-460. [66]

Teshima, H., & Kubo, C. (1984). Changes in immune responses and tumor growth in mice depend on the duration of stress. In B.H. Fox & B.H. Newberry (Eds.), *Impact of psychoendocrine systems in cancer and immunity* (pp. 208-224). Lewiston, NY: Hogrefe. [93]

Teshima, H., Kubo, C., Kihara, H., Imada, Y., Nagata, S., Ago, Y., & Ikemi, Y. (1982). Psychosomatic aspects of skin diseases from the standpoint of immunology. *Psychotherapy and Psychosomatics, 37,* 165-175. [240]

Thomas, C.B., Duszynski, K.R., & Shaffer, J.W. (1979). Family attitudes reported in youth as potential predictors of cancer. *Psychosomatic Medicine, 41,* 287-302. [218]

Thompson, J.K., Jarvie, G.J., Lahey, B.B., & Cureton, K.J. (1982). Exercise and obesity: Etiology, physiology, and intervention. *Psychological Bulletin, 91,* 55-79. [149]

Thompson, S.C. (1981). Will it hurt less if I can control it? A complex answer to a simple question. *Psychological Bulletin, 90,* 89-101. [124, 125]

Timko, C., & Janoff-Bulman, R. (1985). Attributions, vulnerability, and psychological adjustment: The case of breast cancer. *Health Psychology, 4,* 521-544. [115]

Tirrell, I.E. (1987). *Cancer and length of prison term.* Unpublished M.A. Thesis, Kent State University. [217, 227]

Tomporowski, P.D., & Ellis, N.R. (1986). Effects of exercise on cognitive processes: A review. *Psychological Bulletin, 99,* 338-346. [149]

Tracey, K.J., Beutler, B., Lowry, S.F., Merryweather, J., Wolpe, S., Milsark, I.W., Hariri, R.J., Fahey, T.J., III, Zentella, A., Albert, J.D., Shires, G.T., & Cerami, A. (1986). Shock and tissue injury induced by recombinant human cachectin. *Science, 234,* 470-473. [90, 92, 210]

Treasure, J., & Ploth, D. (1983). Role of dietary potassium in the treatment of hypertension. *Hypertension, 5,* 864-872. [146]

Tsutsumi, O., Kurachi, H., & Oka, T. (1986). A physiological role of epidermal growth factor in male reproductive function. *Science, 233,* 975-977. [57]

Tucker, D.M., Penland, J.G., Beckwith, B.E., & Sandstead, H.H. (1984). Thyroid function in normals: Influences on the electroencephalogram and cognitive performance. *Psychophysiology, 21,* 72-78. [54]

Turk, D.C., Meichenbaum, D., & Genest, M. (1983). *Pain and behavioral medicine: A cognitive-behavioral perspective.* New York: Guilford Press. [235]

Tversky, A., & Kahneman, D. (1983). Extensional versus intuitive reasoning: The conjunction fallacy in probability judgment. *Psychological Review, 90,* 293-315. [30, 105, 116]

Tyroler, H.A., Haynes, S.G., Cobb, L.A., Irvin, C.W., Jr., James, S.A., Kuller, L.H., Miller, R.E., Shumaker, S.A., Syme, S.L., & Wolf, S. (1987). Task Force 1: Environmental risk factors in coronary artery disease. *Circulation, 76*(No. 1, Part 2, Suppl. 1), 139-144. [184]

Ulrich, R.S. (1984). View through a window may influence recovery from surgery. *Science, 224,* 420-421. [239]

Unanue, E.R., & Allen, P.M. (1987). The basis for the immunoregulatory role of macrophages and other accessory cells. *Science, 236,* 551-557. [79, 80, 81]

Underwood, L.E., & Van Wyk, J.J. (1985). Normal and aberrant growth. In J.D. Wilson & D.W. Foster (Eds.), *Williams textbook of endocrinology* (7th ed.) (pp. 155-205). Philadelphia: W.B. Saunders. [74, 146]

Unger, R.H., & Foster, D.W. (1985). Diabetes mellitus. In J.D. Wilson & D.W. Foster (Eds.), *Williams textbook of endocrinology* (7th ed.) (pp. 1018-1074). Philadelphia: Saunders. [202, 205]

Uphouse, L. (1980). Reevaluation of mechanisms that mediate brain differences between enriched and impoverished animals. *Psychological Bulletin, 88,* 215-232. [152]

Vaernes, R., Ursin, H., Darragh, A., & Lambre, R. (1982). Endocrine response patterns and psychological correlates. *Journal of Psychosomatic Research, 26,* 123-131. [74]

VanderPlate, C., & Aral, S.O. (1987). Psychosocial aspects of genital herpes virus infection. *Health Psychology, 6,* 57-72. [199]

Van Itallie, T.B. (1979). Obesity: Adverse effects on health and longevity. *American Journal of Clinical Nutrition, 32,* 2723-2733. [146]

Vena, J.E., Graham, S., Zielezny, M., Swanson, M.K., Barnes, R.E., & Nolan, J. (1985). Lifetime occupational exercise and colon cancer. *American Journal of Epidemiology, 122,* 357-365. [222, 229]

Verbalis, J.G., McCann, M.J., McHale, C.M., & Stricker, E.M. (1986). Oxytocin secretion in response to cholecystokinin and food: Differentiation of nausea from satiety. *Science, 232,* 1417-1419. [54]

Verrier, R.L. (1987). Mechanisms of behaviorally induced arrhythmias. *Circulation*, *76*(No. 1, Part 2, Suppl. 1), 48-56. [186]

Verrier, R.L., & Lown, B. (1984). Behavioral stress and cardiac arrhythmias. *Annual Review of Physiology, 46*, 155-176. [186]

Vickers, R.R., Jr. (1988). Effectiveness of defenses: A significant predictor of cortisol excretion under stress. *Journal of Psychosomatic Research, 32*, 21-29. [107]

Visintainer, M.A., Volpicelli, J.R., & Seligman, M.E.P. (1982). Tumor rejection in rats after inescapable or escapable shock. *Science, 216*, 437-439. [20, 213]

Viti, A., Muscettola, M., Paulesu, L., Bocci, V., & Almi, A. (1985). Effect of exercise on plasma interferon levels. *Journal of Applied Physiology, 59*, 426-428. [149]

Vollhardt, B.R., Ackerman, S.H., Grayzel, A.I., & Barland, P. (1982). Psychologically distinguishable groups of rheumatoid arthritis patients: A controlled, single blind study. *Psychosomatic Medicine, 44*, 353-362. [234]

Von Lichtenberg, F. (1984). Infectious diseases. In S.L. Robbins, R.S. Cotran, & V. Kumar, *The pathologic basis of disease* (3rd ed.) (pp. 273-398). Philadelphia: Saunders. [152]

Voudouris, N.J., Peck, C.L., & Coleman, G. (1985). Conditioned placebo responses. *Journal of Personality and Social Psychology, 48*, 47-53. [121]

Wagner, P.J., & Curran, P. (1984). Health beliefs and physician identified "worried well." *Health Psychology, 3*, 459-474. [24, 166]

Waldmann, T.A. (1986). The structure, function, and expression of interleukin-2 receptors on normal and malignant lymphocytes. *Science, 232*, 727-732. [85]

Wallston, B.S., Alagna, S.W., DeVellis, B.M., & DeVellis, R.F. (1983). Social support and physical health. *Health Psychology, 2*, 367-391. [162, 171]

Ward, M.M., Chesney, M.A., Swan, G.E., Black, G.W., Parker, S.D., & Rosenman, R.H. (1986). Cardiovascular responses in Type A and Type B men to a series of stressors. *Journal of Behavioral Medicine, 9*, 43-49. [188]

Watkins, L.R., & Mayer, D.J. (1982). Organization of endogenous opiate and non-opiate pain control systems. *Science, 216*, 1185-1192. [16, 53, 237]

Watson, D. (1988). Intraindividual and interindividual analyses of positive and negative affect: Their relation to health complaints, perceived stress, and daily activities. *Journal of Personality and Social Psychology, 54*, 1020-1030. [171]

Watson, D., & Clark, L.A. (1984). Negative affectivity: The disposition to experience aversive emotional states. *Psychological Bulletin, 96*, 465-490. [108]

Watson, D., & Pennebaker, J.W. (1989). Health complaints, stress, and distress: Exploring the central role of negative affectivity. *Psychological Review, 96*, 234-254. [24, 108, 166]

Weary-Bradley, G. (1978). Self-serving biases in the attribution process: A reexamination of the fact or fiction question. *Journal of Personality and Social Psychology, 36*, 56-71. [106]

Weight disturbances. (1986). *Medical Sciences Bulletin, 8*(10), 3-4. [141, 155, 159]

Weinberg, R.A. (1985). The action of oncogenes in the cytoplasm and nucleus. *Science, 230*, 770-776. [209]

Weinberger, M., Hiner, S.L., & Tierney, W.M. (1986). Improving functional status in arthritis: The effect of social support. *Social Science & Medicine, 23*, 899-904. [235]

Weiner, B. (1985). An attributional theory of achievement motivation and emotion. *Psychological Review, 92*, 548-573. [104]

Weiner, H. (1977). *Psychobiology and human disease*. New York: Elsevier. [23, 39, 158, 162, 180, 181, 240]

Weiner, H. (1985). The concept of stress in the light of studies on disasters, unemployment, and loss: A critical analysis. In M.R. Zales (Ed.), *Stress in health and disease* (pp. 24-94). New York: Brunner/Mazel. [14, 21, 109]

Weinstein, N.D. (1984). Why it won't happen to me: Perceptions of risk factors and susceptibility. *Health Psychology, 3*, 431-457. [106]

Weiss, B. (1983). Behavioral toxicology and environmental health science: Opportunity and challenge for psychology. *American Psychologist, 38,* 1174-1187. [147]

Weiss, J.M., Glazer, H.I., & Pohorecky, L.A. (1976). Coping behavior and neurochemical changes: An alternative explanation for the original "learned helplessness" experiments. In G. Serban & A. Kling (Eds.), *Animal models in human psychophysiology* (pp. 141-173). New York: Plenum. [67, 124, 125]

Weiss, S.J., Lampert, M.B., & Test, S.T. (1983). Long-lived oxidants generated by human neutrophils: Characterization and bioactivity. *Science, 222,* 625-628. [81]

Weitz, J. (1970). Psychological research needs on the problems of human stress. In J.E. McGrath (Ed.), *Social and psychological factors in stress* (pp. 124-133). New York: Holt, Rinehart and Winston. [17]

White, J.R., & Froeb, H.F. (1980). Small airways dysfunction in non-smokers chronically exposed to tobacco smoke. *New England Journal of Medicine, 302,* 720-723. [137]

Whitehead, W.E., & Bosmajian, L.S. (1982). Behavioral medicine applied to gastrointestinal disorders. *Journal of Consulting and Clinical Psychology, 50,* 972-983. [240]

Williams, N.A., & Deffenbacher, J.L. (1983). Life stress and chronic yeast infections. *Journal of Human Stress, 9,* 26-31. [200]

Williams, R.B., Jr. (1984). Type A behavior and coronary heart disease: Something old, something new. *Behavioral Medicine Update, 6*(3), 29-33. [64, 183, 190]

Williams, R.B., Jr. (1985). Neuroendocrine response patterns and stress: Biobehavioral mechanisms of disease. In R.B. Williams, Jr. (Ed.), *Perspectives on behavioral medicine. Volume 2. Neuroendocrine control and behavior* (pp. 71-101). New York: Academic Press. [66, 75, 183]

Williams, R.B., Jr., Haney, T.L., Lee, K.L., Kong, Y.-H., Blumenthal, J.A., & Whalen, R.E. (1980). Type A behavior, hostility, and coronary atherosclerosis. *Psychosomatic Medicine, 42,* 539-549. [190]

Wills, T.A. (1981). Downward comparison principles in social psychology. *Psychological Bulletin, 90,* 245-271. [111]

Wilson, J.D., & Foster, D.W. (Eds.). (1985). *Williams textbook of endocrinology* (7th ed.). Philadelphia: Saunders. [47, 57, 151]

Wilson, J.F. (1985). Stress, coping styles, and physiological arousal. In S.R. Burchfield (Ed.), *Stress: Psychological and physiological interaction* (pp. 263-281). Washington, D.C.: Hemisphere. [110, 115]

Wing, R.R., Epstein, L.H., Nowalk, M.P., & Lamparski, D.M. (1986). Behavioral self-regulation in the treatment of patients with diabetes mellitus. *Psychological Bulletin, 99,* 78-89. [205]

Witkin, H.A., & Goodenough, D.R. (1977). Field dependence and interpersonal behavior. *Psychological Bulletin, 84,* 661-669. [108]

Wittenberg, M.T., & Reis, H.T. (1986). Loneliness, social skills, and social perception. *Personality and Social Psychology Bulletin, 12,* 121-130. [129]

Woloski, B.M.R.J., Smith, E.M., Meyer, W.J., III, Fuller, G.M., & Blalock, J.E. (1985). Corticotropin-releasing activity of monokines. *Science, 230,* 1035-1037. [90]

Woods, S.C., & Burchfield, S.R. (1980). Conditioned endocrine responses. In J.M. Ferguson & C.B. Taylor (Eds.), *The comprehensive handbook of behavioral medicine* (vol. 1) (pp. 239-254). New York: Spectrum. [121]

Wyler, A.R., Masuda, M., & Holmes, T.H. (1968). Seriousness of illness rating scale. *Journal of Psychosomatic Research, 11,* 363-374. [166]

Young, S.N., Smith, S.E., Pihl, R.O., & Ervin, F.R. (1985). Tryptophan depletion causes a rapid lowering of mood in normal males. *Psychopharmacology, 87,* 173-177. [146]

Yunis, J.J. (1983). The chromosomal basis of human neoplasia. *Science, 221,* 227-236. [209]

References 283

Zack, J.A., Cann, A.J., Lugo, J.P., & Chen, I.S.Y. (1988). HIV-1 production from infected peripheral blood T cells after HTLV-I induced mitogenic stimulation. *Science*, *240*, 1026-1029. [197]

Zajonc, R.B. (1980). Feeling and thinking: Preferences need no inferences. *American Psychologist*, *35*, 151-175. [153]

Zajonc, R.B. (1984). On the primacy of emotion. *American Psychologist*, *39*, 117-123. [109]

Zarski, J.J. (1984). Hassles and health: A replication. *Health Psychology*, *3*, 243-251. [167]

Zegans, L.S. (1982). Stress and the development of somatic disorders. In L. Goldberger & S. Breznitz (Eds.), *Handbook of stress: Theoretical and clinical aspects* (pp. 134-152). New York: Free Press. [162]

Zezulak, K.M., & Green, H. (1986). The generation of insulin-like growth factor I-sensitive cells by growth hormone action. *Science*, *233*, 551-553. [60]

Zimbardo, P.G. (Ed.) (1969). *The cognitive control of motivation: The consequences of choice and dissonance*. Glenview, IL: Scott, Foresman. [117]

Zimbardo, P.G., Cohen, A., Weisenberg, M., Dworkin, L., & Firestone, I. (1969). The control of experimental pain. In P.G. Zimbardo (Ed.), *The cognitive control of motivation: The consequences of choice and dissonance* (pp. 100-125). Glenview, IL: Scott, Foresman. [138]

Zuckerman, M., Buchbaum, M.S., & Murphy, D.L. (1980). Sensation-seeking and its biological correlates. *Psychological Bulletin*, *88*, 187-214. [108]

Author Index

Linn, B.S., 239
Linn, M.W. (Edelstein, Linn)
Linsk, R.L. (Goodenow)
Linville, P.W., 170
Linwick, D. (Dess)
Lipowski, Z.J., 8
Lippman, M. (Levy)
Lipsitt, D.R. (Lipowski)
Lipton, J.M. (Murphy)
Lipton, M. (Ciaranello)
Little, R.E., 144
Liu, S.C. (Shekelle)
Lloyd, R., 93
Locke, S.E., 95, (Jemmott)
Loevinger, B.L. (Kalin)
Lombardo, T., 188, 189
Longo, D.J., 200
Loo, R. (De Quattro)
Lorig, K. (O'Leary)
Loucks, A.B., 74
Lown, B., 184, 186, (Verrier)
Lowry, S.F. (Tracey)
Lucas, C.P., 179
Lugo, J.P. (Zack)
Lumpkin, M.D., 62
Lundstrom, K. (Larsson)
Lunzer, M. (Diamond)
Luria, S.E., 193
Lusk, E.J. (Cassileth)
Maas, J.W., 53
MacDougall, J.M., 190, (Dembroski)
Mack, T.M. (Henderson)
MacLennan, A.J., 20
Madden, J.E., 214, (Newberry)
Maddi, S.R. (Kobasa)
Magnus, K., 185
Magnusson, D. (Endler)
Mahler, H.I.M. (Kulik)
Maier, S.F., 125, 126, (Laudenslager, MacLennan, Seligman)
Majerus, P.W., 49
Majewska, M.D., 53
Major, B. (Crocker)
Maliza, C. (Shekelle)
Maloney, M.C. (Haughey)
Malott, J.M. (McCaul)
Maluish, A.M. (Levy)
Mandel, J.S. (Coates)
Mandler, G., 109
Mandrup-Poulsen, T. (Bendtzen)
Manuck, S.B. (Krantz)
Marco, C.A. (Suls)
Marković, B.M. (Janković)
Markovits, D.M. (Gartner)
Markovits, P. (Gartner)

Marniemi, J. (Hyyppa)
Marshall, J.R., 223, 229
Martin, F.C. (Shavit)
Martin, J.E., 149, 186
Martin, R.A. (Lefcourt)
Martinović, J.V. (Milenković)
Marx, J.L., 49
Mason, J. (Kosten)
Mason, J.W., 16, 20, 21, 65, 72, 75, 120
Mason, K.A. (Peters)
Mastrangelo, M.J. (Chirigos)
Masuda, M. (Wyler)
Masur, F.T., III (Anderson)
Matarazzo, J.D., 109
Matroos, A.W. (Magnus)
Matsumoto, K. (Monden, Nakashima)
Matthes, T., 213
Matthews, K.A., 111, 187, 188, (Cottington, Haynes)
Matthysse, S. (Bunney)
Maxwell, C.A. (Foldes)
May, H.J. (Revicki)
Mayer, D.J. (Watkins)
McArthur, D. (Levor)
McCallum, R.W. (Sowers)
McCann, I.L., 149
McCann, M.J. (Verbalis)
McCann, S.M. (Lumpkin)
McCants, T.R. (Stern)
McCarron, D.A., 147
McCaul, K.D., 111, (Glasgow)
McClelland, D.C., 96, 126
McCormick, C.R. (Leaverton)
McCrae, R.R. (Costa)
McCranie, E.W., 191
McCubbin, H.I., 122
McCubbin, J.A., 179
McDaniel, L.K. (Anderson)
McEwen, B. (Lehman)
McGinley, H., 153
McGinley, P. (McGinley)
McGlynn, E.A. (Stewart)
McGrath, J.E., 16
McHale, C.M. (Verbalis)
McKinney, M.E., 183, 187
McKusick, L. (Coates)
McMurry, J.F., Jr. (Peyrot)
Mechanic, D., 24, 166
Medley, D.M. (Cook)
Medniecks, M. (Maas)
Meehan, S.M. (Newberry)
Mefford, I.N. (Bandura)
Meichenbaum, D. (Turk)
Meites, J. (Euker)

Swan, G.E. (*Ward*)
Swank, R.T. (*Shaffer*)
Swann, W.B., Jr., 106
Swanson, M.K. (*Vena*)
Sweet, D.M. (*Temoshok*)
Syme, S.L., 162, (*Tyroler*)
Sytinski, I.A. (*Andreev*)
Taché, J. (*Taché*)
Taché, Y., 74, 75, (*Du Ruisseau*)
Talbott, E. (*Cottington*)
Tanaka, H. (*Monden*)
Tapp, J.T., 8, (*Schneiderman*)
Tapp, W.N., 153
Targan, S., 149
Tarter, R.E., 152
Tateno, M. (*Cheng-Mayer*)
Taylor, C.B. (*Bandura*)
Taylor, P., 144, 147
Taylor, S.E., 111
Taylor, S.P., 154
Telner, J.I., 126
Temin, H.M. (*Blattner*)
Temkin, N.R., 240
Temoshok, L., 33, 216, 225, 226, 230, 231
Tennes, K., 66
Terman, G.W. (*Shavit*)
Teshima, H., 93, 240
Test, S.T. (*Weiss*)
Therrell, T. (*Arnetz*)
Thomas, C.B., 218
Thompson, J. (*Greene*)
Thompson, J.K., 149
Thompson, L. (*Friedman*)
Thompson, S.C., 124, 125
Thoreson, C.D. (*Friedman*)
Tierney, W.M. (*Weinberger*)
Timko, C., 115
Tirrell, I.E., 217, 227
Tokuda, S. (*Rowland*)
Tomporowski, P.D., 149
Tracey, K.J., 90, 92, 210
Treasure, J., 146
Tross, S. (*Holland*)
Tsutsumi, O., 57
Tucker, D.M., 54
Turk, D.C., 235, (*Flor*)
Tversky, A., 30, 105, 116
Tyroler, H.A., 184
Ulmer, D. (*Friedman*)
Ulrich, R.S., 239
Unanue, E.R., 79, 80, 81
Underwood, L.E., 74, 146
Unger, R.H., 202, 205
Uozumi, T. (*Monden, Nakashima*)

Uphouse, L., 152
Ursin, H. (*Hansen, Murison, Overmier, Vaernes*)
Usher, P. (*Flier*)
Vaernes, R., 74
Vaillant, G.E. (*Peterson*)
Valdimarsdottir, H. (*Stone*)
VanCamp, S.P. (*Kasch*)
VanderPlate, C., 199
Vandongen, R. (*Puddey*)
Van Itallie, T.B., 146
Van Kammen, D.P. (*Rogentine*)
Van Thiel, D.H. (*Tarter*)
Van Treuren, R.R. (*Hull*)
Van Wyk, J.J. (*Underwood*)
Vena, J.E., 222, 229
Verbalis, J.G., 54, (*Stricker*)
Verrier, R.L., 186
Vickers, R.R., Jr., 107
Vinters, H.V. (*Koyanagi*)
Virnelli, S. (*Hull*)
Visintainer, M.A., 20, 213
Viti, A., 149
Vogel, J.M. (*Goodenow*)
Vogel, W.H. (*Steplewski*)
Vollhardt, B.R., 234
Volpicelli, J.R. (*Visintainer*)
Von Engelhardt, B. (*Blohmke*)
Von Lichtenberg, F., 152
Voudouris, N.J., 121
Wagner, P.J., 24, 166
Wahby, V. (*Kosten*)
Waldmann, T.A., 85
Walker, L.S. (*Greene*)
Wallace, J.P. (*Kasch*)
Wallston, B.S., 162, 171
Waltz, M.E. (*Baltrusch*)
Ward, M.M., 188, (*Carmelli*)
Ware, J.E., Jr. (*Lau, Stewart*)
Warner, R. (*Tapp*)
Wasserman, J. (*Arnetz*)
Watkins, L.O. (*McCranie*)
Watkins, L.R., 16, 53, 237
Watson, D., 24, 108, 166, 171
Watson, F.M.C. (*Henry*)
Watson, M. (*Morris*)
Weary-Bradley, G., 106
Webster, J. (*Brett*)
Weinberg, R.A., 209
Weinberger, M., 235
Weiner, B., 104
Weiner, H., 14, 21, 23, 39, 109, 158, 162, 180, 181, 240
Weingand, K.W. (*Clarkson*)
Weinstein, N.D., 106

Subject Index

299

Abbreviations and Acronyms

ABS	Affect Balance Scale	con A	concanavalin A	
ACTH	adrenocorticotropic hormone	CRF	corticotropin releasing factor	
ADCC	antibody-dependent cell-mediated cytotoxicity	CSF	colony-stimulating factor	
		CT	calcitonin	
ADH	antidiuretic hormone AVP)	CTL	cytotoxic T-lymphocyte (T_c)	
AdX	adrenalectomized			
AIDS	acquired immunodeficiency syndrome	DDT	dichlorodiphenyltrichloro-ethane	
ANF	atrial natriuretic factor			
AS	atherosclerosis	DG	diacylglycerol	
AT-III	antithrombin-III	DNA	deoxyribonucleic acid	
ATP	adenosine triphosphate	DOC	deoxycorticosterone	
AVP	arginine vasopressin (ADH)	EBV	Epstein-Barr virus	
		EGF	epidermal growth factor	
BCDF	B-cell differentiation factor	EKG	electrocardiogram	
B-cell	B-lymphocyte	ß-END	ß-endorphin	
BP	blood pressure	EP	epinephrine	
		EPO	erythropoetin	
Ca	calcium			
CAD	coronary artery disease	FSH	follicle-stimulating hormone	
cAMP	cyclic 3',5' adenosine monophosphate	GABA	gamma-aminobutyric acid	
CBP	chronic back pain	GH	growth hormone (STH)	
CCK	cholecystokinin	GIP	gastric inhibitory peptide	
CCl_4	carbon tetrachloride	GnRH	gonadotropin releasing hormone (LHRH)	
cGMP	cyclic 3',5' guanosine monophosphate			
		GSR	galvanic skin response	
CHD	coronary heart disease (IHD)	HDL	high-density lipoprotein	
CMV	cytomegalovirus	HgA	glycosylated hemoglobin	
CNS	central nervous system	HIV	human immunodeficiency virus	
CO	carbon monoxide			

Ho	hostility (Cook-Medley)	MG-	macrophage-granulocyte
HR	heart rate	CSF	colony stimulating
HSV	herpes simplex virus		factor
HT	hypertension	MHC	major histocompatibility
HTLV-	human T-cell leukemia		complex
III	virus-III (HIV)	MI	myocardial infarction
HZV	herpes zoster virus	MIF	macrophage migration
	(varicella-zoster)		inhibiting factor
		MMPI	Minnesota Multiphasic
			Personality Inventory
IDDM	insulin-dependent diabetes	α-MSH	α-melanocyte-stimulating
	mellitus		hormone
IFN	interferon	Na	sodium
Ig	immunoglobulin	NE	norepinephrine
IGF	insulin-like growth factor	NGF	nerve growth factor
IHD	ischemic heart disease	NIDDM	non-insulin-dependent
	(CHD)		diabetes mellitus
IL-1	interleukin-1	NK cell	natural killer cell
IL-2	interleukin-2		
ITP	inositol triphosphate	O_2	oxygen (molecular)
		OA	osteoarthritis
JAS	Jenkins Activity Survey	onc	onco(gene)
LAV	lymphadenopathy virus	PCB	polychlorinated biphenyl
	(HIV)	PDE	phosphodiesterase
LDL	low-density lipoprotein	PDGF	platelet-derived growth
leu-	leucine enkephalin		factor
ENK		16PF	16 Personality Factor
LGL	large granular lymphocyte		Questionnaire
LH	luteinizing hormone	PFC	plaque-forming cell
LHRH	luteinizing hormone	PGE	prostaglandin E
	releasing hormone	PGF	prostaglandin F
β-LPH	β-lipotropic hormone	PGI_2	prostacyclin I_2
LPS	lipopolysaccharide	PHA	phytohemagglutinin
LR	lymphoreticular	PKC	protein kinase C
LTE	leukotriene	PLC	phospholipase C
		PNMT	phenylethanolamine
			N-methyltransferase
MAF	macrophage activation	PPD	purified protein derivative
	factor		(of tuberculin)
M-CSF	macrophage colony	PR	proliferative retinopathy
	stimulating factor	PRIF	prolactin release-inhibiting
met-	methionine enkephalin		factor
ENK		Prl	prolactin

PSC	private self-consciousness
PTH	parathyroid hormone
PZ	pancreozymin
RA	rheumatoid arthritis
RNA	ribonucleic acid
SAM	sympathoadrenomedullary
SHR	spontaneously hypertensive rat
SI	structured interview (for TABP)
SM	somatomedin
SNS	sympathetic nervous system
SP	substance P
SRIF	somatostatin
STH	somatotropin (GH)
T_3	triiodothyronine
T_4	thyroxine
TABP	Type A behavior pattern
T_c-cell	cytotoxic T-lymphocyte (CTL)
T-cell	T-lymphocyte
T_h-cell	helper T-lymphocyte
TMD	temporomandibular pain disorder
TMI	Three Mile Island
TNF	tumor necrosis factor
TRH	thyrotropin releasing hormone
T_s-cell	suppressor T-lymphocyte
TSH	thyroid-stimulating hormone
TXA	thromboxane
VIP	vasoactive intestinal peptide

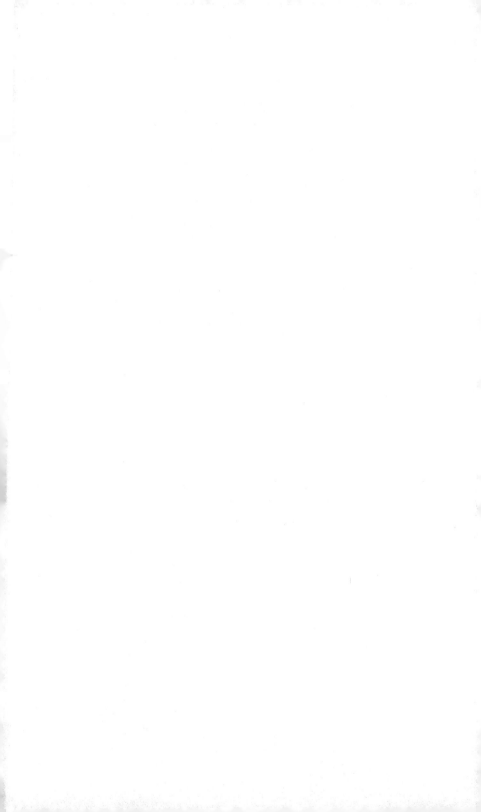